Milestones in Drug Therapy
MDT

Recombinant Protein Drugs

Edited by P. Buckel

Springer Basel AG

Editors

Peter Buckel
Xantos Biomedicine
Fraunhoferstr. 22
D-82152 Martinsried
Germany

Library of Congress Cataloging-in-Publication Data

Recombinant protein drugs / edited by P. Buckel.
p. cm. — (Milestones in drug therapy)
Includes bibliographical references and index.
ISBN 978-3-0348-9527-9 ISBN 978-3-0348-8346-7 (eBook)
DOI 10.1007/978-3-0348-8346-7
1. Protein drugs. 2. Protein engineering. 3. Recombinant proteins—Therapeutic use.
I. Buckel, P. (Peter), 1945- II. Series

RS431.P75 R43 2001
615'.3—dc21 2001025646

Deutsche Bibliothek Cataloging-in-Publication Data

Recombinant protein drugs / ed. by P. Buckel. - Basel ; Boston ; Berlin : Birkhäuser, 2001
(Milestones in drug therapy)
ISBN 978-3-0348-9527-9

Originally published by Birkhäuser Verlag in 2001
Softcover reprint of the hardcover 1st edition 2001

Printed on acid-free paper produced from chlorine-free pulp. TFC ∞
Cover illustration: The genome of hepatitis B virus. The heavy lines represent the partially double-stranded DNA molecule. The arrows show the extent of the four open reading frames, those for HBcAg and HBsAg being marked (see also p. 50).

ISBN 978-3-0348-9527-9

9 8 7 6 5 4 3 2 1 www.birkhasuer-science. com

Table of contents

List of contributors VII

Preface IX

Pioneers and business

Charles Weissmann
Recombinant interferon – the 20th anniversary 3

Peter Hans Hofschneider and Kenneth Murray
Combining science and business: from recombinant DNA to vaccines against hepatitis B virus 43

First generation proteins

George G. Brownlee and Paul L.F. Giangrande
Clotting factors VIII and IX 67

Karl Welte and Erich Platzer
Colony-stimulating factors: altering the practice of oncology 89

Désiré Collen and H. Roger Lijnen
Tissue-type plasminogen activator: helping patients with acute myocardial infarction 107

Proteins with new functions: protein engineering

Stephen D. Gillies
Designing immunocytokines: genetically engineered fusion proteins for targeted immune therapy 129

Further improvement of protein drugs

Paul A. Burke and Scott D. Putney
Improving protein therapeutics: the evolution of the modern pharmacopoeia 151

Theodore Friedmann
Principles of gene transfer and foreign protein expression for human gene therapy 169

Short biographies 181

List of approved "recombinant protein drugs" 189

Subject index 199

List of contributors

George G. Brownlee, Chemical Pathology Unit, Sir William Dunn School of Pathology, University of Oxford, South Parks Road, Oxford OX1 3RE, UK; e-mail: george.brownlee@path.ox.ac.uk

Peter Buckel, Xantos Biomedicine GmbH, Fraunhoferstr. 22, D-82152 Martinsried, Germany; e-mail : p.buckel@xantos-bio.de

Paul Burke, Department of Pharmaceutics and Drug Delivery, Amgen, MS 8-1-C, One Amgen Ctr. Dr., Thousand Oaks, CA 91320, USA; e-mail: pburke@amgen.com

Désiré Collen, Center for Transgene Technology and Gene Therapy, Flanders Interuniversity Institute for Biotechnology, Campus Gasthuisberg O&N, Herestraat 49, B-3000 Leuven, Belgium; e-mail: desire.collen @med.kuleuven.ac.be

Theodore Friedmann, Center for Molecular Genetics, UCSD School of Medicine and Program in Human Gene Therapy, La Jolla, CA 92093, USA; e-mail: tfriedmann@ucsd.edu

Paul L.F. Giangrande, Oxford Haemophilia Centre, The Churchill Hospital, Headington, Oxford OX3 7LJ, UK; e-mail: paul.giangrande@clinical-medicine.oxford.ac.uk

Stephen D. Gillies, Lexigen Pharmaceuticals Corp., 125 Hurtle Ave., Lexington, MA 02173, USA ; e-mail: sgillies@lexigenpharm.com

Peter Hans Hofschneider, Max-Planck-Institut für Biochemie, D-82152 Martinsried, Germany; e-mail: hofschne@biochem.mpg.de

H. Roger Lijnen, Center for Molecular and Vascular Biology, Katholieke Universiteit Leuven, Campus Gasthuisberg O&N, Herestraat 49, B-3000 Leuven, Belgium; e-mail: roger.lijnen@med.kuleuven.ac.be

Kenneth Murray, Institute of Cell and Molecular Biology, University of Edinburgh, Kings's Buildings, Edinburgh EH9 3JR, Scotland

Erich Platzer, Novuspharma SpA, Viale G.B. Stucchi, 110, I-20052 Monza, Italy; e-mail: erich@platzernet.de

Scott D. Putney, Eli Lilly and Co., Lilly Corporate Center, Indianapolis, IN 46285, USA; e-mail: sputney@lilly.com

Charles Weissmann, Neurogenetics Unit, Imperial College School of Medicine at St. Mary's, Norfolk Place, London W2 1PG, UK; e-mail: c.weissmann@ic.ac.uk

Karl Welte, Kinderklinik der Medizinischen Hochschule, Konstanty-Gutschow-Str. 8, D-30625 Hannover, Germany; e-mail: welte.karl@mh-hannover.de

Preface

"The Century of Biology Begins with 369 Biotechnology Medicines in Testing for More than 200 Diseases." Under this headline Alan F. Holmer, President and CEO of the Pharmaceutical Research and Manufacturers of America (P*h*RMA[1]), presented and commented on a survey by his organization that was intended to introduce new medicines in development at the beginning of a new millennium. The fairly unusual term "biotechnology medicines" is defined by proteins and other substances that originate from the human body and are produced to counter disease. The "other substances" mentioned encompass important concepts like antisense DNA, indicating an increasing use of the knowledge derived from gene discovery in the future of medicine. In this book we will concentrate on proteins as drugs because we are convinced that their role in the future will become even more important than is realized today.

In spite of their young age and short time of development, three generations in the field of recombinant protein drugs can already be distinguished. The first generation comprised proteins that occurred naturally, and only their production made use of recombinant DNA methods. The well-known and widely publicized examples are human insulin, growth hormone and erythropoietin (EPO), but there are many more proteins of that kind, many of which are mentioned in this book, for instance, clotting factors, colony-stimulating factors and tissue plasminogen activator (tPA).

Already before the manufacture of these proteins as drugs was well under way, researchers thought of improving the products of given genes by exploiting the concept of evolution. Natural selection can only optimize the normal physiological function of a given protein, and it is thus rather likely that its performance can be improved if one selects for a different (therapeutic) goal, e.g., for activating the immune response against metastatic cancer.

One way of generating improved proteins consists of recombining DNA regions from different genes, thereby producing a "fusion protein" that combines several functions in one molecular structure. Examples of this second generation of recombinant protein drugs are immunocytokines, new hepatitis vaccines or engineered tPAs.

But there is also work on a third generation. The starting point in this case is the observation of the many disadvantages for the patient if proteins have to be administered from the outside. There is a great chance of the proteins being digested, only a slight chance to enter the appropriate body cell and hardly a chance to regulate the protein drug, as is the case with naturally present pro-

[1] www.phrma.org/pdf/charts/biotech2.pdf

teins. The solution would be to change the pharmacokinetic properties of proteins or to supply the body with the medicine, not by taking in the active agent itself but by delivering its genetic instructions. In this book two possible approaches are presented to address some of these opportunities, namely, slow release formulations and gene therapy. Sustained release formulations help reduce the requirement for frequent injections or enable delivery of the protein locally to a particular tissue, thereby lowering overall systemic exposure.

Though gene therapy is encountering hard times in its early days, one should not lose sight of the fact that this technique possesses the possibilities first to get to the root of a genetic disease and second to deliver the right protein at the right time in the right place at the right concentration.

It is obvious that medicine is changing its face rapidly. In the future health problems will find more and more molecular solutions. The promise of breakthroughs on the biotechnology frontier is bright, as Alan Holmer points out in his essay mentioned at the beginning. He expresses his hope that the century of biology will turn out to be a "century of cures". It will definitely be a "century of new cures" and biotechnology companies are providing them.

Peter Buckel
München, January 2001

Pioneers and business

Recombinant Protein Drugs
ed. by P. Buckel

Recombinant interferon – the 20th anniversary[1]

Charles Weissmann

Neurogenetics Unit, Imperial College School of Medicine at St. Mary's, London, UK

On the merits of strolling

In the summer of 1977 at a Gordon Conference I took my annual walk with Peter Lengyel, and, as he described the complexities of the mode of action of mouse IFN and of the control of its expression, it became evident that cloning of the chromosomal IFN gene would lead to a wealth of information unattainable by any other means. Moreover, the undertaking was a challenge, since pure IFN was extremely hard to come by, its structure was unknown and would probably not be elucidated for years to come, no good antibodies to IFN were known to be available, and the mRNA was presumably present at a very low level. However, as Peter explained to me, there did exist a very sensitive assay for IFN mRNA: the injection of about 50 ng of poly(A)$^+$ RNA from IFN-producing cells into each of a dozen *Xenopus* oocytes led to synthesis of easily measurable amounts of IFN [1]. It occurred to me that an assay for cloned IFN cDNA might be based on a hybridisation procedure in connection with this IFN mRNA assay (see Figs 1 and 2). Assume you already possess an IFN cDNA clone and that you immobilise the denatured DNA on a solid support such as a Millipore filter. If this filter is annealed with poly(A)$^+$ RNA containing IFN mRNA and then washed, you would expect it to retain the IFN RNA but none of the other mRNAs. If the filter is subsequently heated in water, the RNA-DNA hybrids will be denatured and the IFN mRNA can be washed off and assayed for in the oocyte test. If any other hybrid cDNA is attached to the filter, some other mRNA will be bound and subsequently recovered, but the oocyte assay will be negative for IFN. This procedure would thus allow the identification of an IFN cDNA plasmid (or, with appropriate modifications, other plasmids of interest, as was reported a year later for rat growth hormone [2]), but it is so time-consuming and labour-intensive that then screening of thousands or even only hundreds of clones would be an overwhelming task.

[1] When asked to contribute an essay on the cloning of interferon (IFN) alpha, I decided to update an article entitled "The Cloning of Interferon and Other Mistakes" (*In*: I Gresser (ed.): *Interferon 1.* Academic Press, London and New York, 101–134)which I had written 1981, at a time when the events were still fresh in my mind. I left the original text largely unchanged, but added retrospective comments in the form of footnotes and appended a summary of some developments following the writing of the original article.

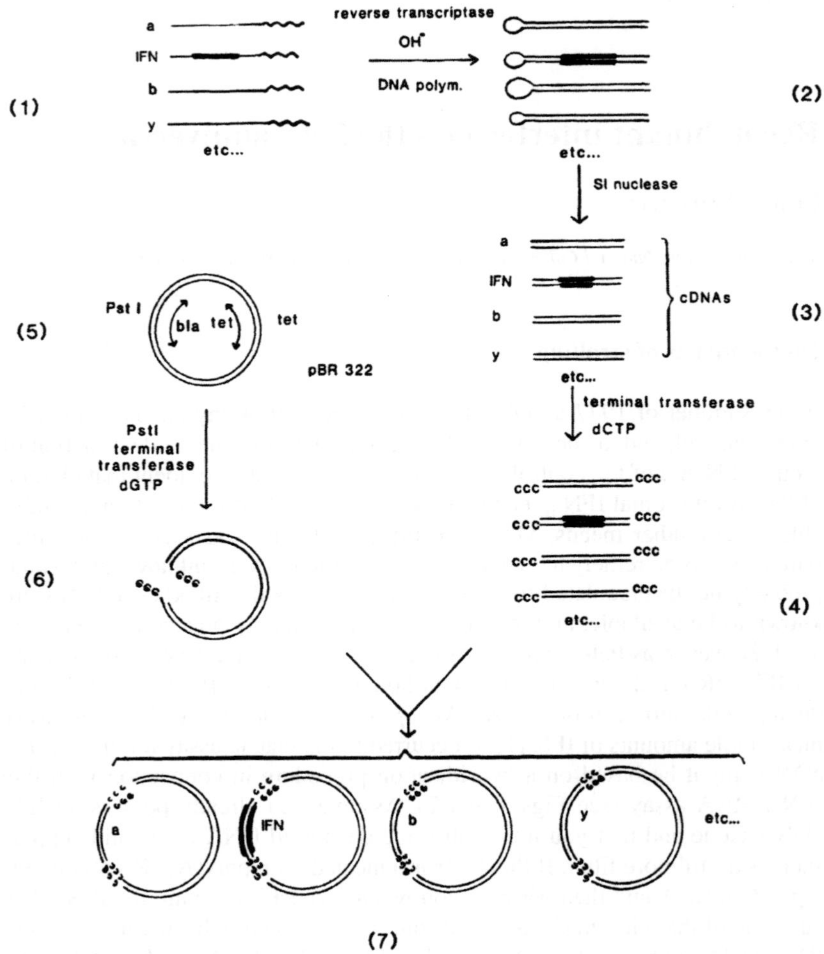

Figure 1. Shot-gun cloning of cDNA sequences derived from leukocyte poly(A)$^+$ RNA·poly(A)$^+$ RNA from Sendai virus-induced leukocytes, which contain a variety of mRNAs, a, b,... y, etc., and a small amount of interferon (IFN) mRNA, was centrifuged through a sucrose gradient and the 12 S fraction (1) copied into single-stranded cDNA using reverse transcriptase. After removal of the RNA by alkali treatment, this DNA was converted to double-stranded DNA using DNA polymerase, which attaches to the 3' end of the template and thereby generates a DNA loop (2). After cleavage with nuclease S1, which is specific for single-stranded DNA (3), the 3' ends were elongated with dCMP residues, using terminal transferase and dCTP (4). Plasmid pBR322 (bla, β-lactamase gene; tet, tetracycline resistance gene) (5) was cleaved with endonuclease PstI, the 3' ends were elongated with dGMP residues, using terminal transferase and dGTP (6), and hybridised with the dCMP-elongated cDNA. The hybrids (7) were introduced into *E. coli* and 10,000 tetracycline-resistant bacterial colonies were picked into the wells of microtiter plates.

However, if one were to examine the plasmid DNA from pools of, say, 1000 clones at a time, then one could rapidly screen 10,000 clones, identify a posi-

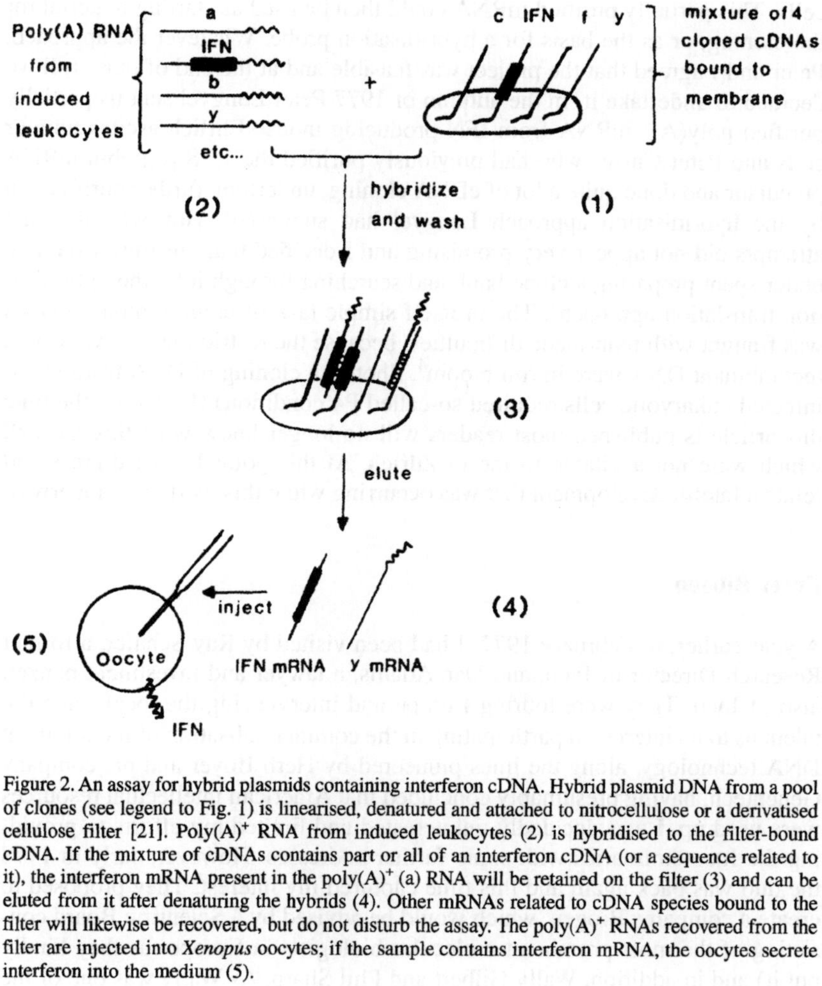

Figure 2. An assay for hybrid plasmids containing interferon cDNA. Hybrid plasmid DNA from a pool of clones (see legend to Fig. 1) is linearised, denatured and attached to nitrocellulose or a derivatised cellulose filter [21]. Poly(A)$^+$ RNA from induced leukocytes (2) is hybridised to the filter-bound cDNA. If the mixture of cDNAs contains part or all of an interferon cDNA (or a sequence related to it), the interferon mRNA present in the poly(A)$^+$ (a) RNA will be retained on the filter (3) and can be eluted from it after denaturing the hybrids (4). Other mRNAs related to cDNA species bound to the filter will likewise be recovered, but do not disturb the assay. The poly(A)$^+$ RNAs recovered from the filter are injected into *Xenopus* oocytes; if the sample contains interferon mRNA, the oocytes secrete interferon into the medium (5).

tive group and then rescreen the clones of that group in subgroups of 100 each. This procedure, known in genetics as subculture cloning, would be repeated with decreasing group size, until the IFN cDNA clone was identified. Peter proposed a different approach, namely, that one make use of the fact that only induced, but not non-induced cells produce IFN mRNA. Thus, one could, for example, make cDNA from non-induced cells, hybridise an excess of it with mRNA from induced cells and separate the non-hybridised RNA – which should consist mainly of mRNA present in induced[2] but not in non-induced

[2] Cells can be induced to secrete IFN by exposure to virus or double-stranded RNA.

cells. This partially purified mRNA could then be used as starting material for the cloning, or as the basis for a hybridisation probe. Whatever the approach, Peter and I agreed that the project was feasible and at the end of our stroll we decided to undertake it. In the autumn of 1977 Peter Lengyel sent us partially purified poly(A)$^+$ mRNA from IFN-producing mouse Ehrlich ascites tumour cells and Peter Curtis, who had previously purified the 15 S β-globin mRNA precursor and done quite a lot of cDNA cloning, undertook further purification by the hybridisation approach Lengyel had suggested. However, the first attempts did not appear very promising and I decided that our time would be better spent preparing a clone bank and searching through it by the hybridisation-translation approach[3]. The in itself simple task of cloning mouse cDNA was fraught with man-made difficulties, because the restrictions on work with recombinant DNA were in full bloom[4]. Shot-gun cloning of DNA from virus-infected eukaryotic cells required so-called P4 conditions (I hope by the time this article is published most readers will no longer know what this means), which were not available to me in Zürich. At this point I must digress and relate a fateful development that was occurring while this work was underway.

Enter Biogen

A year earlier, in February 1977, I had been visited by Ray Schäfer, a former Research Director of Inco, and Dan Adams, a lawyer and investment banker, also of Inco. They were touring Europe and interviewing the local scientific talent as to its interest in participating in the commercialisation of recombinant DNA technology, along the lines pioneered by Herb Boyer and his company Genentech, having presumably concluded that American intellectual resources were used up. I was decidedly uninterested and limited my efforts to providing the Inco emissaries with some further addresses. However, early in 1978 the duo was back again and this time captured my interest. They proposed to create a company, Biogen, which would be advised by a Scientific Board consisting of the most prominent molecular biologists in Europe (as they kindly put it) and in addition, Wally Gilbert and Phil Sharp. As Wally was one of the molecular biologists whom I admired unreservedly, both for his superb mind and his capacity for promoting achievement, it seemed to me that whatever drawbacks my involvement with a commercial venture might bring, an association with Wally would be a redeeming feature[5]. I was thus receptive to an invitation to what was coyly described as "First European Microbiology Conference", but in fact constituted a meeting of the members designate of the

[3] Wrong once again. Two years later Tada Taniguchi was successful in cloning human IFN β cDNA using this approach.

[4] The well-intentioned Asilomar Conference launched mind-numbing discussions such as whether cloning human DNA in *E. coli* was more dangerous than cloning mouse DNA, but it was a boon to the manufacturers of safety cabinets and high-containment hoods.

[5] In the years to follow I came to appreciate to an equal extent Phil's uncanny insight into biology and

Biogen Scientific Board: Wally Gilbert (Harvard University), Brian Hartley (Imperial College), Peter-Hans Hofschneider (Max-Planck Institute, München), Philippe Kourilsky (Institut Pasteur, Paris), Bernard Mach (Institute of Microbiology, University of Geneva), Ken Murray (University of Edinburgh), Ray Schäfer (Inco), Heinz Schaller (University of Heidelberg), Phil Sharp (MIT, Boston) and myself – listed alphabetically and not necessarily by merit. (About a year later Kourilsky had to leave the group because of his commitments to the Pasteur Institute, and I brought in Walter Fiers from Ghent, an old friend and competitor in the RNA phage field, to replace him).

We were received in Geneva, in the Hotel Richmond[6], in surroundings of unmatched luxury (unmatched above all in Biogen meetings subsequent to our signing up) and were pampered from breakfast to bedtime. Our discussions revolved around the possible structure of the company, as well as the feasibility and profitability of a project list I had drawn up and to which some additional possibilities were added. To the delight of our hosts, I revealed that our laboratory was already working on the cloning of mouse IFN-α and that I would be prepared to extend our efforts to the human system. We disbanded, agreeing to meet some weeks later and communicate our decision as to whether we would go ahead to form a company. At this meeting in Paris, on March 25–27, 1978, we were amazed to discover that all of us had decided to join Biogen. Considerable time was devoted to discussing the structure of the proposed company. Briefly, the Scientific Board would provide the scientific direction and members of the Board would undertake projects in their laboratories according to their possibilities. Except for a modest *per diem* fee for attending meetings, all services were to be compensated by shares – both for serving on the board and for undertaking and accomplishing determined research goals. Indeed, the only expenses to Biogen would be for supplies, support of postdoctorals and technicians, and overheads to the universities. The pay–off for the scientist (other than the occasional good meal and the annual January Board Meeting on a Caribbean island) (Fig. 3) would come about when the shares became negotiable, after seven years or upon "going public", whichever came first, while the universities would benefit from royalties, if ever they materialised. The scientists stipulated that one-third of the Directors would be appointed by the members of the Scientific Board, to ensure that the interests of the scientists were being represented at all levels. One such interest was to prevent a sell-out of the company to a large corporation; our major concern, however, was to conserve full freedom of publication and scientific communication, clearly a difficult position to reconcile with

business; it was Phil who visited Genentech at its very beginnings, concluded that their plans to produce insulin in *E. coli* would be successful and recommended to Inco to invest in the company. I was also favorably impressed by the fact that Phil fully supported my strategy for cloning IFN. It would seem that the Nobel committee shared my views on Phil inasmuch as it awarded him its prize for his codiscovery of splicing in 1993. Wally received the Nobel prize for the invention of DNA sequencing, together with Fred Sanger, in 1980.

[6] Now, alas, defunct.

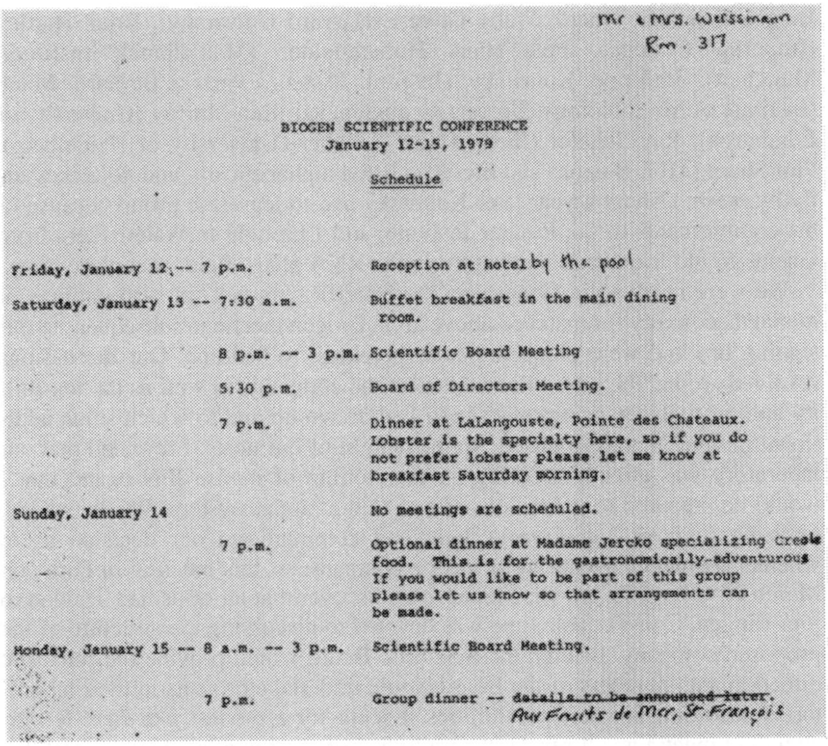

Mr & Mrs. Weissmann
Rm. 317

BIOGEN SCIENTIFIC CONFERENCE
January 12-15, 1979

Schedule

Friday, January 12 -- 7 p.m.	Reception at hotel by the pool
Saturday, January 13 -- 7:30 a.m.	Buffet breakfast in the main dining room.
8 p.m. -- 3 p.m.	Scientific Board Meeting
5:30 p.m.	Board of Directors Meeting.
7 p.m.	Dinner at LaLangouste, Pointe des Chateaux. Lobster is the specialty here, so if you do not prefer lobster please let me know at breakfast Saturday morning.
Sunday, January 14	No meetings are scheduled.
7 p.m.	Optional dinner at Madame Jercko specializing Creole food. This is for the gastronomically-adventurous. If you would like to be part of this group please let us know so that arrangements can be made.
Monday, January 15 -- 8 a.m. -- 3 p.m.	Scientific Board Meeting.
7 p.m.	Group dinner -- ~~details to be announced later~~. Aux Fruits de Mer, St. François

Figure 3. Program of a typical Scientific Board meeting of early Biogen.

demands for patent protection and protection of know-how demanded by commercial partners. We eventually hammered out an arrangement which was to prove satisfactory to the scientists, reasonably so to Biogen but a source of occasional irritation to our future commercial partners. In essence, the scientists undertook to do their best to secure patent applications for all commercially useful achievements prior to publication, but they were not under constraint to secure Biogen's permission for publication. The decision on how to handle our scientific results, including the distribution of strains, thus became our responsibility, and I suppose each of us reacted according to his nature. Those of us who were naturally secretive or uncommunicative could continue to be so to the satisfaction of the commercial partners, while the extroverts would be essentially free to disseminate their own data to their hearts' desire. However, in these same hearts they had to know that a failure to safeguard patent applications or technical know-how might run counter to the interests of the company they were trying to create. There is no denying that a new incentive had appeared to diminish the flow of information, but I am not sure whether it was stronger than the all-pervading pre-existing motivation of being the first to discover and publish and out-doing his colleagues and competitors. The scale of communication even in the "pre-commercial" days ranged from the absolute openness of Tom Maniatis, who provided his rivals with material and methods that helped them compete with their benefactor, to the total secretiveness of colleagues working in the same building who interdicted their "postdocs" to talk to each other.

The faith of the Scientific Board members in the ultimate success of their undertaking ranged from moderate (my own) to Phil Sharp's calm confidence and Wally Gilbert's infectious enthusiasm and prediction that Biogen would become a billion-dollar company, the IBM of biotechnology[7]. It is worth remembering that in 1978 we only knew by word of mouth that the mammalian polypeptide chains, insulin A and B, could be produced as fusion proteins in *E. coli*[8], using chemically synthesised coding sequences [4], while the direct expression in *E. coli* of the first larger protein, growth hormone, was only to be reported in 1979 [5]; whether these recombinant products were biologically active remained unknown for quite a while.

You never can tell

The nascent Scientific Board officially commissioned me to clone human IFN cDNA as a Biogen project and decided to support the mouse projects as well, since I believed that a mouse IFN clone could be used to screen for a human clone by non-stringent colony hybridisation (this assumption proved to be correct, inasmuch as we ultimately used human IFN-α cDNA to identify mouse IFN-α clones). Brian Hartley arranged for the permission of the British Genetic Manipulation Advisory Group to clone mouse cDNA in his C3 containment suite at Imperial College, which solved a major problem for us – the first benefit of the "Biogen network". Since our lab had no experience with induction and measurement of IFN and Peter Lengyel had no source of human IFN mRNA, I had to find a partner who would collaborate with us on the human IFN project. A quick survey of the literature had made it clear that the ideal partner would be Kari Cantell in Helsinki, who had transformed IFN from a laboratory curiosity into a potential clinical tool. IFN, it should be realised, is produced only in minute quantities by virus-induced leukocytes; after a decade of improvements, 10^{10} cells incubated in 1 litre of medium were brought to produce about 50×10^6 units, that is, about 250 μg of IFN. Kari was able to produce 2.5×10^{11} units (about 1 gram's worth) of crude IFN per year, using leukocytes from 90,000 blood donors [6]. This IFN, at a purity level of 0.5–1%, was the first and until that time the only IFN available for human tri-

[7] In February 2000 the market value of Biogen was 15.4 billion and of IBM 198 billion dollars.

[8] In 1977 Genentech prepared minute amounts of somatostatin by cleaving a biosynthetic somatostatin β-galactosidase fusion protein chemically, thereby showing that a mammalian peptide could, in principle, be produced in *E. coli* [3].

als, and Hans Strander had used it in the treatment of osteosarcoma, a type of bone cancer. It was, in fact, the overoptimistic interpretation of these early results that had led to the hope that IFN might be a potent anti-cancer drug and encouraged the American Cancer Society and the National Cancer Institute to sponsor IFN trials in the USA (The Wall Street Journal, December 6, 1979). In this connection, the high price of IFN, purportedly between five and 50 million dollars per gram, became widely known, and probably encouraged the belief that the compound must be highly effective.

I telephoned Kari Cantell, fully expecting to hear that he was already collaborating with one of the many potent cloning groups I knew to be interested in IFN. To my surprise he was not, and in fact I even realised that he was not aware of the potential of the emerging recombinant DNA field. Worse yet, he had never heard of me and was certainly not interested in coming to Zürich to give a seminar, but yes, he would be interested in hearing more about the cloning project[9]. I flew over to see him the day after next, not only because of my hurry to get started but also to impress on him the urgency of our undertaking. This was the second advantage of my association with Biogen: I did not have to apply for funds or justify their use when a trip or some other unexpected expenditure seemed appropriate to me. Not that the university and the national granting agencies had not always been very generous to our lab – I was just reluctant to spend public funds carelessly, and I had a different feeling in regard to money provided by venture capitalists. If they wanted to risk their money I had no qualms about aiding them.

Kari Cantell became very interested in the project and pledged his full support, although I gained the impression that he did not believe that the undertaking would be successful – but then again, neither did I. We started out by determining the relative IFN mRNA levels of leukocytes at different times after induction and the sedimentation coefficient of the RNA. Peter Curtis flew to Helsinki for a day, with distilled phenol, recrystallised sodium dodecylsulfate and all other reagents required to extract the RNA from the leukocytes Kari prepared and returned with the samples for further processing and oocyte injections; the analysis of IFN levels was again carried out in Helsinki. We discovered an unexpected advantage of leukocytes: the level of poly(A)$^+$ RNA was about one-tenth that of normal growing cells, presumably because the leukocytes, as non-growing cells, did not synthesise much protein. Therefore, the IFN mRNA constituted a larger fraction of the poly(A)$^+$ RNA than it would in growing cells, such as lymphoblastoid cells. On the basis of indirect calculations, such as estimating the number of IFN mRNA molecules from the amount of IFN produced in oocytes injected with a known amount of poly(A)$^+$ RNA, and using the relationship found for globin as reference, we concluded that the IFN mRNA might constitute 10^{-3}–10^{-4} of the poly(A)$^+$ RNA and took the lower number as the basis for our further projections. In fact, the higher number ultimately proved to be closer to the correct one. Peter Curtis spent a

[9] The view from the other side of the fence is related in the charming memoirs of Kari Cantell [7].

month or two trying to purify the IFN mRNA by polyacrylamide gel electrophoresis, but although substantial enrichment could be attained, the yields of biologically active RNA from the gels were very variable. I decided that we would carry out the cloning with the 12 S fraction of sucrose gradient-purified poly(A)$^+$ RNA, which was about ten-fold enriched in IFN mRNA, rather than spend much more time on purification. Peter Curtis, who had accepted a position at the Wistar Institute, left in October 1978 and Tada Taniguchi, one of the most gifted students to graduate from our department, who had up to then been pursuing the mouse IFN project, and Shigekazu Nagata, like Tada a veteran of site-directed mutagenesis in QβRNA, continued to work with the human mRNA. In addition, Lorraine Johnsrud, a former student of Wally Gilbert, who had done some elegant work on insertion sequences, joined us in September 1978. Unfortunately Tada was about to leave, and even more unfortunately he intended to continue cloning IFN cDNA in Japan, albeit fibroblast IFN. Since after Tada's departure none of my colleagues had experience in making large-scale RNA preparations, I went to Helsinki, and Kari and I spent a long night making leukocyte RNA from 10^{11} leukocytes, which I then purified in Zürich with Lorraine Johnsrud. Nagata prepared cDNA from the 12 S poly(A)$^+$ RNA fraction, tailed it with dC residues, and joined it to the plasmid pBR322, which had been cleaved with PstI and elongated with dG residues (Fig. 1). This approach[10] was chosen because the PstI site is located in the β-lactamase gene of pBR322 and I hoped that insertion of cDNA into this position could give rise to IFN as a fused protein, as was the case for proinsulin [8].

Casing the bank

Ten thousand clones of *E. coli* z 1776[11], transformed with hybrid plasmids, were picked individually under P3 conditions (the Recombinant DNA Guidelines had meanwhile been somewhat relaxed) into microtiter plates by Nagata and Michel Streuli, an undergraduate student from Tufts University, who had joined us for a year to gain exposure to the vicissitudes of research. We pooled groups of 512 clones, Josef Ecsödi prepared the plasmid DNA from 12 such groups, and Nagata carried out the hybridisation assay described in Figure 2. The eluted RNA had to be treated with DNase (to remove DNA leaching from the filter), purified over oligo(dT) cellulose and concentrated to a few microlitres before injection into oocytes. This lengthy procedure entailed a substantial risk that the RNA might be damaged and for this reason give a negative result. We therefore added some rabbit β-globin cDNA to each filter and rabbit globin mRNA to the leukocyte poly(A)$^+$ RNA, and monitored the production of globin in the injected oocytes whose extracts were assayed in

[10] At the time this was the most sophisticated approach to cloning cDNA.

[11] This was considered to be a "safe" strain because it could only grow in the presence of diaminopimelic acid. It was also difficult to clone anything at all in it, an additional safety feature.

Helsinki. Time and again, one particular group of 512 clones gave a positive result, followed by several negative ones. Each experiment, from hybridisation to the phone call from Finland, took about three weeks. We decided (and what choice did we have?), that in the case of discrepancies we would consider a positive result as the correct answer, and a negative one as a failure of the assay. Thus, four of the groups of 512 clones (see Tab. 1) were broken up into subgroups of 64 clones each and the hybrid DNAs were analysed. While these analyses were going on we tried a short cut: Lorraine prepared bacterial extracts from about 100 pools of 64 bacterial clones each and Kari assayed them for IFN activity. Some pools gave a slight reduction of plaques in the assay but the results were not reproducible and were impaired by a toxic effect of the extracts on the tissue culture cells. Since we did not really believe that this approach would be successful, we dropped it after a few weeks. As we were to realise later, had the assay been more sensitive, or had we used smaller pools of clones, we would indeed have found an IFN-producing clone – a year earlier. We also undertook a further approach, in which we hybridised duplicate colony-carrying filters with cDNA probes made on poly(A)$^+$ RNA from either induced or non-induced cells. Werner Boll, formally a technician

Table 1. mRNA selection hybridisation assay for the detection of IFN cDNA in hybrid DNA from pools of transformed *E. coli*

DNA sample	Interferon activity
Expt 1: Pool of 512 clones	
I	<60 (<60); *110* (<20); <110 (<110); <110 (<110); <35 (<35)
δ	*20* (<20)
N	35 (<20); <110 (<110); *200* (<110)
λ	<60 (<60); *60* (<20); <110 (<110); <110 (<110)
8 other groups negative	
Expt 2: Pool of 64 clones from sample λ	
λ-I	<35 (<35); <35 (<35)
λ-II	*130* (<30); <45 (<45)
λ-III	*225* (<35); *35* (<30); *35* (<30); *600* (<30); <20 (<20)
λ-IV	*85* (<35); <25 (<25)
λ-V to VIII negative	
Expt 3: Pool of 8 clones from sample λ-III	
λ-III-I	<20 (<20); <20 (60); *35* (<30)
λ-III-2	<35 (<35); <30 (<30); *150* (<20); *600* (<35); *110* (60)
λ-III-3	<25 (<25); <30 (<30)
λ-III-4	*30* (<30); <20 (<20); <20 (60)
λ-III-5 to -8 negative	
Expt 4: Single clones from sample λ-III-4	
λ-III-4-C	35 (60); *60* (<35); *111* (<11); <11 (<11); *20* (<20)

The number of bacterial clones indicated in the Table were transferred from the microtiter plates (see legend of Fig. 1) to agar plates, incubated for 24 h and washed off with medium. This suspension was used to inoculate 1-L cultures from which plasmid DNA was prepared. The hybridisation-translation assay was carried out as described in the legend of Figure 2. The values represent the interferon concentration (IU/ml) in the oocyte supernatants. The control values (in parentheses) were obtained with filters carrying only pBR322 DNA. Italicised values are considered positive. From Nagata et al. [21].

but in reality a highly competent research scientist, spent considerable time on this approach, but the hybridisation results were not reproducible and we could not decide which colonies were specifically hybridising with "induced" cDNA.

The Biogen Scientific Board, which met every few months, patiently listened to my inconclusive reports, but other problems were arising which had to be dealt with urgently. For one, the co-founder and president of Biogen, Dan Adams, left the company abruptly at the beginning of 1979 following a disagreement with Inco, an important minority stockholder of Biogen, and the administration of Biogen remained in total disarray. For another, our financial resources were exhausted and at a certain point the company was technically bankrupt (Fig. 4). Nonetheless, plans were being elaborated to set up a Biogen laboratory in Geneva and commitments were made in this direction[12]. Luckily Wally Gilbert, who had been elected chairman of the Scientific Board, took over the duties of a chief executive officer and Moshe Alafi, one of the original venture capitalists backing Biogen, managed to interest Schering-Plough in our company. Thanks in large part to these efforts, Biogen survived the crisis and on June 28, 1979, Schering invested eight million dollars in the company, obtaining in return the rights to leukocyte and fibroblast IFN, as well as an observer seat on the Scientific Board which allowed them to look over our scientific shoulder. The investment permitted us to created the Biogen laboratory in Geneva and intensify research in the universities.

Meanwhile rumours were abounding: in turn, Michel Revel, Lee Hood, Sydney Pestka, Genentech, Dupont or Derek Burke were said to have cloned IFN cDNA; as experience had taught me, I discounted all rumours and hoped for the best. Lorraine left in August 1979 and Table 1 records the arduous progress of Nagata on his own. The subgroups of I, δ and N were negative (although the groups themselves had been positive), but λ-III was repeatedly positive and was therefore subdivided into sub-subgroups of eight. To our surprise, three of these gave positive results. We realised only later that this high frequency of positive sub-subgroups was due to the fact that the frequency of IFN cDNA clones was ten times greater than we had estimated. Most likely each group contained at least one clone and several substantially more than one, but the assay was not sensitive enough to detect groups containing only one or two clones, Thus, to our good fortune, my overestimation of the sensitivity of the assay and underestimation of the IFN mRNA content of leukocyte poly(A)$^+$ RNA cancelled out, allowing us to reach our goal despite my flawed judgement.

---

[12] Bernard Mach had championed Geneva and I Zürich. I was pretty upset when the Board sided with Bernard and, announcing that I was quitting Biogen, stormed out of the meeting held in Davos. Moshe Alafi, ever the mediator, worrying that my resignation might spoil the impending deal with Schering-Plough, followed me out in the street and, entreating me to stay on, asked me which concessions would sway me. I thought up a condition which I considered sufficiently absurd as to be unacceptable, namely to be appointed perpetual member of the Board of Directors. After conferring for a few minutes with the Board, Moshe re-emerged and, grinning, informed me that if I were dumb enough to want this, I should have it. I accepted, in the expectation that this would be galling to Bernard.

zuerich

urgent
biogen s.a.
one new york plaza
suite 3700
new york, n.y. 1004 usa

attn of daniel adams
unable to pay biogen postdocs due to lack of funds
and heavy indebtedness. will have to discontinue biogen
project by end of month unless funds in hand by
feb 25th at latest. regards charles

+
510aq tgptt ch
54354 ehopz ch
+
54354 ehopz ch
517zt tgptt ch

zczc
tax tg jaca1P36 15/1431 newyork fr 69.00
nnnn

+
54354 ehopz ch
517zt tgptt ch

Figure 4. A telegram in an hour of need.

In September Taniguchi wrote from Japan to say that he had identified a fibroblast IFN clone by differential hybridisation and by the same hybridisation-translation analysis we were using, but I was disinclined to believe it because I considered the vagaries of the assay too great to warrant a conclusive identification[13].

The eight clones of λ-III-4 (the first sub-subgroup to give a positive result) were examined singly. At about this time we switched from Millipore to DBM

[13] A nice example of the power of denial.

(dibenzyloxymethyl) paper as support for the DNA and this resulted in recovery of cleaner RNA and lower unspecific backgrounds. Clone λ-III-4C was positive several times – but also negative on occasion. We used the cDNA insert of this clone as a radioactive probe and identified several cross-hybridising clones in sub-subgroups λ-III-1, -2, -3 and -7, although some of these had never been positive in the hybridisation-translation assay. I became very worried about these results – could it be that λ-III-4C had nothing to do with IFN cDNA and was binding IFN mRNA because it contained specially long dC or dG sequences, which might react with complementary sequences in the mRNA? Hapless Nagata (who was convinced he had the correct clone all along) had to carry out further control experiments in which he added oligo(C) to block the putative interactions – with no effect. Finally, Michel Streuli started doing the IFN determinations in our own lab by the cytopathic effect assay[14], and when I saw the protective effect of the oocyte supernatants with my own eyes I too became a believer in λ-III-4C – to an extent.

A merry christmas and a happy new year

Although hybrid DNA responding in the hybridisation-translation assay fulfilled the criteria required of IFN-cDNA containing plasmids, the assay did not provide sufficient proof of identity because any cDNA fortuitously sharing some sequences with IFN mRNA, perhaps even in a non-coding region, could give a positive hybridisation-translation assay. There were only two lines of proof I considered satisfactory. One was to determine the nucleotide sequence of the cloned DNA and compare the amino acid sequence derived from it with that of authentic leukocyte IFN. There was a rumour that Michael Hunkapiller and Lee Hood, using microgram quantities of lymphoblastoid IFN purified by Cathy Zoon and her colleagues [10], had determined the first 15 amino acids of the protein; however, the sequence was not available to us at the time. The other proof would be to get expression of IFN in *E. coli* carrying the hybrid plasmid, a possibility I considered unlikely because I worried that IFN, like other secreted proteins, would be synthesised as a preprotein in which the mature protein was preceded by a signal sequence and thus might be biologically inactive. In addition, leukocyte IFN was considered to be a glycoprotein,

[14] In the summer of 1979 Kari Cantell prepared a large batch of crude nucleic acids from induced leukocytes and shipped it to Zürich for further purification of poly(A)$^+$ RNA before closing down his lab for vacation. While shaking 5 liters or so of the solution with phenol, Lorraine Johnsrud dropped the separatory funnel and the entire preparation, which should have lasted us for the next two months, was lost. I desperately searched for another source of virus-induced human leukocytes – and found it, so to speak, at our doorstep, in the Red Cross laboratory in Bern, which was producing IFN by the Cantell method for the American Cancer Society. While we were working in Bern we were taught the cytopathic assay for IFN, which, while less precise than Cantell's plaque reduction assay, was more sensitive, more rapid and could be carried out in 96-well plates. We then started determining IFN in our own lab, which allowed a greatly reduced turn-around time. Thus, Lorraine's disaster proved to be a blessing in disguise [9].

and we could not expect *E. coli* to glycosylate correctly a eukaryotic polypeptide. Therefore, if activity were contingent on correct glycosylation (although published data suggested the contrary [11–13]), the specific activity of IFN synthesised in *E. coli* might be too low for detection[15].

In any event, we needed a full-length cDNA, and since the insert in the original clone λ-III-4C was only about 3200 nucleotides in length, we searched among cross-hybridising clones for hybrids containing longer cDNAs. λ-III-2H had an insert of 900 nucleotides, which we thought might correspond to the full-length IFN sequence. Hideharu Taira, a "postdoc" from Peter Lengyel's lab, the only person still working on the cloning of mouse IFN cDNA in our lab, abandoned his project and also joined the "human" group to characterise the λ-III-2H DNA by hybridisation-translation. I talked Alan Hall, who had recently joined us, into preparing extracts of *E. coli* containing λ-III-2H DNA and other hybrid plasmids and test them for IFN activity. It was now around December 20, 1979, and after returning to the lab from our institutional Christmas party, Alan reported on the negative outcome of the assay. However, close inspection of the assay plate showed that some extracts had given a barely perceptible protection against the cytopathic effect of the virus. On further enquiry I learnt that the bacterial extracts had been substantially diluted before assaying, and since Alan had left for the Christmas vacation I now asked Michel Streuli to repeat the assay, but at a much lower dilution. Expecting a confirmation of the negative result, I departed on December 23 for a couple of days of skiing with my family. The next day I called Nagata from a phone booth on the top of the Alps and was thunderstruck by the news: a number of bacterial extracts had given strong antiviral protection at several dilutions! My comment: as Nagata recalls it, was simply "fantastic"! I rushed back to Zürich, stopping only to call Nagata a few times more to reassure myself of experimental details, and to call Moshe Alafi in Berkeley asking him to send over Biogen's patent attorney, Jim Haley, with whom I had already drafted the outline of a patent application several months earlier, based on the results accumulated up to that time.

Indeed, the assay plate (Fig. 5) was beautiful, and as I looked at it I experienced the feeling of utter bliss that comes only rarely in a scientific lifetime[16]. I knew with certainty that we had achieved what I had hardly dared hope for, even though we still had to formally prove that the protective agent in the bacterial extracts was indeed an IFN-like substance. Since I had to leave for a meeting in Miami on January 4 and for the Biogen Scientific Board Meeting in Martinique on January 12, we were on a tight schedule. Nagata, Taira and I,

---

[15] In the event, some alpha IFNs, in particular IFN-α2, proved to be glycosylated; however, glycosylation was not essential for activity, at least on cultured cells. It may however play a role in the pharmacokinetics of injected IFN, a possibility that to my knowledge has not been explored.

[16] In my case, six times in 50 years of research. Beside the cloning and expression of IFN: *in vitro* synthesis of infectious Qβ RNA from non-infectious minus strands [14], the first site-directed mutagenesis of Qβ RNA [15], discovery of viral quasi-species [16], infectious Qβ phage produced from cloned Qβ RNA [17] and generation of scrapie-resistant PrP knockout mice [18].

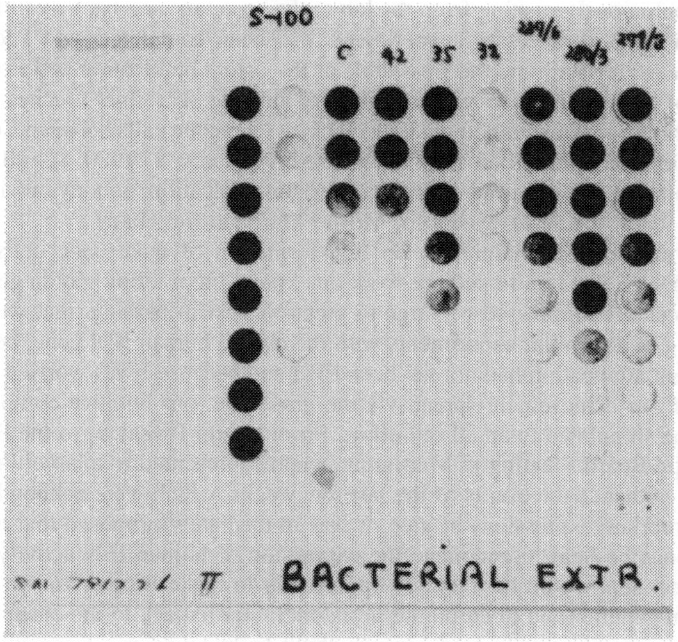

Figure 5. Antiviral activity of crude extracts of bacteria containing interferon cDNA hybrid plasmids. Two hundred bacterial strains containing interferon cDNA hybrid plasmids were identified by a colony hybridisation assay [72] using the first interferon cDNA plasmid isolated (λ-III-4C) as radioactive probe. Bacterial cultures were centrifuged, the bacterial pellet was resuspended in a small volume, digested with lysozyme and the cells lysed by repeated freezing and thawing. The supernatants were assayed by the cytopathic effect reduction assay, using human cells changed with Mengo virus. (a) control cells; (b) cells challenged with Mengo virus; (c) cells pre-treated with 100 units/ml natural leukocyte interferon, serially diluted 1:3 or (d) to (i) with supernatants from the *E. coli* strains SN42, SN35, SN32, 287-2h-AH6, 280-2h-AH3 and 279-2h-AH8, serially diluted 1:3. Assay carried out by Michel Streuli.

the only ones left in the lab, characterised the IFN activity as being due to a trypsin-sensitive, acid-stable substance having almost the same elution profile on Sephadex as authentic leukocyte IFN. However, the critical test was the response of the bacterial activity to antibody directed against human leukocyte IFN. First I, then Taira (and two weeks later Kari Cantell) carried out the titration and to our delight found that the activity was neutralised by leukocyte IFN antibody we had obtained from Mogenson, through Kari Cantell, but not by fibroblast IFN antibody. While these experiments were going on, Jim Haley (who arrived on Christmas Day) and I were writing up the patent application and adding results to it as they came in. A secretary willing to type[17] during the holidays had to be supplied with the hand-written pages in her home, and we

[17] PCs and Macs were still things of the future for us.

were continuously rushing from the lab to the secretary and back at all hours. On January 3 all necessary experiments had been completed, and I left for Miami carrying with me the final draft of the patent application and Polaroid slides of the results to show at the Biogen meeting. The final touches to the application were transmitted via long distance telephone calls between London and Miami, and Jim filed the documents on January 8, 1980. As all these developments had occurred during the Christmas vacation, nobody outside the lab had learnt the news, except for Moshe Alafi and Jim Haley.

The meeting in Miami was on transformation of eukaryotic cells with cloned DNA, and I presented our work on expression of rabbit globin genes in mouse cells. I suppressed my urge to mention, just in passing, that we were planning to do similar experiments with the cloned human IFN gene, because the patent application had not yet been filed and because I was worried that if news of our achievement spread via the grapevine, our putative competitors might be stimulated to an all-out effort. From Miami I went on to the Biogen Scientific Board Meeting in Martinique where I presented to a largely unsuspecting audience the events of the last few weeks, which were acknowledged by appropriate expressions of glee. It was immediately proposed that a press conference be held to announce the expression of human IFN activity in *E. coli*, since this would be a unique opportunity to make Biogen known to the world in general (and to corporate investors in particular). In the ensuing discussion some of us expressed concern about an announcement preceding the publication of a paper, but we were all aware that if we waited until Genentech were successful, we could be sure that they would not hesitate to inform the press and pre-empt Biogen. A compromise was reached: I would give a seminar at MIT and thereafter participate in a news conference. This approach seemed reasonable to me because the scientific aspects or our work would be subjected to critical scrutiny by my peers, prior to appearing in the lay press, not unlike what frequently occurs at a congress, where the speaker is interviewed by the press after an interesting presentation, following which the usual more or less inaccurate accounts appear.

Interferon hits the fan

Since I had to leave for Zürich to start my lecture course at the latest by the night of January 16, i.e., in four days, a flurry of activities developed to organise my seminar and the news conference for January 16, no mean task in view of the difficulties inherent in placing a phone call from the hotel to even the local airport. Transportation to Boston was another problem, and we were finally reduced to chartering a small four-seater plane to take us from Martinique to San Juan. I immediately bought a small typewriter (courtesy of Biogen) and started typing the manuscript for publication, since I wanted to be able to hand out copies to those colleagues or reporters interested in the more technical aspects. Typing in all spare moments, including the wait at the airport, I finished the paper during the trip back to Boston on January 15. The next day, in the early afternoon, I gave my seminar at MIT, coyly entitled something like "Expression of eukaryotic genes in eukaryotic and prokaryotic cells". Despite the title the auditorium was overflowing, and I suspected that some news had preceded me. I spent half the talk on the globin gene transformation work and then, showing my improvised slides, I reported on the cloning and expression of IFN cDNA. Judging by the nature of the questions asked, it was clear that the data had convinced the audience at MIT as they had convinced me, my collaborators and the Biogen Board. In the best of spirits I then went on to the Park Plaza Hotel, to which a number of reporters had been enticed by a somewhat vague invitation promising news of great portent, issued by the Schering-Plough public relations department. I was accompanied by Wally Gilbert, who was going to participate in the presentation for reasons I was to appreciate only later, and Phil Sharp. In a somewhat dingy meeting room, overheated by lights and by a crowd of steaming reporters, Rob Cawthorn, chief executive officer and President of Biogen since several months, started the presentation by introducing Biogen and outlining its relationship to Inco and Schering-Plough. Wally then talked about Biogen's scientific plans and prior achievements, in particular the cloning of hepatitis virus DNA and the expression of hepatitis virus antigens by Ken Murray and his colleagues. He then introduced the subject of IFN, mentioning its scarcity and its potential therapeutic effect. Regarding the putative anti-tumour activity of IFN he said (and this is the complete quote from a transcript; anon. 1980):

"Secondly, at the moment there is a great, great interest in the use of IFN in the treatment of tumour; however again it is not known whether or not the leukocyte IFN is in fact truly a tumor-active agent. There is enough encouragement in the current literature that there are wide-spread clinical trials in this country of IFN as an anti-cancer agent. Those trials will take several years. There is no answer yet from them yet as to whether or not it is a truly effective agent, but the sort of the level of the problem posed by IFN, I can illustrate to you by pointing out to you that the American Cancer Society is spending some two million dollars on those trials and will only manage to treat some one hundred or so people."

Wally's syntax may have left something to be desired, but the description of the potential use of IFN was level-headed and accurate; nevertheless, we were subsequently often misquoted as having touted IFN as an anti-cancer agent in order to promote Biogen. Following Wally, I described the cloning and expression of IFN and then awaited what I expected to be an awe-struck response. However, one of the first questions was whether I had any reason for announcing our results to the press before publishing them in a scientific journal. A transcript of the press conference (Anon., 1980) records for posterity my suave response which started by "Yes, I think, I mean, I don't – " and continued in a similar vein to explain our motivation for the announcement. As the question grew more hostile, Wally Gilbert gently unclenched my fist from the microphone and took firm control of the press conference. Eventually, all important aspects were dealt with accurately; we made it clear that the IFN produced in *E. coli* was most likely not chemically identical to natural IFN, in that it was somewhat larger (presumably because it had a signal sequence or was a fused protein), that it was produced at a level about a thousand times lower (about 20,000 units per litre) than was available from leukocyte cultures and – in response to a specific question – that we were convinced that we were the first to synthesise a compound with human IFN activity in *E. coli*, while others (and this referred to Tada albeit without naming him) had at most identified IFN cDNA-containing clones by hybridisation procedures. With what turned out to be amazing insight, Wally predicted that within one to two years we would be able to manufacture IFN for clinical trials.

I left the press conference somewhat shaken and realised that had Wally, who was well known to the science writer community, not been present to put the full weight of his reputation and authority behind me, the claims of an unknown, seedily clad (despite a tie borrowed from a press agent) foreigner would not have carried much weight. Rob Cawthorn and I took the night plane and emerged bleary-eyed in Zürich[18] to learn that the news had hit the fan with a vengeance, making the front page of most major newspapers in the USA, Japan and Europe. In the first few days, fascination with the achievement (which was, to my annoyance, frequently attributed to "a Biogen scientist" or worse yet, to Wally Gilbert accompanied by his photograph) predominated. The immense response was in part due to the American press having been heavily primed for this forthcoming feature, the bacterial production of a priceless miracle drug; the stage had been set, largely by West Coast entrepreneurs, and when the curtain rose – albeit on the wrong cast – the success of the event was guaranteed. After some weeks, however, interest in the popular scientific features had worn off and a new aspect gained prominence in the newspaper – namely the news conference and my relationship to Biogen (Fig. 6). I was surprised at the negative response to what in other fields had a long tradition in Switzerland and probably elsewhere, namely the underwriting of university research to a significant extent by commercial companies and the issuing of patents to university scientists or the companies themselves. In any event, I experienced no discomfort as I had duly disclosed my commercial relationship with Biogen to the university when it was initiated, and a satisfactory agreement between myself, Biogen and the university, covering the commercially oriented activities of my lab, was formalised soon thereafter[19]. The concerns of part of the scientific community were expressed in a scale

[18] As we walked down the hallway at the Zürich airport, Rob Cawthorn, who was continuing on to Geneva, remembered to repossess the portable typewriter purchased with Biogen funds. Despite this demonstration of fiscal responsibility, Rob was eventually replaced as CEO by Bob Fildes. Bob later became CEO of Cetus and presided over its final downfall.

[19] Up to that time, royalties collected by university professors on inventions carried out during their tenure remained their property. Our agreement was the first ever in Switzerland to provide for participation of the university in royalties; in fact, all royalties flowed to the university and neither my laboratory nor I benefited from them. But not to worry, I reaped a handsome reward from the Biogen shares I was assigned and the lab was supported by Biogen with generous grants for many years.

Cloning Gold Rush Turns Basic Biology into Big Business

Cloning a gene can help raise $50 million for your company. Will the laboratory suffer?

The date on which molecular biology became big business was 16 January 1980. Reporters had been notified by telegram that a "major announcement" in molecular biology would be made by the company Biogen and two members of its scientific advisory board, Charles Weissman of the University of Zurich and Walter Gilbert of Harvard. The news delivered at the Boston Park Plaza Hotel was that Weissman had cloned and got expression of the human leucocyte interferon gene in biologically active form.

"should not be interpreted to mean that it has any significant advantage in either technology or patent protection. Achieving expression of the [interferon] gene is only the first of many steps required to demonstrate a commercial process."

By all accounts, neither Weissman nor Gilbert exaggerated the significance of the news to the assembled reporters. Nonetheless, the mere context of the occasion, which linked the recombinant DNA technique with the possibility of manufacturing a promising anti-cancer

pany's paper value at $50 million. A few months before the January press conference, Biogen had decided to raise more capital on the basis of a self-assessed paper value of more than $100 million. Biogen president Robert Cawthorn says that the purpose of the press conference was not primarily to help raise more capital for the company. "The intent was to draw attention to Biogen. The day may come when we want to go public. So it is better that the public knows something about Biogen." But Cawthorn confirms

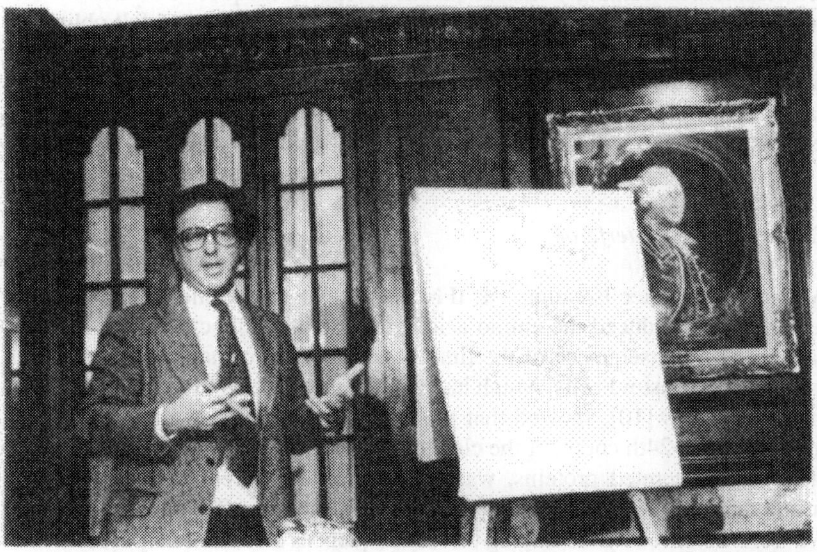

Photo by Julie Miller

Charles Weissman at Biogen's $50 million press conference.

Figure 6. Cloning of interferon as featured in Science magazine. Fragment from an article by Nicholas Wade [19].

ranging from thoughtful and balanced, as in an article by Science reporter Nicholas Wade [19], to plaintive and ill-informed, as in a threnody by Spyros Andreopoulos [20] from the News Bureau of Stanford University, whose attempt to publicise Stanford's gene cloning achievements had fallen short of his aspirations, or emotional and vindictive, as in a pamphlet by a gifted microbial geneticist (but mediocre essayist) at the University of Geneva, which so far has failed to see the light of day but may doubtless be obtained in a plain brown wrapper from the author[20]. Many of the problems raised in these articles are real and will have to be dealt with when the dust has settled and emotions have cooled.

Life after cloning

Upon returning to Zürich I submitted our paper to Nature where it appeared on March 27, 1980 [21], the first report on the production of a human IFN-like protein in *E. coli*. In the meantime, pre-prints describing all essential features of the work, including detailed data on the restriction map of the IFN cDNA, had been sent to all scientists I knew to be working in the field (excepting only some commercial competitors)[21]. Our lab was flooded with requests for IFN, often in the form of desperate letters, all of which I answered in an appropriately apologetic fashion. A seemingly endless stream of reporters requested interviews and information, and feeling guilty of having initiated the publicity, I felt obligated to clarify and explain the cloning of IFN to one and all. In the midst of this bedlam we intensely pushed ahead with the IFN project in four directions: elucidation of the structure of IFN, isolation of the chromosomal IFN gene, high-level expression of a mature IFN, and fermentation and purification of IFN.

The structure of interferon

Within weeks after isolating the IFN cDNA, we determined its nucleotide sequence and deduced the amino acid sequence of "leukocyte IFN". A comparison with the sequence of the first 20 amino acids of natural IFN purified from lymphoblastoid cells, which had just been published by Zoon, Hood and their colleagues [10], showed that the first amino acid of natural IFN corresponded to the 24th codon of the cloned sequence, suggesting that IFN, like so many other secreted proteins, was synthesised as a preprotein and that an amino terminal segment with 23 residues was cleaved off during maturation. We were disturbed by the finding that the sequences determined by Hood's and our group differed in five of 20 positions. A long phone conversation, during which I read off our sequence to Mike Hunkapiller and learnt some additional sequence data from him, led us to the conclusion that neither of us could have made that many errors and that there must exist at least two different genes for

[20] Jeffrey Miller submitted his article to Nature and John Maddox, Editor-in-Chief at the time, after allowing me to respond to the diatribe, decided not to publish it.

[21] It later emerged that Genentech almost immediately obtained the information anyway, as well as the sequence we distributed as pre-prints.

alpha IFN. Michel Streuli therefore started examining other IFN-producing bacterial clones in order to analyse additional IFN cDNAs. In the meantime, I had heard from Tada that he had almost finished the sequence of the cDNA he had isolated and that it encoded an amino acid sequence identical to that of beta IFN from fibroblasts, as far as the latter had been determined [22]. Thus, he could establish the identity of his cloned cDNA, despite the failure to obtain expression of fibroblast IFN in *E. coli* up to that time. Tada and I agreed to publish the two sequences back to front in Gene [23, 24], and Tada came to Zürich (on his way to Harvard, where he was to collaborate with Mark Ptashne on the expression of his clone) so that we could compare the two sequences. Sprawled on the carpet of my living room, we quickly found, to our delight, that alpha and beta IFN were distinctly related, 29% of their residues being identical. We estimated that the two genes must have diverged some 500–1000 million years ago and thus should be as old as the vertebrates. The papers describing these results [23–25] were also widely distributed as pre-prints, and several groups began attempts to synthesise IFN or parts of it chemically, albeit without succeeding in producing biologically active material to the time of writing; others again undertook to synthesise the cDNA chemically. Michel Streuli found a cDNA clone with a restriction pattern distinctly different from that of the first one and when he determined its nucleotide sequence, the two were found to differ in 20% of their residues [26]; again neither of them were identical with the partial sequence described by Zoon et al. [10]. It thus became clear that there had to exist at least three different genes for IFNs of the leukocyte type[22]. We realised that the multiple peaks of IFN activity described by Rubinstein et al. [27] likely corresponded to products of different genes and not to forms of one IFN differing merely in length and in degree of glycosylation, as was commonly thought. We were excited to find that IFN-α1 and -α2 differed in their host-cell specificity, in that IFN-α1 was about ten times less active on human than on bovine cells, whereas IFN-α2 had about the same activity on both cell types [26, 28]. This suggested to us that the IFNs might have different targets within one organism, but no other evidence in favour of this view has yet been reported. In any event it was clear that at least one of the species, IFN-α1, had a number of the properties previously ascribed to the impure mixture of natural IFNs, for example, activation of natural killer cells, inhibition of Daudi cell growth, enhancement of antibody-dependent cell-mediated cytotoxicity and suppression of antigen and mitogen-induced leukocyte migration inhibition [29].

The interferon gene family

Meanwhile I had obtained from Tom Maniatis his human gene bank, which had been prepared by partially cleaving the DNA of a single human embryo

[22] A gene encoding the sequence published by Zoon et al. has never been found, and I believe the sequence represents the composite of two or more IFN species.

with HaeIII and AluI restriction nucleases and cloning the DNA in a phage lambda vector [30]. As the human genome has about 3×10^9 base pairs and the average fragment size of the cloned DNA fragments was about 16,000 base pairs, it was expected that one phage in about 190,000 would contain an IFN gene, if there were one gene per haploid genome. By hybridising 240,000 phage plaques with a labelled IFN cDNA probe, Nagata identified 16 clones containing DNA related to IFN-α1 cDNA, suggesting that there might be 10–15 IFN-related genes per haploid genome [31]. Restriction and sequence analyses of the cloned DNAs, as well as electron microscopic studies carried out by Christine Brack, led to the map shown in Figure 7, in which 15 different alpha IFN genes and pseudogenes are indicated [32]. Altogether, as emerges from the sequence analyses carried out in our laboratories and by David Goeddel and his colleagues at Genentech (Fig. 8) (yes, Genentech eventually did get into the game, and with great vigour, too), there exist at least 12 distinct IFN genes, which we consider to be non-allelic (Tab. 2)[23]. In addition,

Table 2. Interferon genes and pseudogenes

(1) Genes closely related to IFN-α1			
(a)	Sequenced and correlated with Geneentech sequences		
	Zürich		*Genentech Inc. (USA)*
	IFN-α1	=	IFN-D
	IFN-α2	=	IFN-A
	IFN-α3[a]	=	IFN-F
	IFN-α5	=	IFN-G
	IFN-α8	=	IFN-B
	ψIFN-α10	=	IFN-C
(b)	Sequenced but not correlated		
	IFN-α4	=	IFN-E
	IFN-α6	=	IFN-H
	IFN-α7	=	IFN-I
(b)	Not sequenced but different from above		
	G-chr-19		
	G-chr-27		
Altogether at least 12 genes and pseudogenes			
(2) Genes distantly related to IFN-α1			
(a)	Sequenced		
	ψIFN-α9		
	ψIFN-α11		
	ψIFN-α12		
(a)	Not sequenced		
	G-chr-10		
	G-chr-26R		
	G-chr-19R		
	G-chr-16		
Altogether at least 7 genes and pseudogenes			

[a] This designation was originally assigned to the protein sequence of [10]. The gene has not been found in Zürich (or anywhere else).

[23] The final count is 14 alpha-type genes [33].

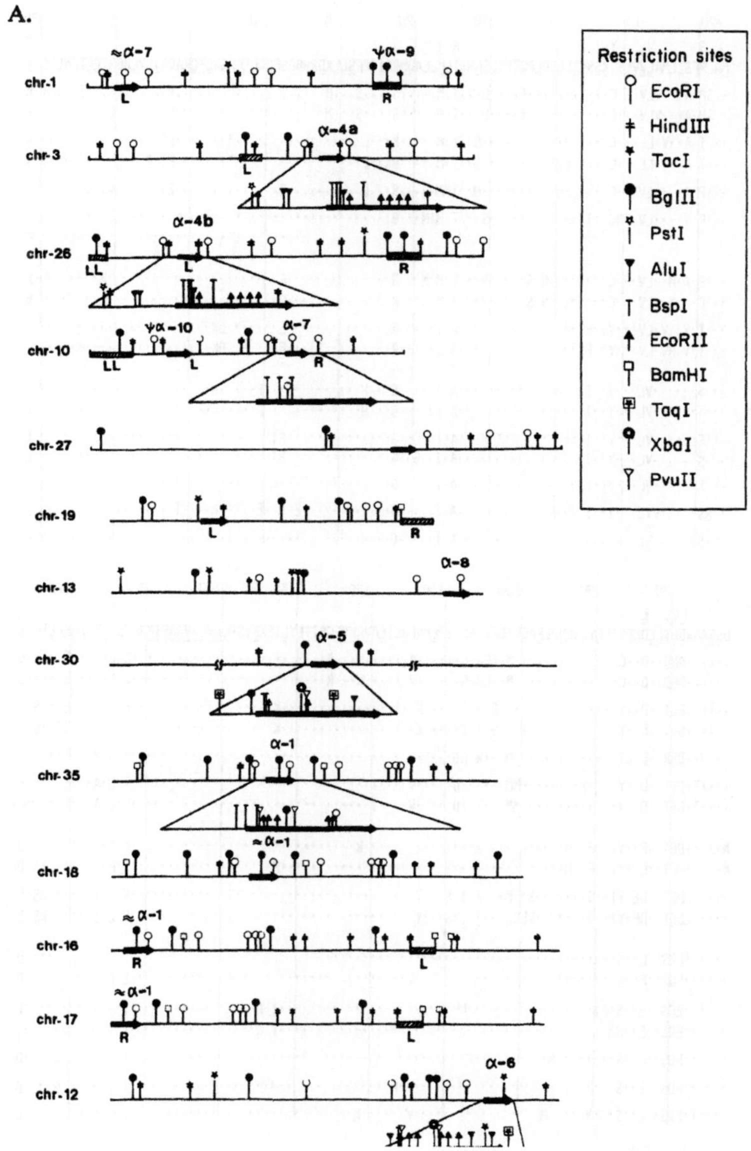

Figure 7. Location of alpha interferon genes and pseudogenes on cloned fragments of human chromosomal DNA. (A) the designation at the left of each line identifies the clone. Arrows indicate the orientation of the gene or pseudogene. Genes designated with α followed by a number have been sequenced; ψ indicates a pseudogene. = means that the gene is identical or very similar (allelic) to the gene with the same designation. Restriction sites are indicated by the key. (B) from the data of (A) and heteroduplex mapping a partial linkage map could be constructed. The 36 kilobase pair DNA segment comprises 6 genes or pseudogenes: α4 and α6 are sequenced genes. ψα-10 and ψα-9 are sequenced pseudogenes. G-chr-10LL and G-chr-26R have not yet been sequenced. From [32].

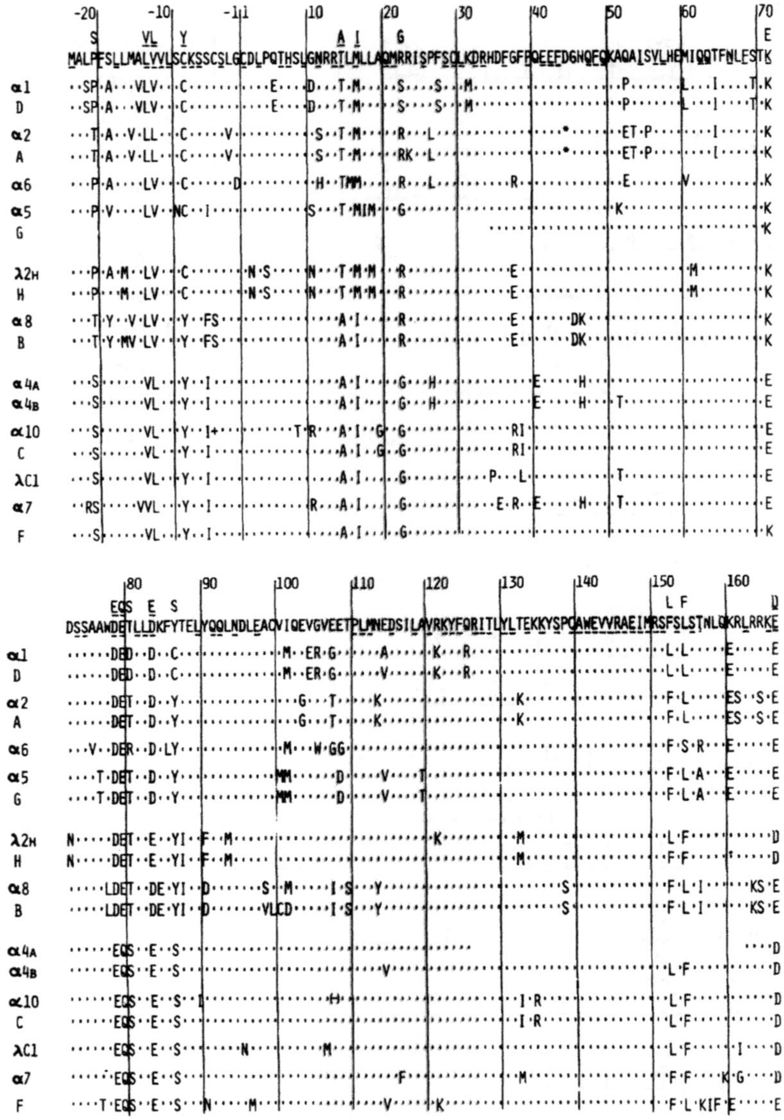

Figure 8. Amino acid sequences of alpha interferons. All sequences have been derived from the nucleotide sequences of cloned cDNAs or chromosomal DNAs. Sequences designated with letters are from work by the Genentech group [34, 73]; the sequences designated with Arabic numerals were determined by Mantei et al. [23] (1980) (IFN-α1), Streuli et al. [26] (IFN-α2), A. Schamböck (IFN-α4a), K. Henco (IFN-α4b), J. Fujisawa (IFN-α5), J. Schmid (IFN-α6), T. Kovacic (Biogen SA, Geneva) (IFN-α7), M. Pasek (Biogen SA, Geneva), (IFN-α8), and J. Hochstadt and J. Brosius (Harvard University Biological Laboratories (IFN-α10)[24].

[24] For a more complete survey of IFN genes and sequences, see refs. [33, 50].

several allelic variants of these genes were identified. Probably ten or more genes are expressed in man, as judged by the fact that they give rise in *E. coli* to biologically active IFNs and that in many cases the corresponding mRNAs occur in IFN-producing cells [34]. Allen and Fantes [35] have, by amino acid sequence analysis, shown that IFN preparations from lymphoblastoid cells contain at least five different IFN species, of which one corresponds to IFN-α2, and another most likely to IFN-α1.

Besides the genes which have an intact coding sequence, a large number of so-called pseudogenes were identified, i.e., DNA sequences which are clearly related to functional genes, but whose coding sequences contain mutations which prevent the expression of a full-length IFN-like protein. These mutations range from a single nucleotide substitution which introduces a premature termination signal into the coding region, to multiple, extensive insertions and deletions that mutilate the gene to virtual unrecognisability.

It seems that the gene family arose by duplication of an ancestral alpha IFN gene some 20–80 million years ago and that further duplications occurred up to recent times; concurrently, genes were constantly degenerating as a consequence of deleterious mutations. The IFN gene family thus seems to be in a state of flux, with genes being created and destroyed over the millennia. We wonder if the maintenance of all these different genes has a purpose. Are different genes turned on in different tissues or in response to different stimuli? Are they directed to different target cells or are we witnessing an evolutionary quirk, for which there is no selective advantage? All these questions can and will be answered: most probably there is a reason for the existence of multiple leukocyte IFNs because the mouse, which probably diverged from the human line before the divergence of the leukocyte IFN genes, also possesses a family of such genes (N. Mantei, unpublished results)[25], while the gene coding for fibroblast IFN-β1[26] is, at least in the human, a solitary gene [39, 40]. I should note, however, that the data could also be explained differently, namely by assuming that the IFN-α gene family arose before human and mouse diverged, and that the genes of the IFN-α family were subsequently rendered more similar to each other by gene conversion.

A further surprise emerged from the sequence analysis of the IFN genes: none of them is interrupted by an intervening sequence (or intron) [31] as are almost all genes of higher eukaryotes. This brings a great advantage to the gene cloners, because it means that all chromosomal IFN genes can be directly expressed in *E. coli*, which is not the case for genes containing an intron in the coding sequence.

The further bonus of this work came quite recently, when Ned Mantei introduced the cloned human IFN-α1 gene into mouse cells and showed that the

[25] [36]

[26] The (transient) designation IFN β1 for the cDNA isolated by both Taniguchi and Fiers came about because Michel Revel claimed to have isolated an cDNA from fibroblasts whose expression product showed antiviral activity and which he called IFN β2 [37]. However, no other lab could confirm the antiviral activity and "IFN β2" was finally identified as congruent with IL-6 [38].

integrated gene is under host cell control, i.e., it is expressed correctly only when the mouse cells are induced to produce their own IFN [41]. This system will probably allow us to determine which part of the DNA is responsible for the control of IFN expression, one of the goals which initially enticed us into the field[27].

Expression and purification of mature interferon from E. coli

The strain of *E. coli* containing the IFN-α1 cDNA is the PstI site of the plasmid pBR322 which had relatively low levels of IFN activity, only a few molecules of the active protein per cell. The yield was rapidly increased about 1000-fold by inserting a DNA fragment containing the lac promoter of the β galactosidase gene [42] in front of the IFN cDNA. The IFN polypeptide produced by this and similar constructions was preceded by part of the signal sequence and by a few amino acids of β galactosidase; in no case was the signal sequence cleaved off correctly in *E. coli*. Having anticipated this problem, we had already undertaken more elaborate constructions, in which the signal sequence of IFN-α2 cDNA was removed and a lac or β-lactamase promoter fused to the latter (M. Mishina, W. Boll and A. Hall, unpublished results) (Fig. 9), such that the sequence coding for the mature protein was preceded by an AUG (initiator) triplet only. The resulting strains produced about 2×10^8 units (about 1 mg) of IFN per litre of culture. This IFN differed from authentic IFN only in that about half of the molecules carried a supernumerary amino terminal methionine residue. In October 1980 David Goeddel and his colleagues [43] reported that they too had cloned and expressed human leukocyte IFN in a similar fashion and had obtained enough of it to inject three squirrel monkeys and demonstrate protection against viral infection. I was impressed[28] (and stimulated) by the speed and efficiency with which the Genentech team had caught up with us in regard to the expression and preparation of IFN. Since Schering-Plough was not yet in a position to ferment *E. coli* on a large scale, I undertook to work out a procedure for the fermentation and extraction of IFN which was compatible with the NIH Recombinant DNA Guidelines and could be applied on an industrial scale. The major problem we had to solve was how to kill the bacteria before removing them from the fermentor in such a way that IFN could still be extracted in an active form. Cathy Schein, Josef Ecsödi and I worked on this – once again man-made – problem for several months and finally came up with an elegant solution which allowed us to scale up fermentation first to the 3000 litre level in Brian Hartley's pilot plant at Imperial College, and then to the 30,000 litre level in an industrial fermentation plant

[27] We did indeed determine that a 42-nucleotide segment preceding the transcribed sequence contained several elements required for inducible expression but our work never reached the in-depth level of the IFN β promoter analysis carried out by Maniatis, Taniguchi, Hiscott and others.

[28] "depressed" would have been the more accurate term.

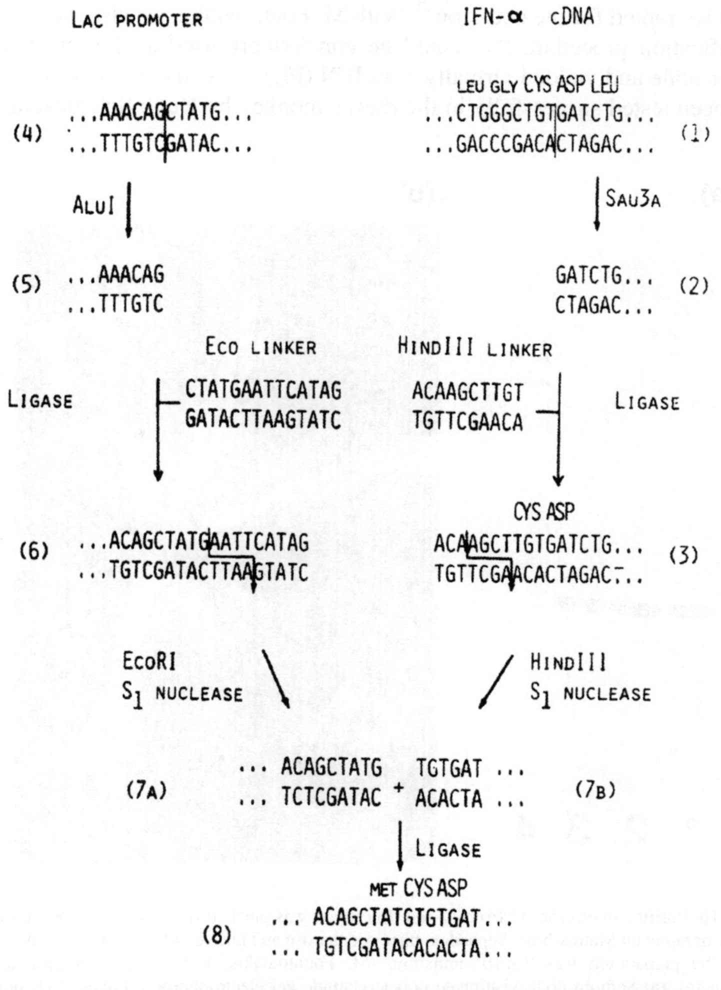

Figure 9. Construction of a hybrid plasmid encoding methionyl-interferon α2. The coding sequence of interferon α2 (1) was cleaved at the Sau3a site (2) located between the codon for the first and second amino acid of the mature interferon sequence, and a synthetic oligonucleotide (HindIII linker) was ligated to the cleavage end, reconstructing the first (cysteine) codon and adding a HindIII cleavage site (3). A bacterial promoter-containing DNA fragment derived from the lac operon (4) was cleaved at an AluI site preceding the AUG initiator triplet by 2 nucleotides (5), and a synthetic oligonucleotide (EcoRI linker) was ligated to the cut end reconstructing the original sequence (3) was digested with HindIII and the single-strand specific nuclease S1 to generate a flush end immediately preceding the cysteine codon (7b). The promoter sequence (6) was digested with EcoRI and S1 nuclease to give a flush end immediately following the initiator AUG codon. The two ends (7b) were joined with DNA ligase to yield a sequence encoding mature interferon preceded by a methionine[29]. When expressed in *E. coli*, about half the interferon molecules lose the methionine residue by post-translation cleavage.

---

[29] If nothing else, the strategy outlined in this figure demonstrates how laborious it was to make precise DNA constructions before the advent and popularisation of PCR technology.

which we rented for the occasion[30]. With M. Fountoulakis we also worked out a purification procedure that could be comfortably used at this or an even greater scale and yielded virtually pure IFN (Figs 10A, B). Such preparations have been tested successfully in the rhesus monkey by Huub Schellekens and

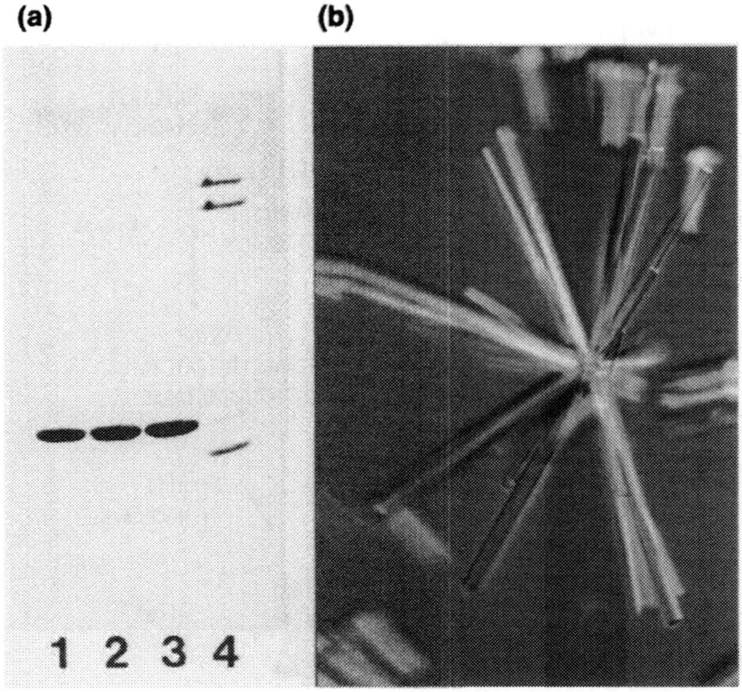

Figure 10. Purified interferon α2 from *E. coli*. Interferon was purified from extracts of *E. coli* using chromatography on Matrex blue, Sephadex, phenylsepharose and DEAE columns. The specific activity of the preparation was 2×10^8 units/mg. (M. Fountoulakis, J. Ecsödi, C. Schein and C. Weissmann). (a) Sodium dodecylsulphate-polyacrylamide gel electrophoresis. Lanes, 1–3, purified IFN-α2. Lane 4, molecular weight markers, from top to bottom: bovine serum albumin (68,000), catalase (60,000), β lactoglobulin (18,000), cytochrome C (13,000). (b) Photomicrograph of interferon α2 crystals (Courtesy of T.L. Nagabhushan, Schering-Plough).

30 The plant, located in Kundl, Austria, belonged to Sandoz and was extremely well run. Schering-Plough, desperate to develop the recombinant IFN, was charged an arm and a leg for the rental.

31 This report led me to believe that our purified recombinant IFN would not show the very unpleasant side-effects reported for partially purified leukocyte IFN. Shige Nagata described the consequences of my misapprehension in his reminiscence 'Happy days in Zürich' [44]: " Several people in the lab produced human IFN-α in *E. coli*. After examination with monkeys, the purified protein was put in small vials for clinical trials. One evening, Charles called me into his office, and said: 'Tomorrow morning, we are shipping this purified IFN-α for clinical trials. I will now inject 10 mg of the recombinant IFN-α into my own vein [in reality, subcutaneously]. If I am dead by tomorrow morning, please do not ship this protein.' I, of course, advised him not to do such a stupid (?) thing.

found to be completely non-toxic[31] at many times the dosage required to fully prevent lesion formation following inoculation with vaccinia [45]. They have recently entered clinical trials. With this, the goals formulated with Biogen in 1978 ("... to clone and express human leukocyte IFN, and develop a product accepted by the human organism...") had been completed[32].

What next?

As discussed above, IFN preparations derived from natural leukocytes or lymphoblastoid cells consist of about ten different species, present in unequal proportions, which are difficult to separate on a preparative scale. The cloning of the genes and their expression in *E. coli* make it possible to isolate each IFN species and examine its properties separately and in combination. One major task is to determine the therapeutic potential of the IFNs. Not only must an effective and safe dosage be determined, but this must be done separately for viral and neoplastic diseases, and for the different IFN species, using appropriate patient control groups. There are basically two approaches to the problem, especially with regard to cancer: either one uses patients in an advanced stage of disease where other treatments are no longer effective, in which case a beneficial effect of IFN may be difficult to demonstrate because of high tumour load and diminished immunological defence, or one has to use IFN in combination with a conventional form of treatment, in which case large patient groups and long follow-ups will be required to discern the additional effect of IFN. Only if and when a distinct beneficial effect of IFN is found, can one substitute it for conventional treatment. If, as some suspect, only a fraction of all cancers were to respond to treatment, it might be possible to screen the response of tumour cells of individual patients in nude mice [46] or even *in vitro* [47] and thus select patients for whom IFN treatment may be beneficial. Should IFN, at least in moderate doses, prove to be innocuous and to cause remission of tumours in a certain proportion of patients, it would be desirable to study the prophylactic effect of IFN, administered periodically for limited time spans, on a group of high-risk cancer patients, for example, heavy smokers or patients previously subjected to irradiation or chemotherapy.

We have shown that it is possible to construct hybrid genes and express the cognate hybrid IFNs in *E. coli*. Figure 11 shows the structure of hybrids

---

But he did. When I came back to the lab from my quick supper, Charles had left the office for a party in town. Next morning I heard from Rose-Marie that Charles suddenly fell down during the party, and could not stand up. He could not come to the lab for three days. This was the first demonstration of the strong side-effects of (pure) IFN-α in man".

[32] Schering-Plough was in the meantime developing better expression systems and a more manageable extraction procedure; one important objection to our lysis method was that it involved penicillin, because even minute residues of penicillin in the final product might lead to anaphylactic shock in sensitive patients. Thanks to a massive effort under the direction of T.L. Nagabhushan a highly purified IFN-α2 was produced by a procedure involving several of the steps we had worked out, followed by crystallisation as final step.

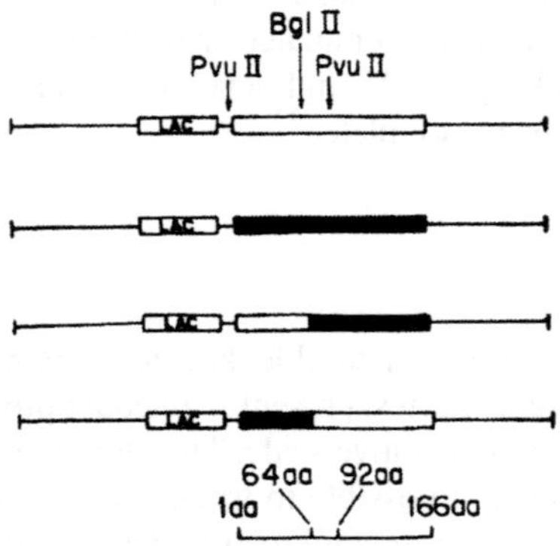

	IFN UNITS PER ML		
	HUMAN WISH	BOVINE MDBK	MOUSE L929
α-1	3500 (20)	17000 (100)	1800 (10)
α-2	25000 (190)	13000 (100)	60 (0.5)
α-1(B)α-2	100 (1.7)	6000 (100)	9 (0.15)
α-2(B)α-1	7000 (100)	7000 (100)	12000 (170)

Figure 11. Target cell specificity of interferon α1, α2 and hybrids of interferons α1 and α2. Hybrid genes were prepared by joining the 5' moiety of one gene with the 3' moiety of another and *vice-versa*. The interferons were expressed in *E. coli* under identical conditions and assayed on different target cells. From Streuli et al. [48].

formed between IFN-α1 and -α2, and some of their biological properties [48]. It is remarkable that some hybrid IFNs have properties different from either parental molecule; for example, both IFN-α1 and -α2 have a lower activity on mouse cells than on human WISH or on bovine cells, but the hybrid molecule consisting of the amino terminal half of IFN-α2 and the carboxy terminal half of IFN-α1 has the highest activity on mouse cells. Using such reconstruction techniques, as well as site-directed mutagenesis, it will perhaps be possible to tailor IFN with specific target specification or even selected functions, although it remains to be seen whether such unnatural compounds are antigenically inert in the human.

On the commercially oriented side, the cost-effectiveness of production must still be optimised, which implies more productive strains (including micro-organisms other than *E. coli*), cheaper media and more effective purification. As regards basic research, we still have to construct a complete map of the IFN gene family, a task which we are collaborating on with Dick Flavell[33]. We have finally isolated a mouse IFN-α gene and are exploring the mouse system with Peter Lengyel. Much of our interest is devoted to identifying the sequences required for expression and control of expression of the IFN genes, using the techniques of reverse genetics [51–54].

[33] See refs. [33, 49, 50].

Epilogue

My decision to perform industrially oriented research in a university laboratory and to participate in the creation of Biogen was taken lightly, as I expected neither project to be successful. I have since asked myself whether I would have acted differently had I anticipated the outcome. On the negative side I count the adverse publicity and the critical attitude of many colleagues (although this consideration is mitigated by most of them having meanwhile also either joined companies or started their own), the very heavy work load I ended up with and the dilution of my interest in purely academic matters. On the positive side, I had the satisfaction of applying my accumulated experience to create a potentially useful product, of learning industrial techniques and procedures I was hitherto wholly unfamiliar with, and helping create a company which might become commercially successful and – a most pleasant prospect – ultimately benefit me and my colleagues. Much of the recent work on strain improvement, fermentation and purification could not have been carried out without the massive financial support by Biogen, since the costs were a multiple of our normal university research budget, and I would not have had the courage to request such sums from public agencies for a project whose ultimate outcome – both medical and commercial – was (and still is) so uncertain[34]. Last but not least, the interferon project generated important spin-offs for the basic research in our laboratory and financial support for the university. In following the path I did, I may have accelerated a controversial development which was taking place anyway, namely the involvement of academic scientists and university laboratories in industrial research. I have not drawn the bottom line on all of this, but it may well be that I would commit all my mistakes over again if given the choice.

Acknowledgements
The research I have described came about thanks to the skill and enthusiasm of as gifted and loyal a group of collaborators as I have ever had the pleasure to work with. My special thanks go to the indefatigable Shige Nagata, Michel Streuli and Josef Ecsödi, and to our dedicated secretary, Rose-Marie von Rotz, whose organisational skill and resourcefulness time and again saved the day. I thank the Kanton of Zürich, the Schweizerische Nationalfonds and Biogen SA for financial support.

Appendix (added July 2000)

Interferon becomes a drug

Interferon had been discovered in 1957 as an antivirally active protein recovered from virus-infected chicken chorio-allantoic membranes [55] and not surprisingly, its possible clinical application in viral infections was explored early on. However, results were not encouraging, not least due to the difficulties in

[34] But see below how IFN-α became an important drug.

preparing sufficient quantities of IFN active in humans, and efforts were virtually suspended in the mid-sixties [56]. As leukocyte IFN, due to the heroic efforts of Kari Cantell, and then lymphoblastoid IFN (prepared from induced lymphoblastoid cells by Wellcome) became available in larger (but as yet limiting) quantities, treatment of hepatitis B patients for several weeks or months became possible and led to transient reductions of disease markers, but not to lasting benefits [57, 58]. In the meantime, the focus of interest was shifting. Because in the mid-sixties it was believed that many human cancers were caused by viruses, studies on the effect of IFN on murine leukaemia (caused by a retrovirus) and other murine tumour models (not known to be caused by virus) were initiated and reported to be successful [59, 60]. However, it was the claim by Strander that leukocyte IFN could arrest the progression of osteosarcoma that sparked a firestorm of enthusiasm, fanned by the indefatigable efforts of Mathilde Krim, a financially and politically well-connected erstwhile geneticist, and led to the commitment of the American Cancer Society to apportion some two million dollars for the purchase of Cantell's leukocyte IFN. The inflated expectations and the publicity generated by these events were at their acme at the time we produced recombinant IFN and they had subsided in the early eighties, when clinical trials with recombinant IFN-α2 as well as with natural IFN as single drugs on a variety of solid tumours failed to demonstrate efficacy and resulted in wide-spread disillusionment and a publicity backlash.

Schering-Plough and Roche nonetheless vigorously and competitively pushed ahead with the development of recombinant IFN-α2 and explored a variety of clinical applications, ranging from warts and the common cold to multiple myeloma and solid tumours. The immediate aim was to obtain FDA approval for at least one application, the hope being that once recombinant IFN could be marketed, off-label use by physicians on a variety of diseases, perhaps in combination with other drugs, would lead to other applications. This climate of despondency was dispelled explosively by the report of Jorge Quesada, in 1984, that 3 complete and 4 partial responses in 7 patients suffering from hairy cell leukaemia, a rare but lethal disease, had been evoked by treatment with partially purified leukocyte IFN [61]. This led to a number of clinical trials with recombinant IFN-α and resulted in the first FDA-approved indication for the products of Schering-Plough (rIFN-α2b, Intron A) and Roche (rIFN-α2a, Roferon), in 1986[35]. The clinical response was dramatic in

[35] rIFN-α2a and rIFN-α2b differ only by a single amino acid in position 23 (lys in α2a, arg in α2b). IFN-α2b, whose cDNA was prepared by us from leukocyte mRNA was identified as a component of natural leukocyte IFN, and the corresponding gene was found [49]. The cDNA for rIFN-α2a was prepared from a T-cell leukaemia line, KG-1; however, a gene encoding this protein was never found in DNA recovered from human tissue, suggesting that it arose by mutation during long-term passaging or that the cell line was derived from an individual with a rare polymorphic variation [62, 63]. Why did both companies develop IFN-α2? IFN-α2 and IFN-α1 are the major species produced by myeloid cells and therefore their mRNAs and consequently their cDNAs were the most abundant. Because IFN-α2 has an about 20-fold higher specific activity on human cells than IFN-α1, our choice was clearly IFN-α2

a large proportion of patients; however, about half the responding patients eventually suffered a relapse. Interferon has now been replaced by purine analogues in the treatment of hairy cell leukaemia; however, the dramatic clinical success and the ready availability[36] of recombinant IFN-α2 paved the way for its further clinical exploration. Beneficial effects, albeit no permanent cures, were attained in a varying proportion of patients with other malignancies, such as non-Hodgkin's lymphomas, chronic myeloid leukaemia, melanoma, AIDS-associated Kaposi sarcoma and renal cell carcinoma. The combination of IFN with chemotherapeutic agents gives an added advantage in some instances. Non-malignant tumours such as life-threatening haemangiomas and genital warts are further indications for IFN-α. However, the obvious application, treatment of viral diseases, took a back seat in the early eighties[37] and surged only by the end of the decade, when it became apparent that prolonged treatment of chronic hepatitis B with IFN-α led to responses in 30–40% of the patients, as shown by loss of viral markers and normalisation of liver enzymes [66]. However, it was only when IFN proved to be effective in chronic hepatitis C, a disease hitherto unresponsive to any treatment, that a major field of application was uncovered, as reflected in an avalanche of reports and a sevenfold or so increase in sales of Intron A between 1990 and 1992, to reach several hundred million dollars per year. Although the initial response rate is 40–50%, sustained responses are only found in 10–20% of patients. Unfortunately hepatitis C virus (Type 1), the most frequent of the six described genotypes, is far more resistant to IFN treatment than the others; there are no clear data as to which of the viral sequences are responsible for this resistance. In recent years the combination of IFN-α with the guanosine analogue ribavirin, which by itself is not a therapeutic agent for hepatitis C [67], more than doubles the response rate found with IFN alone [68]. Pegylated IFN-α, in which polyethylene glycol is covalently linked to the protein at various sites, results in greatly sustained serum levels and increased response rates [69]. The combination of pegylated IFN with ribavirin (or other antiviral drugs) will almost certainly result in further improvement of hepatitis C therapy.

Revolution and evolution in Biogen

I have related how Wally Gilbert, in the hour of need, became CEO of Biogen NV (which was incorporated in the Netherlands Antilles to minimise the tax burden on the greedily anticipated profits) and how Biogen set up a laboratory in Geneva. In 1979 Rob Cawthorn had become CEO of the Geneva subsidiary, Biogen S.A., and in 1980 Julian Davies, a scientist renowned for his

[36] Readily available, yet still expensive; the price of IFN, as provided to the consumer in microgram doses, works out to about 3 million dollars per gram!

[37] One major disappointment was the failure of intranasal IFN treatment of the common cold; it provoked strong local irritation in many patients and led to what Wally Gilbert called a "bloody nose" without discernible benefit. [64, 65].

research on antibiotic resistance, took charge as vice-president of research and began to assemble a scientific staff. Because alpha IFNs, whose genes we had just cloned, were the major priority, Biogen staff undertook to improve expression, devise purification methods and sequence some of the many genes Nagata had isolated. Walter Fiers had in the meantime independently cloned the gene for IFN β and, like Tada Taniguchi, experienced great difficulty in expressing soluble recombinant protein from *E. coli*; this became another project shared with Geneva scientists.

Walter and I set our sights on IFN gamma and I can summarise the outcome by relating that we were beaten to the draw by Dave Goeddel in 1982, while Walter came in second and we in Zürich managed to reisolate one of the IFN-α cDNA plasmids floating around in our lab. Phil Sharp's project, the production of recombinant pig growth hormone, was also placed in the hands of Geneva scientists. I only mentioned in passing the expression of hepatitis B antigen in *E. coli* by Ken Murray, in December of 1978, because when I wrote the earlier part of this essay, the impact of this achievement was not evident to me. However, it emerged that in applying for a patent, Ken had beaten the competition from the Institut Pasteur by a few days and when various companies went on to produce hepatitis B vaccines they found themselves subordinated to Biogen's patent, with felicitous consequences for Biogen's royalty income.

Taking advantage of the prestige I had gained with the Biogen Board and the fact that Schering-Plough was contractually obligated to support our IFN research, I coerced Biogen into setting up an IFN Laboratory in Zürich, in space rented from the Federal Institute of Technology (FIT). In this lab we eventually fermented and purified IFN gamma which was sent to Biogen Geneva for final processing and quality control. Here we also carried out further applied research, resulting in the expression of glycosylated human IFN gamma in eukaryotic cells [70] and IFN-α in yeast [71].

The Scientific Board met at regular intervals and critically evaluated the efforts of the various Biogen groups. Over the years this led to an unhealthy atmosphere in Biogen Geneva; the Biogen staff felt patronised by many of the Board members, foremost probably myself. The Board felt that the staff was not making the progress it had hoped for and quite some of the blame was assigned to Julian whose organisational talents were found wanting. In 1981 a second Biogen laboratory was founded, in Cambridge, Mass., presumably because Wally was getting tired of flying back and forth between Boston and Geneva, but ostensibly to create a presence in the US, essential for eventually going public on a US stock market – there was no chance of going public in Europe at that time. To my surprise, Dick Flavell, a former postdoc who had implemented site-directed mutagenesis in my lab and had embarked on a successful career on his own as head of a laboratory at the National Institute of Medical Research in Mill Hill, accepted the offer to direct Biogen Cambridge. However, the hope that Biogen would gain competitive advantage by extending its research capabilities in different directions on the two sites came to naught. In the event, the two labs competed with each other rather than with the outside world and almost every technical domain was duplicated. It became obvious that having two Research Directors operating independently was untenable and in 1983, at a memorable management meeting in Geneva, this problem was discussed at length. At a certain point, when Julian left for the men's room, Wally turned to Dick and asked him whether he would be willing to assume responsibility for Biogen research "world-wide"; Dick agreed to the proposal without further ado. When Julian returned Wally said to him (and I am, as Dave Barry would say, not making this up): "Oh, by the way, you will now be reporting to Dick Flavell". Not too long thereafter Julian resigned and Flavell ran both laboratories with more or less success.

While Wally's people skills may have been wanting, he developed into a fantastic salesman, capable of off-loading millions of dollars worth of projects, mainly to Japanese pharmaceutical companies. In 1982, despite my naive opposition to doing so before being profitable (at the time a traditional European attitude), the Biogen Board had decided to go public and Wally became the driver in the dog-and-pony show; on March 23, 1983 he succeeded in raising some 70 million dollars at an initial share price of $23, which within a few weeks began its slow but steady decline. Wally, whose goal had always been to evolve Biogen into a "vertically integrated" company, hired as medical director Seth Rudnick, to the glee of Schering-Plough, his previous employer. Rudnick convinced Wally that he could bring to market not only IFN gamma but also tumour necrosis factor for a total investment of about 40 million dollars, which was raised by two limited partnerships. In the event, the funds assigned proved to be woefully inadequate, neither compound showed significant antitumour activity, the projects were dropped and the investment written off.

By 1984, the burn rate of Biogen reached about 35 million dollars per year, the life expectancy of Biogen was down to about a year and the share price reached a nadir of less than $4[38]. In an agitated meeting of the Board of Directors in Geneva, in the autumn of 1984, Wally was charged with drastically reducing the company's personnel and when it became clear during the ensuing months that he had taken no action, an emergency meeting of the Board of Directors was called in New York in December, unbeknownst to Wally, at which the board voted to ask Wally to resign as CEO and Chairman. The vice-chairman, Lou Fernandez, informed Wally of the decision over the phone during the meeting and, despite immense disappointment at the unanimous decision of the board on which he had many personal friends, including myself, he resigned gracefully and continued to serve as member of the Scientific Board for many years. After a search of several months, Jim Vincent was recruited as CEO and Chairman in October 1985. As his first major move, he succeeded in the challenging task of selling Biogen Geneva to Glaxo and

[38] It amuses me to recall that Schering-Plough could probably have bought all of Biogen for less than 150 million dollars, about twice what it ended up paying to Biogen in yearly royalties on IFN sales.

thereby drastically reduced Biogen's running costs. Soon thereafter Jim shut down Biogen Zürich and sold Biogent, a subsidiary that had been created in Ghent under the direction of Walter Fiers, to Hoffmann LaRoche. Jim Vincent's firm leadership and the closure of the Zürich lab convinced me that I had no longer had a useful role to play in Biogen and in 1988 I resigned from all my positions in the company. Biogen responded by prospering; large royalty payments began streaming in from hepatitis antigen and IFN-α sales, and Vincent undertook and ultimately achieved Wally's dream of vertical integration, namely by producing, registering and selling human recombinant IFN beta for the treatment of multiple sclerosis. Biogen is today a multi-billion dollar company, far beyond what had been envisaged by Wally two decades earlier. It is one of the few free-standing and profitable biotech companies in the world. May the power be with it!

References

1 Reynolds FH Jr, Pitha PM (1974) The induction of interferon and its messenger RNA in human fibroblasts. *Biochem Biophys Res Commun* 59: 1023–1030

2 Harpold MM, Dobner PR, Evans RM, Bancroft FC (1978) Construction and identification by positive hybridization-translation of a bacterial plasmid containing a rat growth hormone structural gene sequence. *Nucl Acid Res* 5: 2039–53

3 Itakura K, Hirose T, Crea R, Riggs AD, Heyneker HL, Bolivar F, Boyer HW (1977) Expression in *Escherichia coli* of a chemically synthesized gene for the hormone somatostatin. *Science* 198: 1056–63

4 Goeddel DV, Kleid DG, Bolivar F, Heyneker HL, Yansura DG, Crea R, Hirose T, Kraszewski A, Itakura K, Riggs AD (1979) Expression in *Escherichia coli* of chemically synthesized genes for human insulin. *Proc Natl Acad Sci USA* 76: 106–10

5 Goeddel DV, Heyneker HL, Hozumi T, Arentzen R, Itakura K, Yansura DG, Ross MJ, Miozzari G, Crea R, Seeburg PH (1979) Direct expression in *Escherichia coli* of a DNA sequence coding for human growth hormone. *Nature* 281: 544–8

6 Cantell K (1979) Why is Interferon Not in Clinical Use Today? *In*: I Gresser (ed.): *Interferon I*. Academic Press, London and New York, 1–28

7 Cantell K (1998) *The story of interferon. The ups and downs in the life of a scientist*. World Scientific, London

8 Villa-Komaroff L, Efstratiadis A, Broome S, Lomedico P, Tizard R, Naber SP, Chick WL, Gilbert W (1978) A bacterial clone synthesizing proinsulin. *Proc Natl Acad Sci USA* 75: 3727–31

9 Voltaire F-MA (1747) *Zadig l'ingenue*. Viking Press Paperback, (1978)

10 Zoon KC, Smith ME, Bridgen PJ, Anfinsen CB, Hunkapiller MW, Hood LE (1980) Amino terminal sequence of the major component of human lymphoblastoid interferon. *Science* 207: 527–8

11 Bridgen PJ, Anfinsen CB, Corley L, Bose S, Zoon KC, Ruegg UT, Buckler CE (1977) Human lymphoblastoid interferon. Large scale production and partial purification. *J Biol Chem* 252: 6585–7

12 Fujisawa J, Iwakura Y, Kawade Y (1978) Nonglycosylated mouse L cell interferon produced by the action of tunicamycin. *J Biol Chem* 253: 8677–9

13 Stewart WEd Wiranowska-Stewart M, Koistinen V, Cantell K (1979) Effect of glycosylation inhibitors on the production and properties of human leukocyte interferon. *Virology* 97: 473–6

14 Feix G, Pollet R, Weissmann C (1968) Replication of viral RNA, XVI. Enzymatic synthesis of infectious viral RNA with noninfectious Q-beta minus strands as template. *Proc Natl Acad Sci USA* 59: 145–152

15 Flavell RA, Sabo DL, Bandle EF, Weissmann C (1974) Site-directed mutagenesis: generation of an extracistronic mutation in bacteriophage Q beta RNA. *J Mol Biol* 89: 255–272

16 Domingo E, Sabo D, Taniguchi T, Weissmann C (1978) Nucleotide sequence heterogeneity of an

RNA phage population. *Cell* 13: 735–744
17 Taniguchi T, Palmieri M, Weissmann C (1978) Qβ DNA-containing hybrid plasmids giving rise to QB phage formation in the bacterial host. *Nature* 274: 223–228
18 Büeler H, Aguzzi A, Sailer A, Greiner RA, Autenried P, Aguet M, Weissmann C (1993) Mice devoid of PrP are resistant to scrapie. *Cell* 73: 1339–1347
19 Wade N (1980) Cloning gold rush turns basic biology into big business. *Science* 207: 507
20 Andreopoulos S (1980) Sounding board: gene cloning by press conference. *N Engl J Med* 302: 743–745
21 Nagata S, Taira H, Hall A, Johnsrud L, Streuli M, Ecsodi J, Boll W, Cantell K, Weissmann C (1980) Synthesis in *E. coli* of a polypeptide with human leukocyte interferon activity. *Nature* 284: 316–320
22 Knight E Jr, Hunkapiller MW, Korant BD, Hardy RW, Hood LE (1980) Human fibroblast interferon: amino acid analysis and amino terminal amino acid sequence. *Science* 207: 525–6
23 Mantei N, Schwarzstein M, Streuli M, Panem S, Nagata S, Weissmann C (1980) The nucleotide sequence of a cloned human leukocyte interferon cDNA. *Gene* 10: 1–10
24 Taniguchi T, Mantei N, Schwarzstein M, Nagata S, Muramatsu M, Weissmann C (1980) Human leukocyte and fibroblast interferons are structurally related. *Nature* 285: 547–549
25 Taniguchi T, Ohno S, Fujii KY, Muramatsu M (1980) The nucleotide sequence of human fibroblast interferon cDNA. *Gene* 10: 11–15
26 Streuli M, Nagata S, Weissmann C (1980) At least three human type alpha interferons: structure of alpha 2. *Science* 209: 1343–1347
27 Rubinstein M, Rubinstein S, Familletti PC, Miller RS, Waldman AA, Pestka S (1979) Human leukocyte interferon: production, purification to homogeneity, and initial characterization. *Proc Natl Acad Sci USA* 76: 640–4
28 Stewart WE, Sarkar FH, Taira H, Hall A, Nagata S, Weissmann C (1980) Comparisons of several biological and physicochemical properties of human leukocyte interferons produced by human leukocytes and by *E. coli*. *Gene* 11: 181–186
29 Masucci MG, Szigeti R, Klein E, Klein G, Gruest J, Montagnier L, Taira H, Hall A, Nagata S, Weissmann C (1980) Effect of interferon-alpha 1 from *E. coli* on some cell functions. *Science* 209: 1431–1435
30 Lawn RM, Fritsch EF, Parker RC, Blake G, Maniatis T (1978) The isolation and characterization of linked delta- and beta-globin genes from a cloned library of human DNA. *Cell* 15: 1157–74
31 Nagata S, Mantei N, Weissmann C (1980) The structure of one of the eight or more distinct chromosomal genes for human interferon-alpha. *Nature* 287: 401–408
32 Brack C, Nagata S, Mantei N, Weissmann C (1981) Molecular analysis of the human interferon-alpha gene family. *Gene* 15: 379–394
33 Diaz MO, Bohlander S, Allen G (1996) Nomenclature of the human interferon genes. *J Interferon Cytokine Res* 16: 179–80
34 Goeddel DV, Leung DW, Dull TJ, Gross M, Lawn RM, McCandliss R, Seeburg PH, Ullrich A, Yelverton E, Gray PW (1981) The structure of eight distinct cloned human leukocyte interferon c DNAs. *Nature* 290: 20–26
35 Allen G, Fantes KH (1980) A family of structural genes for human lymphoblastoid (leukocyte-type) interferon. *Nature* 287: 408–11
36 Shaw GD, Boll W, Taira H, Mantei N, Lengyel P, Weissmann C (1983) Structure and expression of cloned murine IFN-alpha genes. *Nucl Acid Res* 11: 555–573
37 Weissenbach J, Chernajovsky Y, Zeevi M, Shulman L, Soreq H, Nir U, Wallach D, Perricaudet M, Tiollais P, Revel M (1980) Two interferon mRNAs in human fibroblasts: *in vitro* translation and *Escherichia coli* cloning studies. *Proc Natl Acad Sci USA* 77: 7152–6
38 Billiau A (1986) BSF-2 is not just a differentiation factor [letter]. *Nature* 324: 415
39 Tavernier J, Derynck R, Fiers W (1981) Evidence for a unique human fibroblast interferon (IFN-beta 1) chromosomal gene, devoid of intervening sequences. *Nucl Acid Res* 9: 461–71
40 Ohno S, Taniguchi T (1982) Inducer-responsive expression of the cloned human interferon beta 1 gene introduced into cultured mouse cells. *Nucl Acid Res* 10: 967–977
41 Mantei N, Weissmann C (1982) Controlled transcription of a human alpha-interferon gene introduced into mouse L cells. *Nature* 297: 128–132
42 Roberts TM, Kacich R, Ptashne M (1979) A general method for maximizing the expression of a cloned gene. *Proc Natl Acad Sci USA* 76: 760–4
43 Goeddel DV, Yelverton E, Ullrich A, Heyneker HL, Miozzari G, Holmes W, Seeburg PH, Dull T,

May L, Stebbing N et al (1980) Human leukocyte interferon produced by *E. coli* is biologically active. *Nature* 287: 411–6
44 Nagata S (1997) Happy days in Zürich. *In*: H. Weber (ed.): *What's New in Molecular Biology*, 30th Birthday Celebration of the Institute of Molecular Biology, University of Zürich, 38–39
45 Schellekens H, de RA, Bolhuis R, Fountoulakis M, Schein C, Ecsodi J, Nagata S, Weissmann C (1981) Comparative antiviral efficiency of leukocyte and bacterially produced human alpha-interferon in rhesus monkeys. *Nature* 292: 775–776
46 Balkwill F, Taylor-Papadimitriou J, Fantes KH, Sebesteny A (1980) Human lymphoblastoid interferon can inhibit the growth of human breast cancer xenografts in athymic (nude) mice. *Eur J Cancer* 16: 569–73
47 Salmon SE, Hamburger AW, Soehnlen B, Durie BGM, Alberts DS, Moon TE (1978) *N Engl J Med* 298: 1321–1327
48 Streuli M, Hall A, Boll W, Stewart WE, Nagata S, Weissmann C (1981) Target cell specificity of two species of human interferon-alpha produced in *Escherichia coli* and of hybrid molecules derived from them. *Proc Natl Acad Sci USA* 78: 2848–2852
49 Henco K, Brosius J, Fujisawa A, Fujisawa JI, Haynes JR, Hochstadt J, Kovacic T, Pasek M, Schamböck A, Schmid J et al (1985) Structural relationship of human interferon alpha genes and pseudogenes. *J Mol Biol* 185: 227–260
50 Weissmann C, Weber H (1986) The interferon genes. *Prog Nucleic Acid Res Mol Biol* 33: 251–300
51 Flavell RA, Sabo DL, Bandle EF, Weissmann C (1975) Site-directed mutagenesis: effect of an extracistronic mutation on the *in vitro* propagation of bacteriophage Qbeta RNA. *Proc Natl Acad Sci USA* 72: 367–371
52 Weissmann C (1978) Reversed genetics. A new approach to the elucidation of structure-function relationships. *Trends Biochem Sci* 3: N109–N111
53 Dierks P, van OA, Mantei N, Weissmann C (1981) DNA sequences preceding the rabbit beta-globin gene are required for formation in mouse L cells of beta-globin RNA with the correct 5' terminus. *Proc Natl Acad Sci USA* 78: 1411–1415
54 Weber H, Dierks P, Meyer F, van Ooyen A, Dobkin C, Abrescia P, Kappeler M, Meyhack B, Zeltner A, Mullen EE et al (1981) Expression of β-globin genes modified by restructuring and site-directed mutagenesis. *In*: DD Brown, CF Fox (eds.): *Developmental biology using purified genes*. Academic Press, New York, 347–366
55 Isaacs A, Lindenmann J (1957) Virus interference: I. The interferon. *Proc Roy Soc* 147: 258–267
56 Pieters T (1997) History of the developments of the interferons: from test-tube to patient. *In*: R Stuart-Harris, RD Penny (eds.): *Clinical applications of the interferons*. Chapman and Hall Medical, London, 1–18
57 Greenberg HB, Pollard RB, Lutwick LI, Gregory PB, Robinson WS, Merigan TC (1976) Effect of human leukocyte interferon on hepatitis B virus infection in patients with chronic active hepatitis. *N Engl J Med* 295: 517–22
58 Weimar W, Heijtink RA, ten Kate FJ, Schalm SW, Masurel N, Schellekens H, Cantell K (1980) Double-blind study of leukocyte interferon administration in chronic HBsAg-positive hepatitis. *Lancet* 1: 336–8
59 Gresser I, Bourali C (1969) Exogenous interferon and inducers of interferon in the treatment Balb-c mice inoculated with RC19 tumour cells. *Nature* 223: 844–5
60 Gresser I, Bourali C, Levy JP, Fontaine-Brouty-Boye D, Thomas MT (1969) Increased survival in mice inoculated with tumor cells and treated with interferon preparations. *Proc Natl Acad Sci USA* 63: 51–7
61 Quesada JR, Reuben J, Manning JT, Hersh EM, Gutterman JU (1984) Alpha interferon for induction of remission in hairy-cell leukemia. *N Engl J Med* 310: 15–8
62 Kita M, Tanaka K, Uoshima N, Kobayashi Y, Ozawa M, Kondo M, Imanishi J (1997) Determination of interferon-alpha2 allele composition in the genomic DNA from healthy volunteers and leukemic patients in Japan. *J Interferon Cytokine Res* 17: 135–40
63 Palleroni AV, Aglione A, Labow M, Brunda MJ, Pestka S, Sinigaglia F, Garotta G, Alsenz J, Braun A (1997) Interferon immunogenicity: preclinical evaluation of interferon-alpha 2a. *J Interferon Cytokine Res* 17 Suppl 1: S23–7
64 Tyrrell DA (1986) The efficacy and tolerance of intranasal interferons: studies at the Common Cold Unit. *J Antimicrob Chemother* 18 Suppl B: 153–6
65 Hayden FG, Kaiser DL, Albrecht JK (1988) Intranasal recombinant alfa-2b interferon treatment

of naturally occurring common colds. *Antimicrob Agents Chemother* 32: 224–30
66 Zein NN (1998) Interferons in the management of viral hepatitis. Cytokines Cell Mol Ther 4: 229–41
67 Dusheiko G, Main J, Thomas H, Reichard O, Lee C, Dhillon A, Rassam S, Fryden A, Reesink H, Bassendine M et al (1996) Ribavirin treatment for patients with chronic hepatitis C: results of a placebo-controlled study. *J Hepatol* 25: 591–8
68 Schvarcz R, Glaumann H, Reichard O, Weiland O (1999) Histological and virological long-term outcome in patients treated with interferon-alpha2b and ribavirin for chronic hepatitis C. J Viral Hepat 6: 237–242
69 Lindsay KL (1999) Treatment of chronic hepatitis C: comparative virologic response rates among the different interferons. *J Hepatol* 31 Suppl 1: 232–6
70 Haynes J, Weissmann C (1983) Constitutive, long-term production of human interferons by hamster cells containing multiple copies of a cloned interferon gene. *Nucl Acid Res* 11: 687–706
71 Palva I, Lehtovaara P, Kaariainen L, Sibakov M, Cantell K, Schein CH, Kashiwagi K, Weissmann C (1983) Secretion of interferon by *Bacillus subtilis*. *Gene* 22: 229–235
72 Grunstein M, Hogness DS (1975) Colony hybridization: a method for the isolation of cloned DNAs that contain a specific gene. *Proc Natl Acad Sci USA* 72: 3961–5
73 Lawn RM, Adelman J, Dull TJ, Gross M, Goeddel D, Ullrich A (1981) DNA sequence of two closely linked human leukocyte interferon genes. *Science* 212: 1159–1162

Recombinant Protein Drugs
ed. by P. Buckel

Combining science and business: from recombinant DNA to vaccines against hepatitis B virus

Peter Hans Hofschneider[1] and Kenneth Murray[2]

[1] *Max-Planck-Institut für Biochemie, Martinsried, Germany*
[2] *Institute of Cell and Molecular Biology, University of Edinburgh, Edinburgh, Scotland*

Introduction

Our involvement in research on hepatitis B virus (HBV) really began at a Microbiology Conference in Geneva in February, 1978. For the small group of academics involved this was not at all the sort of conference to which we were accustomed. It was an intensive discussion, convened by Dr. Raymond Schaeffer and Mr. Dan Adams of the venture capital group of the International Nickel Company of Canada (INCO), of the prospects for formation of a European biotechnology company and a review of research projects and products that such a company might pursue. The role model was Genentech Inc., a company that had been formed two years previously and in which INCO had been a significant and well satisfied corporate investor. How about a European analogue? After two fascinating if rather surrealistic days we all agreed to take the matter further at a second meeting in Paris a few weeks later.

Together, the group had assembled a substantial shopping list of products for the proposed company, but the production of a sub-unit vaccine against HBV based upon the viral surface antigen (HBsAg) produced by the new gene manipulation methods was advocated strongly by one of us, P.H.H., who was already interested in the role of HBV in the development of hepatocellular carcinoma (HCC). There was a good case. Hepatitis B was clearly a significant public health problem of major proportions world-wide (Fig. 1) with some 250 million carriers of the disease which could sometimes lead to chronic infections with sequelae of serious liver disease including HCC. The virus was, however, very difficult to work with, because it could not be produced in cell culture, there was no animal model, and it had a very tight host range infecting only a few higher primates, the chimpanzee being the best-known non-human host. HBV was clearly a prime target for gene cloning approaches, and a recent review by Robinson [2] summarised the relevant background information around which experimental approaches could be based. The virus had a very small DNA genome of unusual structure and, in addition to its core and surface antigens, at least one other antigen, the *e* antigen (HBeAg), and a spe-

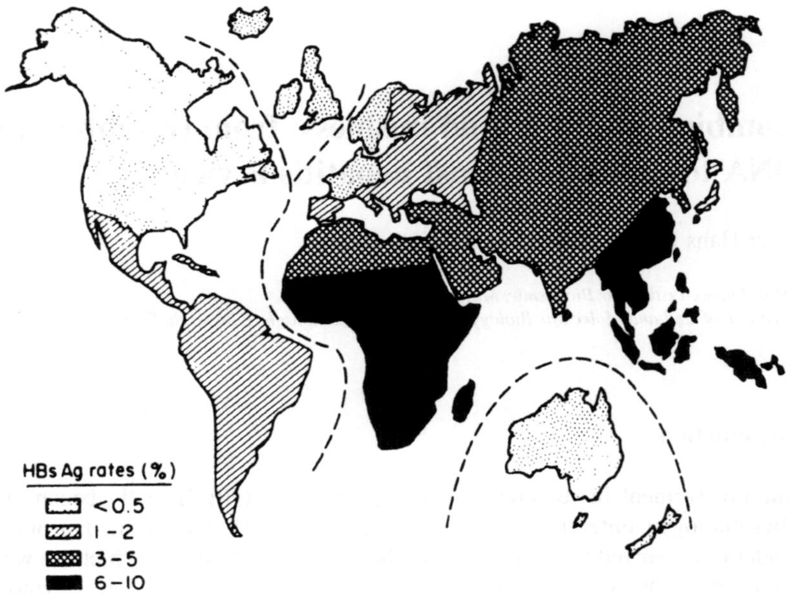

Figure 1. The geographical distribution of HBV based upon HBsAg incidence in blood samples. Reproduced, with permission from Szmuness et al. [1].

cific DNA polymerase were associated with the virus. This complement of proteins at that time was difficult to reconcile with one copy of the viral genome which was equivalent to about 3000 base pairs for a fully double-stranded molecule. Possibly one of the proteins associated with the viral infection was an induced host gene product, or maybe simultaneous infection by two different viruses was needed, as was believed to be the case with some plant viruses, or perhaps introns (which had been discovered quite recently) enabled multiple use of the viral genome in different reading frames?

But a further immediate problem was the concern at the time over possible biohazards that surrounded the cloning experiments involved, for such work with animal viruses was placed in a high-risk category by most of the authorities concerned and, if at all, could only be pursued under the most stringent conditions of physical containment (P4).

And then there was the competition to be considered. Following the landmark demonstration by Krugman et al. [3] that boiled serum containing HBsAg induced protective antibody formation, production of a sub-unit vaccine from HBsAg purified from the plasma of HBV-infected individuals was under development by the international pharmaceutical giant, Merck Inc., and by Maupas et al. at Tours and the Institut Pasteur [4, 5]. These groups and no doubt others would be actively interested in cloning HBV DNA for further analysis and attempts to produce HBsAg by fermentation of appropriately transformed cells.

After a long discussion, in which the recent experience of two of those present (K.M. and Charles Weissmann) in the cloning of polyoma DNA in plasmid and phage vectors as part of a risk-testing experiment sponsored by the European Molecular Biology Organisation (EMBO) played a significant part, it was agreed to add the production of HBsAg for development as a vaccine to the embryonic portfolio of projects for sponsorship by the new company. Soon afterwards Biogen N.V. (incorporated in the Netherlands Antilles) formally came into existence and work on the company's projects began under the direction of the appropriate member (usually the project's proposer) of the company's Scientific Board, and for the most part in their university laboratories.

Getting started

The HBV project soon encountered its first obstacle, even before consideration of physical containment conditions for cloning HBV DNA in plasmids for propagation in *Escherichia coli* to provide sufficient DNA for analysis and further manipulation for expression of genes once identified. Our prospective collaborators in Munich had, to our surprise, become interested in another collaboration and did not supply the serum from HBV-infected patients which was the essential starting material for our experiments. Fortunately, help was soon at hand. Following a serious outbreak of serum hepatitis (as hepatitis B was then described) at a hospital in Edinburgh some ten years earlier, Barrie Marmion, who had just been appointed to the Chair of Medical Microbiology there, initiated a research programme on hepatitis serology. He and his colleagues had just the experience and materials that we needed and readily agreed to collaborate with us.

Experiments began in June on the characterisation of DNA samples prepared by Patricia MacKay from a number of different plasma samples taken from patients who were HBsAg-positive. The work was supported by a research grant from Biogen with an exclusive intellectual property agreement from the University of Edinburgh. HBV DNA was known to be a small, partially double-stranded circular molecule which could be repaired to a fully double-stranded state by the DNA polymerase associated with the virus on incubation with the four deoxynucleoside triphosphates [6]. The quantity of DNA derived from the plasma samples was extremely small, but the endogenous polymerase reaction enabled the samples to be radioactively labelled by inclusion of one (or more) α-^{32}P-dNTPs in the reaction mixtures. Such preparations could be handled safely and legitimately in the recently equipped category 2 containment facility (P2) in one of our university departments (K.M.'s at Edinburgh) while agreement was being sought from the appropriate authorities to pursue DNA cloning operations in the high containment laboratories

(P4) of the U.K. Ministry of Defence Microbiological Research Establishment at Porton Down.

The DNA samples from the various plasma sources did not give identical fragmentation patterns with some of the restriction endonucleases used, and the most abundant sample differed from the others in two significant respects: it came from a source exhibiting the complex serotype *adyw* and it did not contain a target for the restriction enzyme R.*Eco*RI through which it had been anticipated that the molecule would have been linearised [2] to facilitate its cloning in an *E. coli* plasmid such as pBR322. This reinforced our decision to pursue a dual strategy for the project simultaneously. In addition to cloning the entire viral genome for nucleotide sequence determination, followed by selection of appropriate segments for insertion into expression vectors, we would attempt to express sequences for antigenic determinants directly, relying upon the newly developed immunological screening method of Broome and Gilbert [7] for their detection. For this purpose a range of HBV DNA fragments from digestion with various enzymes were prepared for insertion into the single site for the restriction enzyme R.*Pst*I in the plasmid pBR322. This enzyme generates breaks with short 3'-single-stranded projections, which were extended with several guanine residues through reactions with 3'-terminal transferase and dGTP, so that the HBV DNA fragments could be joined to the plasmid DNA after they had been similarly adapted in terminal transferase reactions with the complementary dCTP. This should yield a population of recombinant DNA molecules in which the normal expression of β-lactamase would be replaced by a fusion protein carrying the N-terminal segment of the enzyme followed by a few glycine residues, from translation of the oligo-G linker sequence, and the product of the HBV DNA segment.

The HBV DNA fragments were taken to Zurich where the 3'-tailing experiments were carried out in the laboratory of our colleague, Professor Charles Weissmann, one of very few in Europe with both the enzyme and the relevant experience at that time, and they were then ready for the cloning operations in the P4 suite at Porton. It may be that in the future the Human Genome Project will enable us to characterise molecular biologists from their genotype, but at that time the phenotype was unmistakable; you could pick them out at airports by the small thermos flasks in which they carried their precious enzyme preparations and new vectors for their colleagues (Fig. 2).

Cloning and expression

The director of the research station at Porton, Dr. R.J. Harris, and his staff, particularly Dr. Peter Greenaway, were extremely helpful and sympathetic to our needs. They were no doubt accustomed to visitors unfamiliar with the strict regimes for working safely with truly dangerous pathogens. To the newcomers, however, the fitting and testing of respirators, the strict routine of changing into laboratory clothing before entering the P4 laboratory via an airlock,

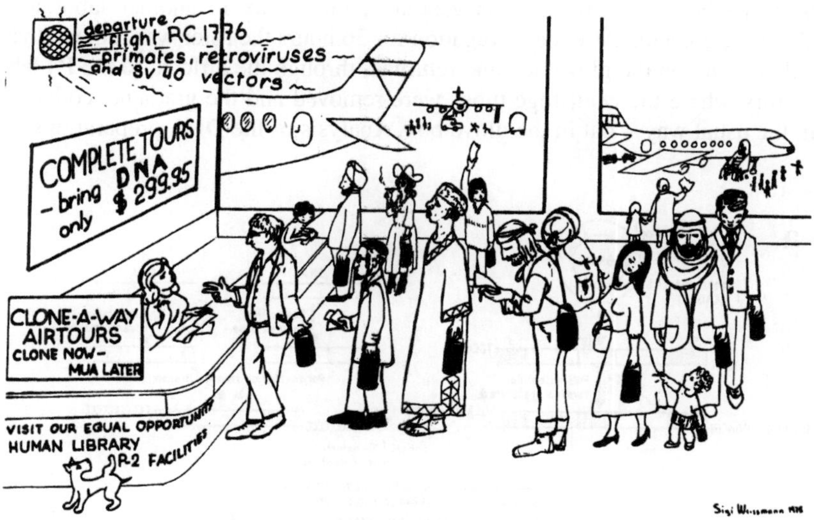
departure
Flight RC 1776
primates, retroviruses
and SV 40 vectors
COMPLETE TOURS
- bring DNA
only $ 299.95
CLONE-A-WAY
AIRTOURS
CLONE NOW -
MUA LATER
VISIT OUR EQUAL OPPORTUNITY
HUMAN LIBRARY
P-2 FACILITIES

Figure 2. Molecular biology on the move. A cartoon drawn by Sigi Weissmann for a lecture given by her husband, Charles, early in 1977, and reproduced here with her permission.

conducting all experiments in glove boxes fitted with air filters, and leaving via a shower and airlock before dressing in one's normal clothing seemed more like preparing for space travel than laboratory work, but this discipline certainly established confidence in the procedures for containment of proven biohazards, let alone potential ones.

Thanks to the care and teaching of our hosts, our experiments progressed well. Since the quantity of HBV DNA for the cloning operations was very limited, phage λ DNA had been added as a carrier prior to digestion with the restriction endonucleases in order to reduce mechanical losses. The cells transformed with the recombinant plasmid preparations and recovered on the basis of their resistance to tetracycline, but sensitivity to ampicillin, had to be screened for the presence of HBV DNA, rather than the carrier DNA, by colony hybridisation with ^{32}P-labelled HBV DNA prepared via the endogenous polymerase reaction. Cells from colonies that gave positive reactions were then grown as colonies on agar plates for antigen screening with ^{125}I-labelled antisera to the major HBV antigens, the core antigen (HBcAg) and HBsAg.

The next step was making plasmid preparations from cells giving positive reactions for antigen expression in order to examine their HBV DNA content. For us, this provided the ultimate challenge in working under P4 containment. The precious DNA samples for purification by equilibrium centrifugation in CsCl gradients were loaded into the tubes for the ultracentrifuge rotor in a glove box in the P4 laboratory, placed in the buckets of the rotor and transferred in a box, via a dunk-tank, to the ultracentrifuge which itself was housed in a specially constructed filter-ventilated glove box in another laboratory along the corridor. After centrifugation for 36 hours the rotor was removed via a dunk-tank on the glove box and returned, through the airlock, to the P4 laboratory where the centrifuge tubes were removed and the gradients collected in the usual way – but in the glove box. Analysis of the DNA preparations by

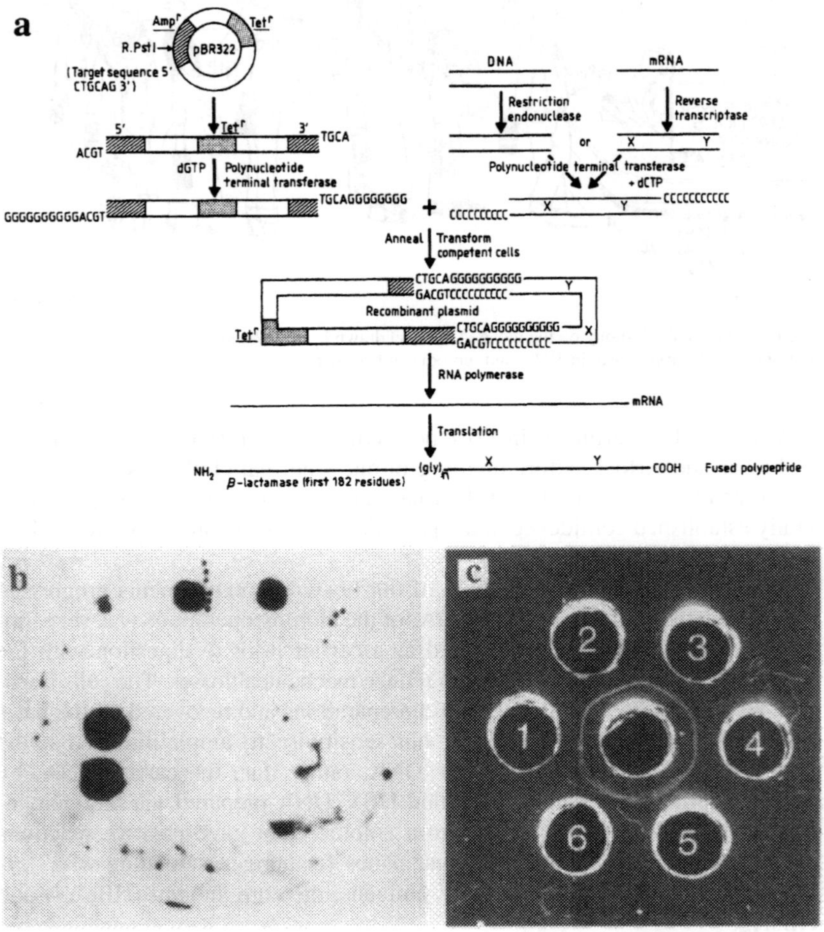

Figure 3. (a) The procedure for insertion of DNA fragments at the R.*PstI* site in the β-lactamase gene of pBR322 for expression as fusion proteins. (b) Autoradiograph showing the detection by radioimmunoassay of the expression of HBcAg in four of the 52 colonies of *E. coli* transformants on a Petri plate [8]. (c) Comparison by immunodiffusion of antibodies induced by HBcAg produced in *E. coli* with those induced by HBV infection [9]. The centre well contained HBcAg from human liver. Wells 1 and 4 contained human anti-HBc, wells 2 and 3 contained serum from rabbits inoculated with an unfractionated extract of bacteria carrying the recombinant plasmid, and wells 5 and 6 contained serum from rabbits inoculated with the same extract after fractionation.

restriction enzyme digestion and gel electrophoresis then seemed very straightforward and showed that the plasmids contained HBV DNA fragments, but none were of full genome length; they could therefore be handled under lower levels of containment. Pursuing such a series of operations under P4 laboratory conditions certainly gave the impression of selection for commitment to one's experiments and objective, but we were well rewarded with the positive indications of expression of antigen products that reacted with antibodies to HBcAg [8]. It was an exciting start to the project, and the first patent applications were filed in December 1978.

Extracts from the transformants that exhibited HBcAg antigenicity were then shown to induce antibodies in rabbits, which in the Ouchterlony immunodiffusion test behaved identically with human anti-HBc-positive sera [9]; fractionated extracts from such cells were later shown to contain particles which in the electron microscope were morphologically indistinguishable from those of HBcAg preparations derived from the liver of a patient with fulminant hepatitis [10]. Figure 3 provides a summary of the project at this stage. Meanwhile, the recombinant plasmids from several of the transformants were propagated (now back in the P2 laboratory) for characterisation of the cloned HBV DNA segments and determination of their nucleotide sequences, which were done in the laboratories of our colleagues, Professors Walter Gilbert and Heinz Schaller.

The viral genome

Our sequence analysis showed how the organisation of the HBV genome accommodated the genes for all the known HBV proteins as uninterrupted, but extensively overlapping, reading frames [9] and is summarised in Figure 4. Partial and complete sequences of cloned HBV DNA were also determined contemporaneously by others [11, 12]. The coding sequence for HBcAg was identified from plasmids that expressed the antigen as an open reading frame (ORF) of 549 nucleotides, giving a polypeptide of 183 amino acids with a molecular mass consistent with that of HBcAg [9]. The viral DNA sequence was therefore numbered from the beginning of this ORF rather than from an arbitrary restriction enzyme target or the point of its linkage to the plasmid. Partial amino acid sequence data on HBsAg [13] enabled its coding sequence to be located in a different reading frame. This was particularly interesting, for although the linear sequence from nucleotides 1437 to 2114 (in the numbering system of Pasek et al. [9]) corresponded with the N- and C-terminal amino acid sequences of HBsAg and gave a polypeptide (226 amino acids) with the molecular mass of the antigen, the ORF began 489 residues upstream at nucleotide 948. The sequence 948 to 1437 later became known as the PreS region and includes methionine or initiation triplets at residues 1164 and 1272. Longer HBsAg molecules (corresponding to N-terminal extensions of the molecule previously regarded as the surface antigen or S polypeptide) carrying either part (PreS2) or the entire PreS sequence (which was therefore split into

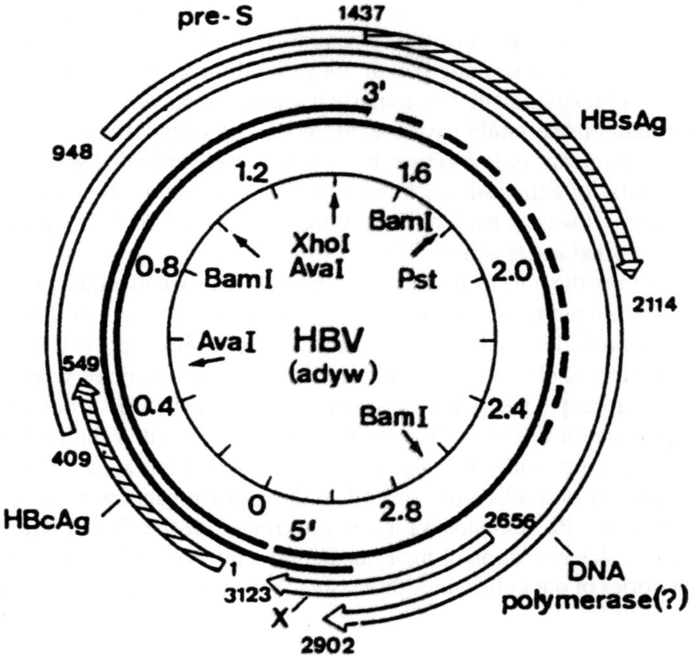

Figure 4. The genome of HBV. The heavy lines represent the partially double-stranded DNA molecule, with the broken line indicating the extent of the single-stranded region (which varies in individual molecules). The nucleotide numbering is that of Pasek et al. [9] and the restriction enzyme targets located in the inner circle refer to the *adyw* serotype of the HBV DNA used in their analysis. The arrows show the extent of the four ORFs, those for HBcAg and HBsAg being hatched.

segments PreS1 and PreS2) were specifically recognised as components of HBV and HBsAg particles derived from serum. They were further characterised by Heermann et al. [14] and are now known to play substantive roles in virus assembly and interaction with hepatocyte receptors. The three polypeptides were described as the short (S), medium (M, i.e., S + PreS2), and long (L, i.e., S + PreS2 + PreS1) surface antigens.

The third reading frame contained a very long ORF (nucleotides 409 to 2902) which overlapped the last 141 residues of the HBcAg ORF, completely covered the L-HBsAg ORF and largely overlapped a fourth ORF (the first 246 residues) which was in frame with the HBcAg ORF, but from residues 2656 to 3123. This long ORF was a candidate for the HBV polymerase coding sequence because bacterial and viral DNA polymerases have molecular masses around 10^5 (see [9] for references). The size of the fourth ORF was suggestive of a coding sequence for HBeAg, but when it was shown that HBeAg reactivity could be derived from HBcAg [15], the ORF was referred to as the *x* coding sequence and its product as the *x* antigen (HBxAg). The *x* ORF was later shown to be transcribed in appropriately transformed mouse L or rat 2 cell cultures [16], and HBxAg was shown by Wollersheim and Hofschneider [17] to be a transactivator, which enhanced levels of HBsAg expression in human hepatoma cell cultures [18].

We could now construct new plasmids for the expression of specific sequences. Several were made to produce HBsAg in *E. coli*, but while some gave material that was antigenic and induced anti-HBs in rabbits [19], the antibody titres were low in comparison with patients' serum levels or those induced by our HBcAg preparations. Others had similar experiences [20–22]. Instead of continuing with *E. coli*, it was time to consider different systems.

Making and testing the vaccine

Looking at animal cell culture systems and yeasts, the latter had more immediate appeal because of the recent development of vectors with controllable expression systems of known nucleotide sequence (and thus more amenable to manipulation) and an anticipated lower eventual production cost through yeast fermentation. Collaborative experiments were set up with Dr. Albert Hinnen at the Friedrich Miescher Institute in Basel, who had cloned the *PHO5* gene of the yeast *Saccharomyces cerevisciae* and shown its expression to be regulated by phosphate concentration [23]. This system was adapted for construction of plasmids for expression of HBsAg in yeast, but gave only low levels of expression upon induction; these, however, were substantially increased by transferring the DNA fragment carrying the coding sequence appropriately linked to the *PHO5* promoter into the multicopy plasmid pJDB207 [24]. Other groups had been pursuing expression of HBsAg in animal cell culture systems and in yeasts. Valenzuela et al. [25] and Hitzeman et al. [26] produced the antigen in yeast with expression from the alcohol dehydrogenase and phosphoglycerate kinase promoters, respectively, and Miyanohara et al. [27] also used the *PHO5* promoter to express HBsAg in yeast. The product precipitated by anti-HBs was particulate, similar in size to particles isolated from patients' sera and induced antibodies in laboratory animals.

The yield of HBsAg from yeast transformed with our new construct (pJDB207/*PHO5*-HBsAgΔ14), as measured by radioimmune assay methods, proved to be enhanced more than tenfold. Such preparations were subsequently examined in the electron microscope and shown to be particulate, closely resembling the 22 nm particles found in the serum of infected individuals (Fig. 5). Sufficient material was obtained in a partially purified form for immunogenicity and efficacy tests in chimpanzees which were pursued in collaboration with Dr. H. Schellekens and his colleagues at the TNO Primate Centre in The Netherlands [28].

The pathological effects of HBV infection are very similar in humans and chimpanzees and are illustrated in a simple form in Figure 6. The viral surface antigen and HBeAg appear in the serum about six to eight weeks after infec-

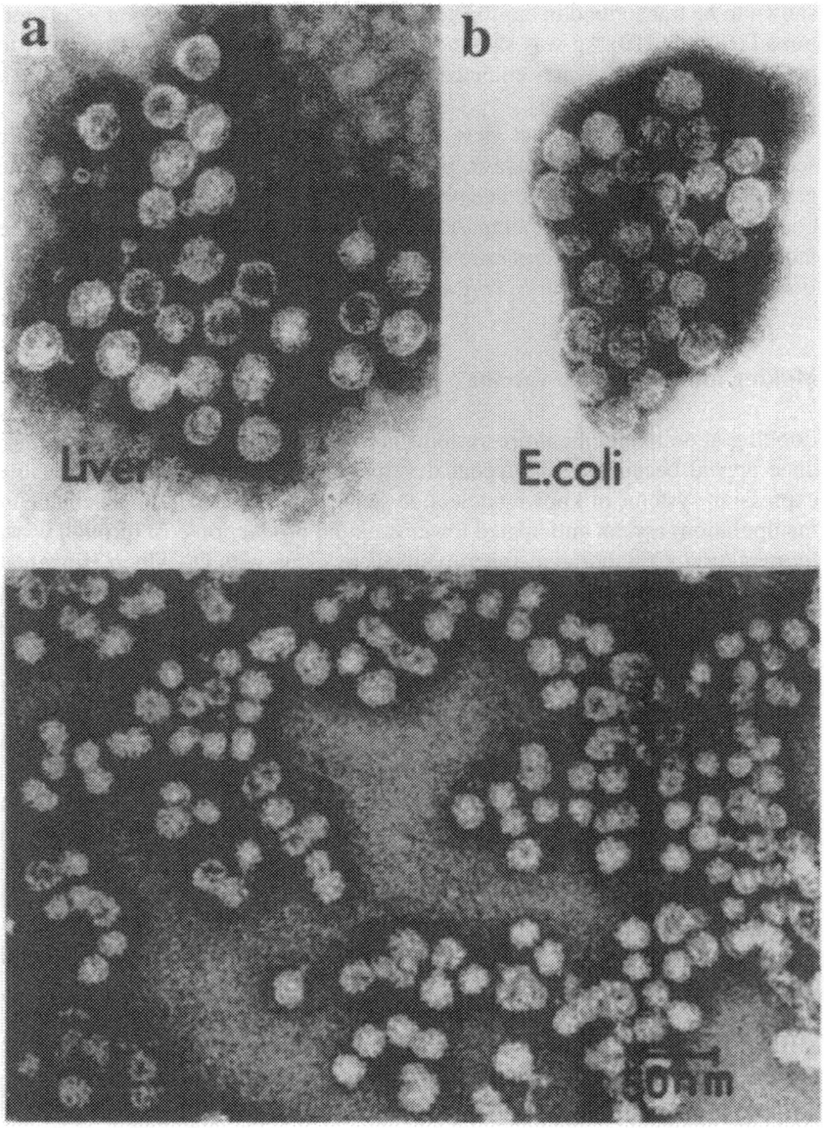

Figure 5. Electronmicrographs of HBcAg particles (upper panels: (a) isolated from the liver of an acutely infected patient, (b) synthesized in *E. coli*) and HBsAg purified from genetically engineered yeast. The photographs of the HBcAg preparations were kindly supplied by Dr. Joan Richmond [10] and that of the HBsAg sample was kindly provided by Drs. H. Arimura and T. Suyama of the Green Cross Corporation, Osaka, and are reproduced with their permission.

tion, and although HBcAg is not manifest in the serum, anti-HBc appears around three months after infection and precedes the formation of anti-HBe or

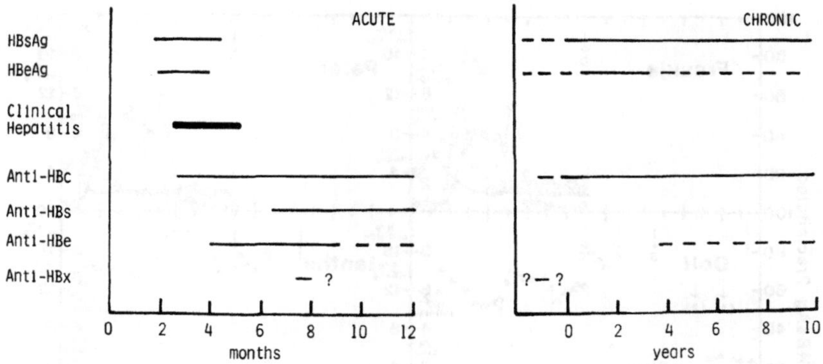

Figure 6. The appearance of HBV antigens and their antibodies in serum during acute and chronic infections. The time at which the various markers are found varies appreciably in individual cases, which is indicated in part by the broken lines.

anti-HBs. A principal clinical manifestation of the infection is a marked elevation of serum levels of liver transaminases which generally occurs around eight to ten weeks after infection and then falls to normal levels by around five months as anti-HBs levels rise, usually generating lasting immunity to further infection, although some 5–10% of cases may become chronic carriers of the disease.

Evaluation of the efficacy of a vaccine candidate thus requires extensive and prolonged monitoring of several serum parameters at regular intervals on the primate species concerned (usually the chimpanzee for HBV) and after challenge with the virus the animals must be kept in isolation until shown to be clear of infection. This is obviously a long and expensive process and in any event such tests were not undertaken lightly. To test the efficacy of our HBsAg preparations, two animals were inoculated with material mixed with an aluminium hydroxide adjuvant which, although less potent than the conventional Freund's adjuvant used in laboratory animal tests, is less toxic and is that which would be used in clinical trials in humans. The animals received booster inoculations in the normal manner and when anti-HBs levels rose and appeared to plateau, the animals were inoculated intravenously with the virus (about 5.10^3 infectious units); two unimmunised animals were similarly inoculated at the same time to serve as controls. In view of the time and expense involved in such operations, these controls served to monitor another vaccination trial simultaneously with two animals that had been inoculated with preparations of HBcAg produced in *E. coli*, even though the conventional view was that this protein, being an internal antigen, was unlikely to have significant protective potential.

The results of these tests [28] (Fig. 7) show clearly that the HBsAg inoculations had completely protected the two chimpanzees against the infection manifest in the control animals. The results of the test on HBcAg were also

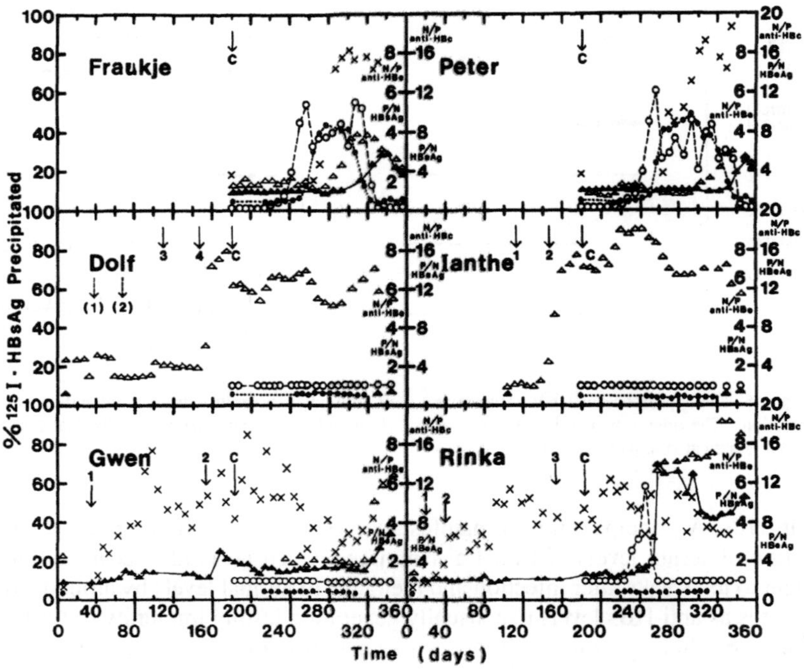

Figure 7. Immunisation of chimpanzees with HBsAg produced in yeast and with HBcAg produced in *E. coli*. The animals Fraukje and Peter were unimmunised controls, Dolf and Ianthe were immunised with HBsAg, and Gwen and Rinka with HBcAg. Vertical arrows show the time of inoculation and C indicates a challenge for all six animals with the virus (5.10^3 I.D.$_{50}$). Serum levels of HBV antigen and antibody levels were determined routinely by solid-phase radioimmune assay with ^{125}I-labelled reagents. O—O, HBsAg:, Δ—Δ anti-HBs; ●—●, HBeAg; ▲—▲, anti-HBe; ×—× anti-HBc. Reproduced with permission from [28].

interesting and encouraging and are discussed further below. Similar results on the immunisation of chimpanzees with HBsAg derived from yeast were also obtained by McAleer et al. [29]. Following the earlier demonstrations of efficacy of HBsAg derived from plasma [4, 5] and a controlled clinical trial in a high-risk population by Szmuness et al. [30], the results of the chimpanzee studies with HBsAg made in yeast provided a sound basis for proceeding to large-scale production of material for the extensive toxicology tests and clinical trials required for registration of a vaccine. Although vaccines based upon HBsAg from human plasma were now in advanced stages of development (and following approval by many regulatory authorities were soon to become widely used), the combination of complex purification regimes for large volumes of highly infectious plasma, particularly following the recognition of the bloodborne human immunodeficiency virus (HIV), with their attendant time-consuming and expensive safety testing, resulted in long and expensive production cycles. These factors reinforced the argument for alternatives to blood as a source of the immunogenic component of vaccines and the case for yeast as a source of HBsAg for vaccine formulation.

For a new and still relatively small biotechnology company with an already diverse range of projects, the only feasible route to commercial development was by licensing to an established pharmaceutical manufacturing company on an appropriate fee and royalty basis. Biogen's first such arrangements were made in 1981 with the Green Cross Corporation for Japan (whose vaccine was approved and in use in 1991) and, shortly thereafter, with two European companies which, however, did not complete the development and so the agreements were terminated. Following the issue of a patent to Biogen by the United States Patent Office in 1987, an exclusive licensing arrangement was completed with SmithKline Beckmann who could sublicense the patent to one other company, which they did: to Merck. In the meantime a number of clinical trials had been reported (see, e.g., [31–33]) and the experience and resources of these two new licensees ensured that the vaccine was approved and in widespread use in a timely manner. For Biogen significant royalty income began in 1989 and grew substantially in 1992 as vaccination programmes for young children and adolescents were put in place in a number of countries in the face of an increasing incidence of HBV infection.

It is often said that from the initial research stage of a new drug, its approval and appearance on the market takes ten years and an investment of some US$ 300 million, the costs escalating rapidly as development reaches its later stages. Biogen's research on HBV began in 1978, and that of others around the same time, and it was almost ten years later that vaccines based upon recombinant DNA technology were introduced to the market. The very extensive and thorough clinical trial described by André and Safary [33], which represents a late stage in the drug development process, provides a good illustration of significant components of the development time and costs, in addition to production facilities. For a newly formed organisation such a development prospect is formidable, but the long time lag between the initial fees of a licensing agreement and the beginning of a royalty income stream can also generate severe problems, sometimes putting the survival of the company at risk. In Biogen's case the focused strategies and economies introduced by Mr. James Vincent on his appointment as C.E.O. of the company in 1985 enabled the company to survive until royalty income from its α-interferon (initiated by Professor Charles Weissmann and licensed to Schering-Plough) and HBV projects contributed to a revenue stream that supported the transition of the company into a fully operational biopharmaceutical company and the development of its first drug, Avonex (β-interferon), for the treatment of multiple sclerosis.

Hepatitis B under control?

Our HBV project, then, has served Biogen well and contributed to the development of an effective vaccine against a major infectious disease of worldwide importance. There is already evidence that the introduction of mass vaccination of children in Taiwan is leading to the anticipated decrease in the incidence of HCC as the rate of chronic infection falls [34]. It has been said, therefore, that vaccination against HBV is a vaccination against cancer. The attendant business success has also been very beneficial to the University of Edinburgh, through its original agreement with Biogen, and to the Darwin Trust of Edinburgh, a charitable foundation established in 1983 to support education and research in science. And no less importantly, the project also catalysed much continuing basic research on HBV by ourselves and our colleagues and several others.

The end of our story? Unfortunately no, or at least not yet. In spite of effective vaccines against pathogenic agents, the combination of antigenic variation and chronic infection result in the emergence of mutants that escape the immune defences of vaccinated populations. The combination of a more permissive society, increasing affluence and the jumbo jet may be good for the global economy, but not for public health. There will be a continuing need for new vaccines and therapeutic agents; the control of tuberculosis, at least temporarily, in many parts of the world emphasises the importance of multiple approaches, including multiple drug therapy, in containing the emergence of resistant strains [35]. An escape mutant of HBV in a vaccinated population in Italy was reported by Carman et al. in 1990 [36], as arising from a glycine to arginine substitution at residue 145 of HBsAg, which lies in the immunodominant region of the antigen; this same mutant also has arisen in three other locations as far apart as New York, London and Singapore. In cases such as this, where the mutation can be quickly identified by means of the polymerase chain reaction, it is clearly straightforward to construct derivative plasmids for production of the new variant HBsAg in yeast for the preparation of another vaccine against the new strain, which in principle could be used in combination with the original material, and such derivatives have been made. These are certainly useful modifications, but obviously can only be developed after the event. In addition to new therapeutic approaches for use in both acute and chronic infections, might it be possible to develop vaccines based on multiple epitopes and which could, in effect, anticipate at least some of the mutants before they arise? Inclusion of PreS sequences of HBsAg (Fig. 4) is one approach that has been used with the intention of improving the vaccine and may help to prevent infection by inhibiting, at least in part, association of some types of escape mutant with hepatocyte receptors.

For some alternative approaches we turn to the results obtained with HBcAg in chimpanzees [28]. Figure 7 shows that of the two animals involved, one suffered a mild, brief infection that was followed by a rapid appearance of a high level of anti-HBs, while the other was essentially uninfected, as judged by the range of serological markers used, but began to produce anti-HBs several months after challenge with the virus. In a second experiment [37] with two more animals, one was completely protected from infection upon challenge with HBV and the other developed a very weak and short-lived HBsAg level followed immediately by a strong anti-HBs response. With the same HBcAg preparation, Iwarson et al. [38] also demonstrated protection of a chimpanzee against infection with HBV. The results were tantalizing: the experiments had not been as successful as those with HBsAg, nor had they altogether failed.

The influenza virus nuclear antigen stimulates T-cell responses [39, 40] and the specificity of cytotoxic T-cells for hepatocytes in chronic HBV infections [41] indicated that HBcAg could be involved in the cell-mediated response to HBV infection. The results of Milich et al. [42] on the stimulation of T-lymphocyte proliferation in inbred strains of mice by peptides representing parts of HBcAg provided compelling evidence for this view and explained the results from vaccination of the chimpanzees with HBcAg [43]. Importantly, the experiments of Milich et al. with inbred strains of mice primed with HBcAg or their strain-specific epitope peptide (from the HBcAg sequence) and challenged with HBV (which cannot replicate in the mouse), showed production of antibodies not only to HBcAg, but also to HBsAg, including the PreS, S and sub-type epitopes, whereas equivalently primed animals challenged with a mixture of HBcAg and HBsAg generated only anti-HBc. Thus, challenge with a molecule or particle comprising other epitopes *physically linked* to that used for priming the immune system induced a response to all the epitopes present in the challenging particle because these would all be taken up by a single antigen-presenting cell.

Adding more epitopes to HBcAg

In experiments to improve the yield of HBcAg in *E. coli*, substitution of the two N-terminal residues of HBcAg by the N-terminal eight residues of β-galactosidase and a linker sequence of three amino acids did not impair particle formation or stability [44]; yields were further enhanced by truncation of the HBcAg polypeptide at amino acid 144, again without impairing particle formation or immunogenicity. The robust structure of HBcAg together with its immunological potency make it an attractive prospect as a carrier for additional epitopes and, in principle, the construction of multicomponent vaccines by cross-linking additional immunogenic components chemically or by incorporating relevant coding sequences at appropriate positions in plasmids expressing HBcAg.

Fusion or insertion of several polypeptide sequences to the major segment of HBcAg have now been described and together with the properties of the products have been summarised [45] and reviewed more extensively by Ullrich et al. [46].

Several of the experiments involved addition of segments of HBsAg to HBcAg. Immune responses of HBsAg, however, are complex; in addition to epitopes within the PreS sequences and the immunodominant *a* region, subtype determinants have been assigned to the other segments of HBsAg close to the *a* epitope. Analysis of DNA cloned from sera of different sub-types showed corresponding differences in amino acid sequences of HBsAg. However, single mutations of candidate residues did not effect a simple switch from one sub-type (*y*) to another (*d*), but induced a gradual change with both *y* and *d* characteristics displayed from the same molecule, and further single mutations changed the phenotype further, giving a molecule with only *d* immunogenicity, but both antigenicities [47]. This gradual change implied that small conformational changes in the relevant region of HBsAg altered the sub-type specificity and suggested that fusion of HBsAg segments to HBcAg could, in a similar way, change the conformation of the *a* epitope, and perhaps thereby broaden the cross-reactivity of anti-HBs antibodies induced by this epitope.

The escape mutation of HBV with glycine$_{145}$ in HBsAg changed to arginine [36], was therefore made in a segment of HBsAg (residues 111–156) and fused via a short linker sequence to HBcAg truncated at residue 144. The product had HBcAg antigenicity and immunogenicity, and in immunoblotting experiments after electrophoresis in acrylamide gels under denaturing conditions, it reacted strongly with a rabbit anti-HBs serum. Rabbits immunised with this mutant fusion protein exhibited strong T-cell proliferation on exposure to HBcAg or the fusion protein, with the latter exhibiting a higher stimulation index than HBcAg itself. The rabbit sera gave a positive anti-HBs response when tested against the normal HBsAg, showing that the HBcAg fusion carrying the arginine 145 mutant induced antibodies with a broad *a* determinant specificity [48].

The antigenic determinants of HBcAg were located by Salfeld et al. [49]; other studies with a range of HBcAg fusion proteins explored the impact of the position of fusion, or insertion, of the additional sequence [50, 51] and the effect of multiple epitope sequences [45]. Fusion at or close to the N-terminus of HBcAg was disadvantageous unless part of the pre-core sequence or a flexible linker was included [51, 52]. Substitution of the major HBcAg epitope residues with other segments [51, 53] imparted the antigenic and immunogenic characteristics of these sequences at the expense of the HBcAg characteristics without impairing particle formation.

These and other results were completely consistent with the structure of HBcAg particles revealed at 7.4 Å resolution by electron cryomicroscopy and image analysis [54, 55] and the alignment of the amino acid sequence with the fold of the protein by Böttcher et al. [54]. Icosahedral particles of two sizes, with triangulation numbers T = 3 and T = 4, are assembled from 90 or 120 dimers of HBcAg, respectively, which form spikes protruding from the surface of the capsid shells. Sequences fused to the truncated C-terminus of HBcAg would be buried within the particle and therefore not readily accessible for interaction with antibodies, but nonetheless immunogenic, as had been found by Stahl and Murray [56], while those fused to the N-terminus are likely to be severely sterically hindered in the troughs between spikes unless they include a flexible linker sequence [52]. The major epitope of HBcAg itself (residues 78–82) is located at the tip of the particles' spikes and therefore prominently displayed on the outermost surface of the particle, while the T-cell epitopes reside in the α-helices (Fig. 8).

The structure of HBcAg at 3.3 Å resolution deduced very recently from X-ray diffraction analysis by Wynne et al. [57] now offers an excellent guide to the many points for attaching other sequences. Peptides, each containing one or more epitopes, may be fused at the N-terminus, at a truncated C-terminus, substituted for the major HBcAg epitope and attached to the particles by chemical crosslinking; these modifications may be made combinatorially to one HBcAg molecule or particle. The selection from fd fusion phage libraries [58] of peptides that bind to HBcAg and block its association with HBsAg [59] offered a pathway for crosslinking any peptide sequence to HBcAg, because the free peptide sequences identified from fusion phage that bind HBcAg also bind to the particles and could be crosslinked quite simply, and were shown by electron cryomicroscopy to be located at the tip of the nucleocapsid spikes [60]. Synthetic peptides in which these binding sequences are linked to the N- or C-terminus of other peptide epitopes, including the short linear epitope of the PreS1 region of HBsAg, have been synthesised and crosslinked, separately and as mixtures, to HBcAg, to give products that are precipitable by antibodies to all of the new epitopes involved and will then further cross-react with other relevant antibodies (K. Murray, unpublished work).

There is thus proof of principle for the modification of HBcAg to carry a large number of different epitopes, including non-peptide epitopes attached to a binding peptide, on a single particle (there are 90 or 120 spikes on each particle) to take advantage of the multiple powerful T-cell epitopes of HBcAg. Whether some such particles will find use as vaccines is a different question.

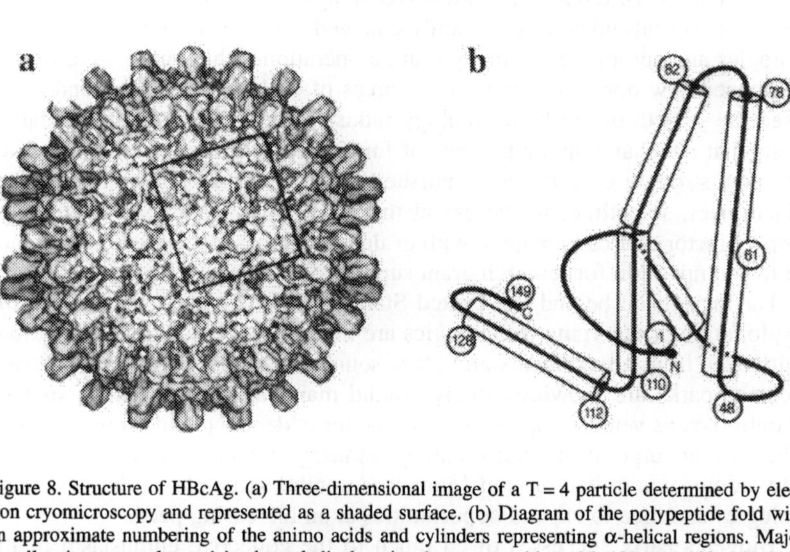

Figure 8. Structure of HBcAg. (a) Three-dimensional image of a T = 4 particle determined by electron cryomicroscopy and represented as a shaded surface. (b) Diagram of the polypeptide fold with an approximate numbering of the animo acids and cylinders representing α-helical regions. Major T cell epitopes are located in the α-helical region between residues 85–100 and 120–140 [42]. Reproduced with permission from Böttcher et al. [54].

They face the stern economic test of the time and cost of development and clinical trials, which are formidable if competing with an existing effective vaccine.

In retrospect

It's hard to believe that 20 years have passed since those early Biogen meetings. It was unusual then for academics, particularly in biologically related science, to be closely involved in applied aspects of their research, let alone playing a leading role in developing new companies. At that time, we embarked upon our new adventure with great enthusiasm and curiosity, and a lot of naivety. The thought that Biogen would become one of the leading independent biopharmaceutical operating companies was little more than fantasy for most of us. We hardly knew what venture capital meant, and indeed were staggered by the modest investment upon which the company was founded, but it also represented a new avenue for funding research.

A combination of synergistic discoveries in basic biological science over the preceding few years had opened up a range of new possibilities, such as making insulin or cytokines in *E. coli* or producing viral antigens in yeast, which were so intrinsically exciting that they would have been pursued enthusiastically in our academic departments anyway. That they were of interest as potential projects for commercial development was an added bonus which did not generate conflicts between Biogen's interests and our academic activities, but gave impetus to our research by bringing together academic groups that might otherwise have been competitors.

Our activities did not meet with universal approval in the academic world at the time, but attitudes have certainly changed. The recent advances in technologies and automation of many routine operations which have so effectively opened new opportunities in many areas of biological research and catalysed the growth of the biotechnology industry, have also brought escalating costs that are changing the patterns of funding for basic research. Academics are now strongly encouraged to pursue the commercial exploitation of their discoveries, sometimes to the extent that potential for application is a high impact factor that can compete with evaluation of basic scientific importance in the competition for research grant support.

Having lagged behind the United States for so long, new ventures in the exploitation of emerging technologies are now strongly supported by various initiatives from governments and other sources in many European countries. Science parks are growing rapidly around major academic centres, such as Cambridge, as venture capital becomes better understood and more available. The current surge of the biotechnology industry in Germany with around 30 new companies in and around Munich is another example as the new technologies continue to expand opportunities at an increasing pace.

Biogen's early successes owed much to the collective enthusiasm of the company's founding members and their spirit of collaboration under the inspiring scientific leadership of Walter Gilbert and Charles Weissmann. Within a year Gilbert took an extended sabbatical from Harvard to salvage Biogen and as CEO led both the scientific and business development through both private and public stock offerings as the company expanded its range of projects and opened laboratories first in Geneva and then in Cambridge, Massachusetts.

But overoptimism and commitment to too broad a range of projects following the early licensing agreements and successful financings soon transformed those initial successes into unsustainable levels of expenditure and huge annual financial losses with their attendant hard lessons imposing stringent economies and attrition. Jim Vincent brought the disciplined strategy and focus necessary for survival when he joined the company, by then in severe financial difficulty, towards the end of 1985 (his first meeting with Gilbert was over dinner: "That was a great session, Wally, but next time I'll order the wine!") The Geneva laboratories were facing closure, but recognizing their value, Vincent sold that part of the company to Glaxo and consolidated activities in Cambridge as he built a bridge to survival until further stock offerings and, at last, a surging royalty income stream secured the recovery of the company with a focussed strategy for development of further products, enabling it to become one of the leading independent biopharmaceutical operating companies of today.

Meanwhile, many of our colleagues of those early days have moved to other activities. Walter Gilbert returned to academic life at Harvard, but has since been very active in starting up four other new technology-based companies. Charles Weissmann gradually turned his principal research activities from cytokines to new challenges in the molecular biology of spongiform encephalopathies, and after ten very influential years left Biogen's board and joined that of Hoffmann-La Roche. Heinz Schaller extended and maintained a very active interest in hepatitis B and its variants in other animal species, making major contributions to our understanding of the replication of the virus and its interactions with its host. And we, too, have continued to find HBV fascinating: P.H.H. in studies, particularly in the context of HCC, of the integration of viral DNA into the genome of its host and of transactivation by HBxAg and segments of HBsAg expressed from chromosomally integrated HBV DNA, and K.M. in extending earlier work on HBcAg fusion proteins and using phage display systems to study their interactions and immunological properties.

Finally, we must thank our many friends and colleagues who over the years have shared with us, and indeed made possible, the experiences that we have recounted here. We also thank Ms. Thelma Coutts for preparing the manuscript, and Ms. Sigi Weissmann for Figure 2.

References

1 Szmuness W, Harley EJ, Ikram H, Stevens CE (1978) Sociodemocratic aspects of the epidemiology of hepatitis B. *In*: GN Vyas, SN Cohen, R Schmid (eds): *Viral hepatitis*. Franklin Institute Press, Philadelphia, Pennsylvania, 297–320

2 Robinson WS (1977) The genome of hepatitis B virus. *Annu Rev Microbiol* 13: 357–377

3 Krugman S, Giles JP, Hammond J (1971) Viral hepatitis type B (MS-2 strain) – Studies on active immunization. *J Amer Med Assoc* 217: 41–45

4 Hilleman MR, Bertland AU, Buynak EB, Lampson GP, McAleer WJ, McLean AA, Roehm RR, Tytell AA (1978) Clinical and laboratory studies of HBsAg vaccine. *In*: GN Vyas, SN Cohen, R Schmid (eds): *Viral hepatitis*. Franklin Institute Press, Philadelphia, Pennsylvania, 525–537

5 Maupas Ph Goudeau A, Coursaget P, Drucker J, Barin F, André M (1978) Immunization against hepatitis B in man: a pilot study of two years' duration. *In*: GN Vyas, SN Cohen, R Schmid (eds): *Viral hepatitis*. Franklin Institute Press, Philadelphia, Pennsylvania, 539–556

6 Kaplan PM, Greenman RL, Gerin JL, Purcell RH, Robinson WS (1973) DNA polymerase associated with human hepatitis B antigen. *J Virol* 12: 995–1005

7 Broome S, Gilbert W (1978) Immunological screening method to detect specific translation products. *Proc Natl Acad Sci USA* 75: 2746–2749

8 Burrell CJ, MacKay P, Greenaway PJ, Hofschneider P-H, Murray K (1979) Expression in *Escherichia coli* of hepatitis B virus DNA sequences cloned in plasmid pBR322. *Nature* 279: 43–47

9 Pasek M, Goto T, Gilbert W, Zink B, Schaller H, MacKay P, Leadbetter G, Murray K (1979) Hepatitis B virus genes and their expression in *Escherichia coli*. *Nature* 282: 575–579

10 Cohen BJ, Richmond JE (1982) Electron microscopy of hepatitis B core antigen synthesised in *E. coli*. *Nature* 296: 677–678

11 Valenzuela P, Gray P, Quiroga M, Zaldivar J, Goodman HM, Rutter WJ (1979) Nucleotide sequence of the gene coding for the major protein of hepatitis B virus surface antigen. *Nature* 280: 815–819

12 Galibert F, Mandart E, Fitoussi F, Tiollais P, Charnay P (1979) Nucleotide sequence of the hepatitis B virus genome (subtype ayw) cloned in *E. coli*. *Nature* 281: 646–650

13 Peterson DL, Roberts IM, Vyas GN (1977) Partial amino acid sequence of two major component polypeptides of hepatitis B surface antigen. *Proc Natl Acad Sci USA* 74: 1530–1534

14 Heermann KH, Goldmann U, Schwartz W, Seyffarth T, Baumgarten H, Gerlich WH (1984) Large surface proteins of hepatitis B virus containing the pre-S sequence. *J Virol* 52: 396–402

15 MacKay P, Lees J, Murray K (1981) The conversion of hepatitis B core antigen synthesised in *E. coli* into *e* antigen. *J Med Virol* 8: 237–243

16 Gough NM (1983) Core and E antigen synthesis in rodent cells transformed with hepatitis B virus DNA is associated with greater than genome length viral messenger RNAs. *J Mol Biol* 165: 683–699

17 Wollersheim M, Hofschneider PH (1988) Transactivation by a product of the X gene of hepatitis B virus. *In*: AJ Zuckerman (ed.): *Viral hepatitis and liver disease*. Alan R Liss Inc, New York, 334–340

18 Rossner MT, Jackson RJ, Murray K (1990) Modulation of expression of the hepatitis B virus surface antigen gene by the viral X-gene prouct. *Proc R Soc Lond B* 241: 51–58

19 MacKay P, Pasek M, Magazin M, Kovacic RT, Allet B, Stahl S, Gilbert W, Schaller H, Bruce SA, Murray K (1981) Production of immunologically active surface antigens of hepatitis B virus by *Escherichia coli*. *Proc Natl Acad Sci USA* 78: 4510–4514

20 Charnay P, Gervais M, Louise A, Galibert F, Tiollais P (1980) Biosynthesis of hepatitis B virus surface antigen in *Escherichia coli*. *Nature* 286: 893–895

21 Edman JC, Hallewell A, Valenzuela P, Goodman HM, Rutter WJ (1981) Synthesis of hepatitis B surface and core antigens in *E. coli*. *Nature* 291: 503–506

22 Fujisawa Y, Ito Y, Sasada R, Ono Y, Igarashi K, Marumoto R, Kikuchi M, Sugino Y (1983) Direct expression of hepatitis B surface antigen gene in *E. coli*. *Nucl Acid Res* 11: 3581–3591

23 Meyhack B, Bajwa W, Randolph H, Hinnen A (1982) Two yeast acid phosphatase structural genes are the result of a tandem duplication and show different degrees of homology in their promoter and coding sequences. *EMBO J* 1: 675–680

24 Beggs JD (1981) Gene cloning in yeast. *In*: R Williamson (ed.): *Genetic engineering, Vol 2*. Academic Press, London, 175–203

25 Valenzuela P, Medina A, Rutter WJ, Ammerer G, Hall BD (1982) Synthesis and assembly of hepatitis B virus surface antigen particles in yeast. *Nature* 298: 347–350
26 Hitzeman RA, Chen CY, Hagie FE, Patzer EJ, Liu CC, Estell DA, Miller JV, Yaffe A, Kleid DG, Levinson AD et al (1983) Expression of hepatitis B virus surface antigen in yeast. *Nucl Acid Res* 11: 2745–2763
27 Miyanohara A, Toh-EA, Nozaki C, Hamada F, Ohtomo N, Matsubara K (1983) Expression of hepatitis B surface antigen gene in yeast. *Proc Natl Acad Sci USA* 80: 1–5
28 Murray K, Bruce SA, Hinnen A, Wingfield P, van Erd PMCA, de Reus A, Schellekens H (1984) Hepatitis B virus antigens made in microbial cells immunise against viral infection. *EMBO J* 3: 645–650
29 McAleer WJ, Buynak EB, Maigetter RZ, Wampler DE, Miller WJ, Hilleman MR (1984) Human hepatitis B vaccine from recombinant yeast. *Nature* 307: 178–180
30 Szmuness W, Stevens CE, Harley EJ, Zang EA, Oleszko WR, William DC, Sadovsky R, Morrison JM, Kelner A (1980) Hepatitis B vaccine. Demonstration of efficacy in a controlled clinical trial in a high-risk population in the United States. *N Engl J Med* 203: 833–841
31 Davidson M, Krugman S (1985) Immunogenicity of recombinant yeast hepatitis B vaccine. *Lancet i* 108
32 Hilleman MR (1988) Recombinant hepatitis B vaccine produced in yeast. *Vaccine* 6: 175–183
33 André FE, Safary A (1988) Clinical experience with a yeast-derived hepatitis B vaccine. *In*: AJ Zuckerman (ed.): *Viral hepatitis and liver disease*. Alan R Liss, New York, 1025–1030
34 Chang MH, Chen CJ, Lai MS, Hsu HM, Wu TC, Kong MS, Liang DC, Shau WY, Chen DS (1997) Universal hepatitis B vaccination in Taiwan and the incidence of hepatocellular carcinoma in children. *N Engl J Med* 336: 1855–1859
35 Ryan F (1992) *Tuberculosis: The greatest story never told.* Swift Publishers, Bromsgrove UK
36 Carman WF, Zanetti AR, Karayianni P, Waters J, Manzillo G, Tanzi E, Zuckerman AJ, Thomas HC (1990) Vaccine-induced escape mutant of hepatitis B virus. *Lancet* 336: 325–329
37 Murray K, Bruce SA, Wingfield P, van Erd P, de Reus A, Schellekens H (1987) Protective immunisation against hepatitis B with an internal antigen of the virus. *J Med Virol* 23: 101–107
38 Iwarson S, Tabor E, Thomas HC, Snoy P, Gerety RJ (1985) Protection against hepatitis B virus infection by immunisation with hepatitis B core antigen. *Gastroenterology* 88: 763–767
39 McMichael AJ, Gotch FM, Noble GR, Beare PAS (1983) Cycloskeleton T-cell immunity to influenza. *N Engl J Med* 309: 13–17
40 Yewdell JW, Bennink JR, Smith GL, Moss B (1985) Influenza A virus nucleoprotein is a major target antigen for cross-reactive anti-influenza virus cytotoxic T lymphocytes. *Proc Natl Acad Sci USA* 82: 1785–1789
41 Mondelli M, Miele VG, Alberti A, Vergani D, Portmann B, Eddleston ALWF, Williams SR (1982) Specificity of T lymphocyte cytotoxicity to autologous hepatocytes in chronic hepatitis B virus infection: evidence that T cells are directed against HBV core antigen expressed on hepatocytes. *J Immunol* 129: 2773–2778
42 Milich DR, McLachlan A, Thornton GB, Hughes JL (1987) Antibody production to the nucleocapsid and envelope of the hepatitis B virus primed by a single synthetic T cell site. *Nature* 329: 547–549
43 Murray K (1988) Application of recombinant DNA techniques in the development of viral vaccines. *Vaccine* 6: 164–174
44 Stahl S, MacKay P, Magazin M, Bruce SA, Murray K (1982) Hepatitis B virus core antigen: its synthesis in *Escherichia coli* and application in diagnosis. *Proc Natl Acad Sci USA* 79: 1606–1610
45 Murray K, Shiau A-L (1999) The core antigen of hepatitis B virus as a carrier for immunogenetic peptides. *Biol Chem* 380: 277–283
46 Ullrich R, Nassal M, Meisel H, Krüger DH (1998) Core particles of hepatitis B virus as carrier for foreign epitopes. *Adv Virus Res* 50: 141–182
47 Ashton-Rickardt PG, Murray K (1989) Mutations that change the immunological subtype of hepatitis B virus antigen and distinguish between antigenic and immunogenic determination. *J Med Virol* 29: 204–214
48 Shiau A-L, Murray K (1997) Mutated epitopes of hepatitis B surface antigen fused to the core antigen of the virus induce antibodies that react with the natural surface antigen. *J Med Virol* 51: 159–166
49 Salfeld J, Pfaff E, Noah M, Schaller H (1989) Antigenic determinants and functional domains in core and *e* antigens from hepatitis B virus. *J Virol* 63: 798–808

50 Borisova GP, Berzins I, Pushko PM, Pumpens P, Gren EJ, Tsibinogin VV, Loseva A, Ose V, Ulrich R, Siakkou H et al (1989) Recombinant core particles of hepatitis B virus exposing foreign antigenic determinants on their surface. *FEBS Lett* 259: 121–124
51 Schödel F, Moriarty AM, Peterson DL, Zheng J, Hughes JL, Will H, Leturq DJ, McGee JS, Milich DR (1992) The position of heterologous epitopes inserted in hepatitis B virus core particles determines their immunogenicity. *J Virol* 66: 106–114
52 Clarke BE, Newton SE, Carroll AR, Francis MJ, Appleyard G, Syred AD, Highfield PE, Rowlands DJ, Brown F (1987) Improved immunogenicity of a peptide epitope after fusion to hepatitis B core protein. *Nature* 330: 381–384
53 Borisova G, Arya B, Dislers A, Borschukova O, Tsibinogin V, Skrastina D, Eldarov MA, Pumpens P, Skryavin KG, Grens E (1993) Hybrid hepatitis B virus nucleocapsid bearing an immunodominant region from hepatitis B surface antigen. *J Virol* 67: 3636–3701
54 Böttcher B, Wynne SA, Crowther RA (1997) Determination of the fold of the core protein of hepatitis B virus by electron cryomicroscopy. *Nature* 386: 88–91
55 Conway JF, Cheng N, Zlotnick A, Wingfield PT, Stahl SJ, Steven AC (1997) Visualisation of a 4-helix bundle in the hepatitis B virus capsid by cryoelectronmicroscopy. *Nature* 386: 91–94
56 Stahl S, Murray K (1989) Immunogenicity of peptide fusions to hepatitis B virus core antigens. *Proc Natl Acad Sci USA* 86: 6283–6287
57 Wynne SA, Crowther RA, Leslie AGW (1999) The crystal structure of the human hepatitis B virus capsid. *Molec Cell* 3: 771–780
58 Scott JK, Smith GP (1990) Searching for peptide ligands with an epitope library. *Science* 249: 386–390
59 Dyson MR, Murray K (1995) Selection of peptide inhibitors of interactions involved in complex protein assemblies: association of the core and surface antigens of hepatitis B virus. *Proc Natl Acad Sci USA* 92: 2194–2198
60 Böttcher B, Tsuji N, Takakashi H, Dyson MR, Zhao S, Crowther RA, Murray K (1998) Peptides that block hepatitis B virus assembly: analysis by cryomicroscopy, mutagenesis and transfection. *EMBO J* 17: 6839–6845

First generation proteins

Recombinant Protein Drugs
ed. by P. Buckel

Clotting factors VIII and IX

George G. Brownlee[1] and Paul L.F. Giangrande[2]

[1] *Chemical Pathology Unit, Sir William Dunn School of Pathology, University of Oxford, Oxford, UK*
[2] *Oxford Haemophilia Centre, The Churchill Hospital, Oxford, UK*

Introduction

Haemophilia is the most common congenital disorder of coagulation and affects approximately 1 in 10,000 males around the world. Haemophilia A is due to a deficiency of factor VIII in the circulating blood whilst haemophilia B (also known as Christmas disease) is a clinically identical disorder caused by factor IX deficiency. It is less common than haemophilia A and affects 1 in about 30,000 males. Both factors VIII and IX are essential glycoproteins in the clotting cascade [1] (Fig. 1). The hallmark of severe haemophilia is recurrent and spontaneous haemarthrosis, typically affecting the hinge joints such as the ankle, knee and elbow. The severity of bleeding depends upon the level of factor in the blood.

Severe haemophilia is usually defined by a level of <2 iu/dl (or <2%) of factor VIII or IX in plasma. Moderately severely affected patients have levels varying from 2–5 iu/dl and mild from 5–25 iu/dl. It is unusual for an infant to have spontaneous haemarthroses in the first few months of life, and the first joint to be affected tends to be the ankle as the child learns to crawl. Repeated bleeding into joints may cause permanent damage, with painful arthritis and limb deformity and associated muscle wasting. Bleeding into muscles is also a feature of haemophilia, but this is usually a consequence of direct injury, albeit often minor. Bleeds into certain areas are particularly dangerous because of the risk of compression of neighbouring structures. Bleeds in the tongue can obstruct the airway, and retroperitoneal bleeding within the ilio-psoas muscle may result in femoral nerve compression. Bleeding from the gastrointestinal tract and bleeding into the urinary tract may also occur. There is also a significant risk of intracranial haemorrhage in severe haemophilia which was a significant cause of mortality in the past when treatment was not so readily available. The poor prognosis in the absence of effective treatment is reflected by the fact that the median life expectancy of haemophiliacs in Sweden was only 11 years during the period 1831–1920, but rose to 56.8 years during the period 1961–1980 [2]. It is also interesting to note that a century ago haemophilia affected several members of the royal families of Britain, Spain and Russia,

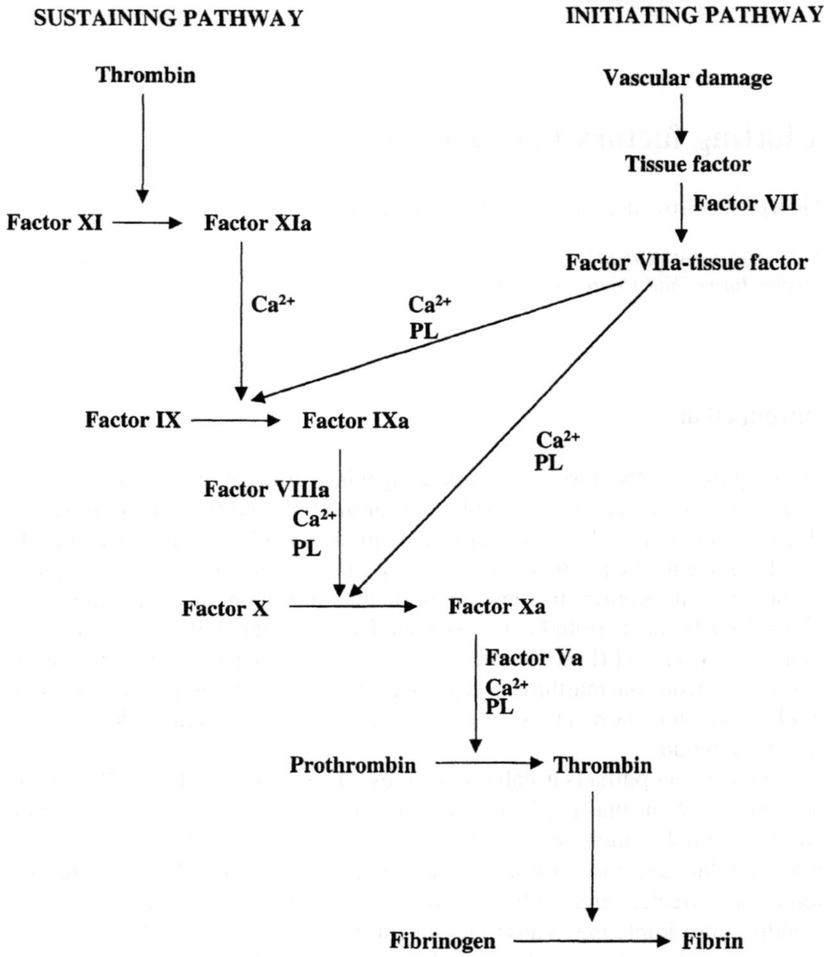

Figure 1. The revised clotting cascade. Thrombin, formed by the action of factor Xa as a result of vascular damage in the initiating (or extrinsic) pathway activates factor XI, thereby sustaining the cascade through the sustaining (or intrinsic) pathway. PL = phospholipid. The scheme is simplified and omits many details for clarity [1].

but, despite the best medical facilities of the age being available, all affected members died in their youth and no surviving descendants are affected.

Approximately 5% of patients with haemophilia A develop inhibitory antibodies to factor VIII at some stage but it is quite likely that this figure underestimates the true prevalence. Inhibitor development in haemophilia B is, by contrast, very rare (<1%). This is a potentially serious complication of therapy, as patients are refractory to conventional doses of coagulation factor concentrates and bleeding can be difficult to control. Family studies suggest that there is a genetic predisposition to the formation of antibodies but no HLA association or other linkages have been conclusively identified. There is some evidence that people of Afro-Caribbean origin are more susceptible to inhibitor formation than other ethnic groups. Certain mutations are undoubtedly associated with a significantly increased risk of inhibitor development, particularly large gene deletions and nonsense mutations resulting in stop codons – presumably because patients lack immune tolerance [3, 4]. There is a weaker association between inhibitor formation and the presence of an inversion in intron 22 of the factor VIII gene [5].

The genes for factor VIII and IX are both located at the telomere of the long arm of the X chromosome and thus haemophilia is inherited as an X-linked, recessive condition affecting males. The daughters of affected males are obligate carriers but sons are normal. A proportion of all cases of haemophilia occurs in the absence of a previous family history and is due to new mutations. Perhaps the most famous example is that of Queen Victoria, who had a haemophiliac son (Leopold) and also two daughters who were carriers. It is not known, however, whether they suffered from haemophilia A or B. There are very rare instances of haemophilia affecting females due to inheritance of the defective gene from both parents or to unequal X-inactivation in carriers [6]. There are also reports of haemophilia in females with Turner's syndrome (XO karyotype) and congenital androgen insensitivity (testicular feminization with XY karyotype).

Molecular basis of haemophilia A

Factor VIIIa is an essential cofactor which is required for the activation of factor X by factor IXa in the clotting cascade (Fig. 1). Factor VIII is a glycoprotein of 2332 amino acids and is synthesized predominantly by hepatocytes of the liver. It is processed intracellularly in the Golgi apparatus by proteolytic cleavage giving rise to a N-terminal heavy chain and a C-terminal light chain. Its domain structure (Fig. 2A) includes a carbohydrate-rich B domain that is not required for activity (see below). Factor VIII is activated to give rise to factor VIIIa by further proteolytic cleavage, probably by thrombin. In plasma, factor VIII circulates as a large glycoprotein complex non-covalently bound to multimers of von Willebrand factor (Fig. 2). The factor VIII gene is about 186 kb in length, with 26 exons, and is situated on the long arm of the X chromosome at Xq28.

Developments in molecular biology have permitted rapid identification of mutations in haemophilia A (and B) patients by various methods. PCR amplification of either genomic DNA or cDNA derived from the reverse transcription of mRNA of patient lymphocytes has superseded older methods based on restriction enzyme digestion and Southern blotting. Although automated DNA sequence analysers have been developed, gene sequencing of the entire factor VIII gene would be both expensive and labour-intensive because of its size.

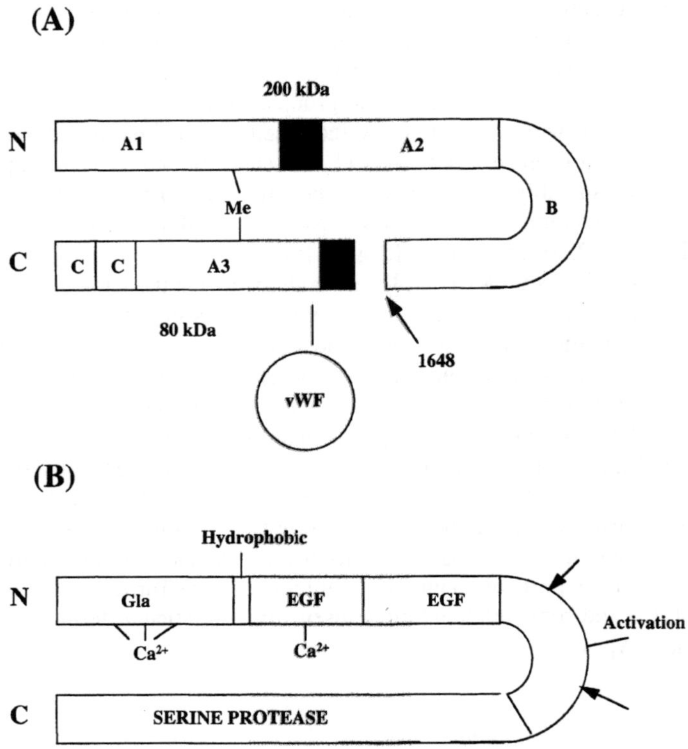

Figure 2. The domain structure of (A) factor VIII and (B) factor IX. In factor VIII (above) the N-terminal heavy chain and C-terminal light chain, formed after proteolysis at amino acid 1648 as shown, are stabilized by a metal (Me) binding site; a proposed site of binding to von Willebrand (vWF) factor is shown. The A1 and 2, B and C domains are marked. In factor IX (below) arrows mark the sites of proteolytic cleavage in the activation domain by either factor XIa or VIIa. For further details, see text.

Thus methods have been developed to initially prescreen the gene or mRNA, in order to define the mutated exon of the DNA, or region of the mRNA, before sequencing to define the actual mutation itself. Chemical cleavage of mismatches in heteroduplexes formed from the mutated DNA and a test DNA is the best current technique for detecting all mutations [7, 8]. Other useful methods are conformation-sensitive gel electrophoresis and denaturing-gradient gel electrophoresis, although these alternatives do not allow all mutations to be detected.

By far the commonest single genetic defect causing haemophilia A is an inversion in intron 22, which is encountered in about 20% of all patients, and in nearly half of all severely affected patients [5]. The inversion mechanism proposed involves homologous, intra-chromosomal recombination between an intronless gene of unknown function, designated F8A, which lies within intron

22 of the factor VIII gene and either of 2 further copies of F8A flanking the factor VIII gene. In either case, the inversion results in a truncated factor VIII gene generating a truncated mRNA and inactive factor VIII protein, thus explaining the severe haemophilia. Recombination with the distal copy of F8A is commoner than with the proximal copy and accounts for approximately 80% of the inversions (reviewed in [9]). It is now recognised that inversion is much more common in a male than a female meiosis.

All other known haemophilia A mutations are summarized in a valuable mutation database [10]. At present, 454 unique mutations are listed, including 92 cases of large deletions. However, it is generally thought that large deletions account for only a minority of cases of haemophilia and the reason that a much higher proportion than 5% is listed in the database reflects an ascertainment bias. Most mutations are point mutants or very short additions or deletions of only a few nucleotides. Nonsense, frameshift and splice-site mutations, caused by point mutations or short additions or deletions, usually cause severe haemophilia. Most other cases are caused by missense mutations causing amino acid substitutions and 218 missense mutations are presently known [10]. They have varying degrees of severity for patients from very mild to very severe [10]. Mutations at CG doublets, giving rise to a TG or CA doublet, are common. As is well known, CG doublets are genomic "hotspots" because of specific methylation of cytosine to 5' methylcytosine and because the methylated cytosine is particularly susceptible to mutation by deamination.

Molecular basis of haemophilia B

Factor IXa is a serine protease required for the activation of factor X in the clotting cascade. Factor IXa is itself formed from factor IX by proteolysis by either factor VIIa-tissue factor complex, which initiates the clotting cascade, or by factor XIa, which sustains it [1] (Fig. 1). Factor IX is a glycoprotein of 415 amino acids and is made up of a N-terminal γ-carboxyglutamic acid-rich sequence (Gla domain), two epidermal growth factor-like (EGF) domains – the first of which binds calcium – an activation domain and finally a C-terminal serine protease or catalytic domain (Fig. 2B). The 12 glutamic acid residues of the Gla domain undergo γ-carboxylation by a vitamin K-dependent γ-glutamyl carboxylase in the endoplasmic reticulum (ER) during the synthesis of factor IX in the liver hepatocyte. This essential post-translational modification is necessary for the correct protein folding and calcium binding of factor IX. The factor IX gene is about 34 kb in length and contains eight exons. Its basic exon structure is similar in organisation to coagulation factors VII, X and protein C and it is likely that they all evolved from a common ancestral gene by gene duplication.

The factor IX gene is considerably smaller than that of factor VIII, and patients with haemophilia B have been studied more extensively than those with haemophilia A. The first defects identified in haemophilia B were large gene deletions detected in patients with inhibitory antibodies by Southern blotting [3]. However, it is now clear that point mutations, or short additions or deletions, account for the vast majority of cases of haemophilia B, and over 689 unique mutations are listed in an extensive mutation database of 1918 families who have been studied from around the world [6, 11]. Most of the unique mutations are point mutants causing missense, nonsense or splicing defects involving all 8 exons. For example, there are at present 425 different missense mutations that cause amino acid substitutions. These include the original case of Christmas disease, which is a G $\rightarrow$ C mutation at nucleotide 30,070 causing an amino acid change from Cys $\rightarrow$ Ser at residue 206 within exon 7 [12]. Many mutations have been observed more than once, even where there is no known kinship. Many of these repeat mutations – as in the case of haemophilia A patients, occur at CG doublets, suggesting they are independent mutation hotspots. However, other repeat mutations do not involve CG doublets, suggesting a founder effect. A good example is the mutation at nucleotide 31,311 where there are 41 examples.

A few patients have been described in whom the factor IX level rises significantly after puberty (the haemophilia B Leiden patients); this is associated with complete clinical recovery. These interesting regulatory mutations have been all localized to a short region of the factor IX promoter and 18 unique mutations are now known [6]. These mutations inhibit the binding of transcription factors, e.g., hepatic nuclear factor 4, which are required for the efficient initiation of transcription. An androgen response element (ARE) in the factor IX promoter, which interacts with the androgen receptor in the presence of testosterone, is responsible for the upregulation of factor IX mRNA at puberty [13]. Consistent with this hypothesis, patients with mutations in the ARE do not recover at puberty [13].

Treatment of haemophilia

Over a century ago, the first effective product available for treatment of bleeding episodes was fresh blood. The preparation of an antihaemophilic factor of bovine origin by Macfarlane in 1954 [14] was a major therapeutic advance, although serious allergic reactions were not infrequent. The use of cold-insoluble cryoprecipitate was introduced in 1965. The subsequent development of lyophilized concentrates of factors VIII and IX in the early 1970s transformed the life of haemophiliacs. The goals of treatment, as stated by the World Federation of Haemophilia, are "to minimise disability and prolong life, to facilitate general social and physical well-being and to help each patient achieve full potential whilst causing no harm" (www.wfh.org). Advances in therapy have certainly resulted in a dramatic increase in the longevity of haemophiliacs in developed countries. A study of 717 Dutch patients documented a calculated life expectancy for these patients of 66 years, compared with 74 year for normal males [15], and the authors of this study concluded that the mortality associated with even severe haemophilia was similar to that associated with cigarette smoking.

Treatment of bleeding episodes involves the intravenous injection of coagulation factor concentrates. The total dose and frequency of treatment is determined by the severity and site of bleeding. Most bleeds resolve with a single infusion, if the bleed is recognised early and treated promptly. There is an increasing move to prophylactic therapy, in which the patient gives himself injections at home of coagulation factors two or three times a week to prevent bleeds rather than just treating on demand when bleeds occur. Patients on prophylactic therapy experience few or even no spontaneous bleeds and thus progressive joint damage and arthritis can be avoided.

The pooling of plasma donations introduced the risk of transmission of viral infections, and many haemophiliacs were infected with HIV and/or hepatitis C in the 1980s. In the UK, 1229 haemophiliacs were infected with HIV, and about 300 were exposed to hepatitis C [16, 17]. The introduction in 1985 of physical methods of viral inactivation, such as heat-treatment or the addition of a solvent/detergent mixture, eliminated the risk of transmission of HIV or hepatitis C. However, other viruses are relatively resistant to these measures and cases of hepatitis A and parvovirus infection have been documented even with these more modern products. More recently, there has been concern about the possibility of transmission of prion disorders, although no cases have yet been described in haemophilia [18]. Recombinant products offer the greatest margin of safety for haemophiliac patients and have been recommended as the treatment of choice for all patients with haemophilia (see below).

Development of recombinant DNA methods

During the late 1970s there was a quiet revolution in molecular biology. Using restriction enzymes and DNA ligase, it became possible to clone copies of mRNA into either bacterial plasmids or into bacteriophages such as phage λ. Such clones could then be sequenced using Sanger's dideoxy chain termination method or Maxam & Gilbert's chemical degradation procedure. Once these mRNAs had been cloned, each cloned cDNA served as a probe in order to isolate from the entire genome its respective gene, which could then in turn be sequenced. Oligonucleotides were starting to be used as primers for the enzymatic synthesis of DNA. The presence of introns in most genes was discovered. Southern had described his blotting technique that was to become so widely used in this field until the development of PCR techniques much later in the 1980s.

Globin, immunoglobulin and ovalbumin mRNA – all mRNA species which could be purified in reasonable quantities from specialized cells or organs – could now be cloned in *E. coli* and sequenced in their entirety for the first time. Moreover, the new cloning methods suggested that mRNA and/or genes of medical interest, such as human insulin and human growth hormone mRNA, might be cloned and the protein expressed artificially in bacteria. This, it was thought, might be a cost-effective and safer alternative to isolating these proteins from natural sources for the treatment of diabetes and pituitary dwarfism.

1980 was a time of optimism and some of us thought that we might be able to clone rare, low-abundance mRNA, if only new methods could be developed. We decided to clone human factor IX mRNA. This would be an ambitious and difficult project because of its low abundance in liver. However, if the project were successful, the benefits for patients with haemophilia B would be considerable.

Recombinant factor IX

The factor IX gene was cloned in 1982 – some 2 years before the factor VIII gene – and this work will be described first. The expression of biologically active recombinant factor VIII, however, proved technically easier than factor IX. Moreover the priority was to produce recombinant factor VIII before recombinant factor IX because of the higher incidence of haemophilia A than B in the population. Consequently recombinant factor VIII was available for the treatment of patients in 1992, much sooner than recombinant factor IX, which was only produced much later in 1997.

Cloning the human factor IX gene in Oxford

It was the availability of the complete amino acid sequence of bovine factor IX [19] that initially led us to think that it might be possible to clone the factor IX gene. We thought that short synthetic oligonucleotides, with their sequence partly predicted from the genetic code and the amino acid sequence of the protein, would probably be the key to cloning rare mRNAs, like the factor IX mRNA. We had previously used oligonucleotides both for our earlier sequencing of regions within the α and β-globin, ovalbumin and immunoglobulin mRNAs [20], as well as for our later influenza cloning [21, 22]. Oligonucleotides were clearly powerful and highly specific reagents for nucleic acids. In particular, they could be used to hybridize to specific sequences in mRNA and prime the synthesis of cDNA by reverse transcriptase.

We first decided to enrich the bovine factor IX mRNA, which we had isolated from a calf liver, by two successive sucrose density-gradient centrifugation steps [23]. We then set up a rabbit reticulocyte *in vitro* translation assay to detect factor IX mRNA, locating it in the 20–22S fraction of the sucrose gradient. We estimated that it had been purified about 10-fold over the starting mRNA. Even so it was unlikely that the factor IX mRNA was >0.1% pure at this stage.

We then synthesized, as a mixture, eight 14-nucleotide (nt) long oligonucleotides (oligo N1 mixture), complementary to the bovine mRNA sequence, whose sequence was predicted from the amino acid sequence of residues 348–352 of bovine factor IX (Fig. 3). This was a particularly favourable region

```
First               348             352
Amino acid          His-Met-Phe-Cys-Ala
sequence
                     U      U   U
mRNA             5'  CA AUG UU  UG  GCN 3'
                     C      C   C

                     A      A   A
Oligonucleo-     3'  GT TAC AA  AC  CG  5'
tides (N1)           G      G   G


Second            70                 75
Amino acid        Glu-Cys-Trp-Cys-Gln-Ala
sequence
                   A   U       U   A
mRNA          5'   GA  UG  UGG UG  CA  GCN 3'
                   G   C       C   G

                   T   A       A
Oligonucleo-  3'   CT  AC  ACC AC  GTT CG   5'
tides (N2A)        C   G       G

                   T   A       A
Oligonucleo-  3'   CT  AC  ACC AC  GTC CG   5'
tides (N2B)        C   G       G
```

Figure 3. Two regions of amino acid sequence of bovine factor IX used to design mixed oligonucleotide sequence primers (N1) or probes (N2A & N2B) [22]. See text for further details.

of amino-acid sequence since the number of alternative possible nucleotide sequences predicted from the genetic code was limited to 8, because the sequence contains a methionine residue which has a unique codon. This oligo N1 mixture of primers was used to prime the synthesis of cDNA from factor IX-enriched bovine mRNA in order to generate a library of cDNA clones. Briefly, after synthesis of cDNA by reverse transcriptase and subsequent removal of mRNA by alkaline hydrolysis, "loop-back" synthesis of double-stranded DNA was catalysed by *E. coli* DNA polymerase I (Klenow subfragment) in the absence of added primer. Cloning of this double-stranded DNA was simplified by restriction digestion of DNA with MboI (GATC-recognition sequence) and ligation into the unique Bam HI site of the classic plasmid, pBR322. An "MboI" cDNA library of about 7000 recombinant clones was thus obtained in *E. coli*.

Bacterial colonies were then screened on Whatman 541 paper [24] using a second mixture (oligo N2A plus oligo N2B) of 16 ^{32}P-labelled 17-nt long oligonucleotides based on the predicted sequence of bovine factor IX mRNA of another favourable region of amino acid sequence between residues 70–75 (Fig. 3). We obtained a single clone, labelled BIX-1, which was sequenced by the Maxam and Gilbert method. This clone encoded bovine factor IX mRNA from amino acids 52 to 139 and predicted an amino acid sequence that was in complete agreement with the literature, except for a single discrepancy changing the amino acid at position 57. This discrepancy was, in fact, confirmed as a correction to the published bovine factor IX sequence, since it was also present in an independent clone in a "dC/dG-tailed" cDNA library of about 10,000 *E. coli* colonies.

Thus the choice of oligonucleotides and our ability to synthesize them in-house were two important factors in our initial success in isolating factor IX cDNA clones. Acting in the hope that the human and bovine factor IX genes would be sufficiently conserved in nucleotide sequence to cross-hybridize, the bovine factor IX probe was then used to probe a Charon 4A bacteriophage λ library of human genomic clones [22]. A positively hybridizing clone, λHIX1b, was isolated and mapped by restriction enzyme cleavage and Southern blotting. A restriction fragment corresponding to the probe was thus identified on Southern blots and sequenced. There was 85% nucleotide sequence conservation between bovine and human factor IX gene in the region initially sequenced. We had thus isolated a clone containing part of the human factor IX gene.

Further cloning and expression of factor IX in mammalian cells

Further cloning Two additional reports from other groups [25, 26] extended our initial work by describing the complete coding sequence of human factor IX, which was found to be preceded by a leader sequence with a potential signal peptide and propeptide sequence. There was uncertainty, however, as to whether the entire coding sequence had been cloned, since the 5' non-coding of the factor IX mRNA was not characterized. There were, also, in one report [26] some 6 differences in the coding nucleotide sequence attributed, incorrectly as it turned out later except for one nucleotide [27], to the presence of polymorphisms. Interestingly, although the details of the cloning procedures differed in these reports from our own work, all of the studies had relied on oligonucleotides to prepare or isolate clones from cDNA libraries.

We concentrated on characterizing the complete factor IX mRNA sequence by cDNA cloning, and independently sequencing all exons in order to define splice points and to check for potential cDNA cloning errors, which are known to occur during reverse transcription and cloning. We defined the mRNA start site precisely and sequenced the entire 3' non-coding region of the mRNA [27]. The factor IX gene turned out to be about 34 kb long with 8 exons. The factor IX mRNA was about 2800 nucleotides long and had a relatively short 5' non-coding region, but a reasonably long 3' non-coding sequence of nearly 1400 nucleotides containing the usual AAUAAA poly(A) signal. Finally, the complete human factor IX gene sequence of 33.5 kb, including all 7 introns, was established by Davie's group [28].

Expression of biologically active factor IX in mammalian cells If cloning the factor IX cDNA and gene sequence were to be a "useful" contribution to medicine, then expression of recombinant factor IX protein would have to be achieved. A major uncertainty was whether *biologically active* factor IX was synthesized, because after synthesis, factor IX has to be post-translationally modified and correctly processed. In particular, after γ-carboxylation of 12 glutamyl residues near the N-terminus of factor IX by a vitamin K-dependent carboxylase, the 18 amino acid residues of the propeptide sequence [29] must be cleaved by a furin protease. Both these processes are essential for factor IX activity. It was conceivable that these essential post-translational events would only occur in liver, the site of factor IX synthesis in the body, and would not occur in hepatic or other cell types derived from other tissues in tissue culture.

We were fortunate that the aim of producing biologically active factor IX in mammalian cells in tissue culture was feasible but it was only achieved after a considerable effort by Don Anson and Ian Jones in the Brownlee laboratory. We published, in 1985, that "we were able to isolate small amounts of biologically active (recombinant) human factor IX" [30]. In particular, factor IX was expressed in rat hepatoma cells that had been stably transfected with a factor IX expression plasmid. Much higher yields of >90% biologically active factor IX were obtained in canine kidney cells (MDCK cells) using a slightly different expression plasmid [31]. Our results were particularly convincing because we purified the recombinant factor IX by immuno-affinity chromatography.

Subsequently, higher yields of recombinant factor IX were achieved by other groups using different expression vectors in different mammalian cells, i.e., baby hamster kidney (BHK), human hepatoma (HepG2) and chinese hamster ovary (CHO) cells [32–34]. But in every case the biological activity of factor IX was less than in our reports. Indeed, in the initial work by Kaufman's group in CHO cells (in which the factor IX gene was amplified in the genome) factor IX was secreted to give as much as 100 mg/ml of factor IX in the medium, yet only 2% was biologically active [34]. This low biological activity in CHO cells was subsequently solved by the introduction of a furin-type protease (see below), suggesting that factor IX propeptide processing must have been limiting.

Development of recombinant factor IX for clinical use

The observation that some, albeit low, biological activity was present in the factor IX expressed in CHO cells was important [34], since this cell line has properties that are particularly suited for large-scale culture needed for the industrial production of recombinant proteins by the biotechnology industry. Therefore, development work was undertaken by Genetics Institute, Boston. This presented a significant challenge since it was essential that propeptide processing and γ-carboxylation, known to be essential for factor IX activity, had to occur. Neither of these processes had been previously required in CHO cells in the production of recombinant proteins for the biotechnology industry.

Initially it was suspected that γ-carboxylation was limiting in the factor IX-expressing CHO cells, thus accounting for the presence of the inactive, incompletely γ-carboxylated factor IX. However, when the cloned γ-carboxylase became available, transient transfection of expression constructs of the γ-carboxylase into factor IX-secreting CHO cells failed to improve factor IX biological activity [35]. By contrast, propeptide processing of factor IX was significantly improved by the co-expression of a furin-like enzyme, specifically a soluble form of PACE (paired basic amino acid cleaving enzyme) introduced stably into the CHO cell line [36]. Finally, Genetics Institute produced factor IX in a form that was fully processed by screening factor IX-expressing CHO clones to identify those with the highest factor IX-processing capacity, by optimizing the concentration of vitamin K added to the defined serum-free culture medium (which lacked any added protein) and by defining the precise conditions of growth of the factor IX-secreting CHO clone in large-scale (2500 l) bioreactors.

A down-stream large-scale purification protocol was developed that did not require the use of monoclonal antibodies for affinity purification, to avoid any risk of introducing viral contaminants. The purified recombinant factor IX showed a slightly reduced γ-carboxylation level of about 11 γ-carboxyglutamyl (Gla) residues per molecule compared to 12 Gla residues in blood-derived factor IX (Tab. 1 and ref. [37]). A new result obtained from the analysis of this recombinant factor IX is that the post-translational modification of Gla residues 36 and 40 are not apparently needed for activity [38]. Other differences between recombinant and human blood-derived factor IX were appar-

Table 1. Comparison of post-translational modifications of plasma-derived and recombinant factor IX

Modification	Plasma-derived	Recombinant
1. γ-carboxyglutamic acid (Gla)*		
12 of 12 Gla residues	100%	60%
11 of 12 Gla residues	0%	35%
10 of 12 Gla residues	0%	5%
2. β-hydroxyaspartic acid 64	37%	46%
3. Carbohydrate		
N-linked glycans		
Asn 157 }	High heterogeneity	Low heterogeneity
Asn 167 }	fully sialylated	<fully sialylated
O-linked glycans		
Ser 53	$(Xyl)_{1-2}$-Glc	$(Xyl)_2$-Glc
Ser 61	NeuAcGalGlcNAcFuc	NeuAcGalGlcNAcFuc
Thr 159, 169 & 172	Classical, partially filled	Classical, partially filled
4. Tyr 155 sulphation	>90%	<15%
5. Ser 158 phosphorylation	>90%	<1%

Footnotes: Adapted from ref. [37] with permission. *The 10 completely modified Gla residues occur at amino acid residues 7, 8, 15, 17, 20, 21, 26, 27, 30 and 33. Gla residues at positions 36 and 40 are incompletely modified, as indicated, in recombinant factor IX.

ent in the extent of N- and O-linked carbohydrate side chains, and in sulphation and phosphorylation levels of particular residues (Tab. 1). The extent of β-hydroxyaspartate modification at serine 64, however, was similar. Fortunately, none of the differences in post-translational modification seemed to affect the biological activity of factor IX, although the differences in sulphation and phosphorylation, it was suggested, may explain the slightly lower recovery (on average about 20% lower) of recombinant, as compared to blood-derived, factor IX seen in patients [37].

In summary, recombinant factor IX is already really a "second-generation" recombinant product because it is prepared from cultured cells and purified under conditions where there is no contact with human or bovine proteins [37]. Thus the product should be free of known blood-borne viral diseases, such as HIV, hepatitis A, B or C and parvoviruses. There should also be no risk from diseases caused by prions, such as Creutzfeldt-Jakob disease (CJD) or the variant CJD, caused by the prion of bovine spongiform encephalitis in cattle. Recombinant factor IX (BenefIX) was approved for sale in the USA and Canada in 1997 and in Europe in 1998.

Recombinant factor VIII

When factor VIII was first cloned and expressed in cultured cells by two competing companies in 1984, this achievement was hailed as one of the most exciting advances to be reported by the biotechnology industry [39]. However, in a Nature editorial in the same week that the factor VIII cloning was announced, we were poignantly reminded that the first deaths had occurred in Australia and in the UK from HIV-contaminated blood. Clearly blood-derived clotting factors were potentially dangerous and would eventually be superseded by recombinant proteins. Not for the first time was the fear of disease driving scientists and biotechnology companies to find improved and safer medicines.

Cloning and expression of factor VIII

The factor VIII gene and its cDNA were cloned by the use of oligonucleotide probes based on the amino acid sequence of peptides isolated from either human or porcine factor VIII, essentially by similar methods to those employed previously to clone factor IX. Due to its low concentrations in plasma, its high molecular weight and extreme sensitivity to proteolytic processing, it was a very difficult protein to purify. The breakthrough came when amino acid sequence information on peptide fragments of human or porcine factor VIII became available [40, 41].

Surprisingly, a unique 36-nt long oligonucleotide, rather than a mixture of oligonucleotides, was successfully used as a probe in one report [40], and in the other [41] two sets of mixed oligonucleotides, either 45-nt long or 15-nt long, were used. Because of uncertainty as to whether factor VIII was synthesized in the liver, both groups initially cloned the factor VIII gene by screening genomic libraries of clones in bacteriophage λ with these probes. The gene turned out to be 180 kb long with 26 exons and at that time was the longest known gene. Human cDNA clones were then subsequently isolated, using genomic probes, by screening appropriate human cDNA libraries. Full-length cDNAs were then used for expression studies by introducing expression plasmids with heterologous viral promoters into BHK [40] or monkey kidney (COS-1) cell lines [41]. Human factor VIII was secreted into the medium of these transfected cells and shown to be active in a clotting assay. Cloning and characterization of the factor VIII gene and its cDNA had been a long task, but its expression was initially surprisingly straightforward.

Development of recombinant factor VIII for clinical use

The subsequent production and purification of recombinant factor VIII from cultured mammalian cells by the biotechnology industry were quite rapid and commensurate with the urgency in producing recombinant factor VIII, which was free of viral contamination for the treatment of haemophilia A patients.

Initially, however, there was some difficulty in the approach developed by Kaufman's group at Genetics Institute in obtaining high yields of factor VIII secreted by CHO cells. Factor VIII cDNA had been introduced into CHO cells by linking it to the selectable, amplifiable marker, dihydrofolate reductase (DHFR). Protein expression levels were, however, much lower than had been observed with other cDNAs, e.g., factor IX, in CHO cells. It emerged that the reason for this was that during intracellular processing of factor VIII in the ER, a significant proportion of the factor VIII became bound to the chaperone, immunoglubulin-binding protein (BiP), through a primary binding site of its A1-domain. Interactions also occurred between factor VIII and 2 other protein chaperones, calnexin and calreticulin, primarily mediated by the B-domain of factor VIII. It was suggested that factor VIII has unique requirements, not shared by the related coagulation factor V, for carbohydrate processing and molecular chaperone interactions that may limit its secretion [42]. In practice the problem of the low yield of secreted factor VIII was initially overcome, at least in part, by the addition of von Willebrand factor (vWF) (the cofactor with which factor VIII is normally associated as a high-molecular-weight complex in plasma) to the tissue culture medium. Thus factor VIII secreted in the absence of vWF appeared to be rapidly degraded. In its presence, however, factor VIII associated with vWF to form high-molecular-weight multimers. This stabilized the factor VIII, protecting it from proteolytic degradation and improving factor VIII yields significantly [43].

Finally, in order to develop a large-scale process for production of factor VIII, the vWF cDNA was introduced into the factor VIII-expressing CHO cells by linking it to a second amplifiable marker, the adenosine deaminase gene. Co-expression of factor VIII and vWF was thereby achieved even in serum-free medium (Fig. 4), improving the factor VIII yields by 1–2 orders of magnitude [44, 45]. Even so, the yield of factor VIII was still significantly lower

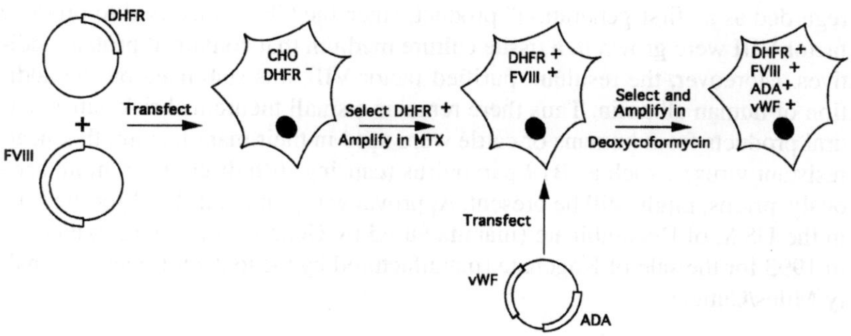

Figure 4. Derivation of factor VIII and von Willebrand factor coexpressing CHO cells used for the manufacture of recombinant factor IX. Adapted from Kaufman [45] with permission. Plasmids encoding DHFR and factor VIII were transfected into DHFR-deficient CHO cells and transformants selected by growth in nucleoside-free medium. Cells were then selected in increasing concentrations of methotrexate to obtain a cell line that had amplified the DHFR and factor VIII genes. These cells were subsequently transfected with a vWF expression plasmid containing an ADA (adenosine deaminase) gene and selected for growth in the presence of cytotoxic concentrations of adenosine with increasing concentrations of 2'-deoxycoformycin. The final cell expressed DHFR, ADA, vWF and factor VIII.

than that of the co-expressed vWF. This suggested that the intracellular regulation of factor VIII mRNA levels and/or regulation of the intracellular folding and processing of factor VIII were still limiting the yields of factor VIII secreted into the culture medium [44]. The factor VIII-expressing CHO cell line is cultured in a defined, serum-free medium in 2500 l bioreactors for the large-scale manufacture of recombinant factor VIII. However, it should be noted that the culture medium is reported to contain (unspecified) added bovine proteins from natural sources, which were, however, tested to minimize the risk of introducing viral contamination [46].

By contrast, a different cell line was used for factor VIII expression in the approach adopted by Genentech/Bayer. A clone of BHK cells was isolated after introducing the factor VIII cDNA, linked to DHFR, into chromosomal DNA followed by amplification of the factor VIII copy number by selection with methotrexate. The BHK clone used for the commercial production of factor VIII contains about 150 copies of the factor VIII cDNA per cell [47]. For the subsequent manufacture of factor VIII in deep-tank stirred suspension fermenters, a proprietary (unspecified), serum-free medium was used [48]. This medium presumably contained some added protein, since there was no requirement to introduce the vWF cDNA to improve the stability of the factor VIII secreted in this BHK cell line, unlike the situation in CHO cells (see above).

Both recombinant factor VIII products (Genetics Institute or Genentech), after purification by immuno-affinity chromatography with monoclonal antibodies, ion-exchange chromatography and other methods, were reported to be essentially indistinguishable from plasma-derived factor VIII [45, 48]. The full-length recombinant factor VIII produced by both companies may be regarded as a "first-generation" product, since the CHO cells used to produce factor VIII were grown in a tissue culture medium that contained protein additives. Moreover, the resultant purified factor VIII was stabilized by the addition of human albumin. Thus there remains a small theoretical risk, since natural products from humans or cattle were used in their manufacture, that heat-resistant viruses, such as B19 parvovirus (causing fifth disease) or, more seriously, prions, might still be present. Approval was granted in 1992 for the sale, in the USA, of Recombinate (manufactured by Genetics Institute/Baxter) and in 1993 for the sale of Kogenate (manufactured by Genentech/Bayer, originally Miles/Cutter).

B-domainless recombinant factor VIII

A second generation, B-domainless factor VIII, recombinant factor VIII SQ ("Refacto": Pharmacia/Upjohn/Genetics Institute), is now (1999) also approved [49]. Early work, both by recombinant DNA and classic protein chemistry methods, had shown that factor VIII with its B domain deleted was active in clotting assays [50–52]. Factor VIII SQ was developed from one particular construct, which retained the factor VIII processing protease cleavage sites at amino acids 740 and 1649 with only 14 residues of the B domain still present. This was almost fully processed when expressed in CHO cells, consistent with its retaining a furin cleavage site preceding amino acid 1649 [53]. An advantage of factor VIII SQ, in comparison to the first-generation full-length factor VIII products, is that it is formulated without the addition of human albumin. However, human albumin is still added to the tissue culture medium in which the CHO-expression construct is grown [49]. Thus, these second-generation products have a reduced theoretical risk of transmission of human viruses [49].

Clinical experience with recombinant factors

Recombinant products offer the greatest margin of safety for haemophilic patients and have been recommended for the treatment of all patients. However, they are significantly more expensive and many patients continue to receive plasma-derived products. In addition to offering an increased margin of safety with regard to viral contamination, recombinant products also offer a solution to the problem of the burgeoning demand for coagulation factors which continues to rise steeply. Thus 62 million units of factor VIII were used in the UK in 1981, but by 1998 consumption had increased to 200 million units. This largely reflects the changing pattern of treatment, with patients now being encouraged to treat themselves at home on a prophylactic basis to prevent joint bleeds. The plasma half-life and recovery of the various recombinant factor VIII products are identical to those observed with conventional plasma-derived products and are typically around 14–16 hours. In contrast to many plasma-derived products, none of the recombinant products contain vWF, and thus they are of no use in the treatment of this different congenital haemorrhagic disorder. The plasma half-lives of recombinant factor IX are approximately 18 hours, which are also the same as those observed with plasma-derived factor IX products [37].

Recombinant factor VIIa

Recombinant factor VIIa (Novoseven, Novo Nordisk) has proved very useful in the clinical management of patients with either haemophilia A or B and inhibitory antibodies, as well as those with acquired haemophilia. It by-passes the requirement for either factor VIIIa or IXa because it activates factor X (see Fig. 1). Control of bleeding episodes in patients with inhibitory antibodies is a major clinical challenge. Most of the clinical experience relating to use of recombinant factor VIIa has been gained outside the setting of formal clinical trials, and this has hindered licensing in the United States [54]. The product is extremely expensive and this is likely to hinder widespread use when other products may be just as effective. It is valuable in patients who have high titres of inhibitory antibodies. It is of particular value, however, in the few patients with haemophilia B and inhibitory antibodies, as administration of either plasma-derived or recombinant factor IX in these cases can result in serious anaphylactic reactions [55]. Factor VIIa has a plasma half-life of only approximately two hours, so that frequent bolus injections are required to control bleeding; it is not licensed for continuous intravenous administration. No specific adverse effects have been identified. The excellent safety profile, including lack of allergic reactions, has encouraged some clinicians to employ this product for first-line treatment of bleeds at home [56]. In the past, physicians were often reluctant to undertake elective surgery in haemophiliacs with inhibitors, but such procedures can now be carried out with confidence with factor VIIa [57].

Safety issues

Concerns about recombinant coagulation factor concentrates have focused on three main issues: viral safety, incidence of inhibitor development and problems with laboratory assays. It is somewhat ironic that several currently licensed preparations of recombinant factor VIII actually contain a considerable quantity of human, plasma-derived albumin that is added to the product as a stabilizer. Furthermore, most recombinant products are not subjected to specific virucidal treatment, such as heat treatment, during manufacture. Alternative stabilizers have been developed and clinical trials with these second-generation recombinant factor VIII products are already underway. Recombinant factor IX does not require the addition of albumin as a stabilizer. Bovine proteins are incorporated in growth media used in the manufacture

Table 2. Recombinant factor concentrates

Product and manufacturer	Viral inactivation	Human albumin	Bovine protein
Recombinate (Baxter)	No	Yes	Yes
Kogenate[1] (Bayer)	Yes	No[2]	No
Refacto (Wyeth)	Yes	No[2]	No
BeneFIX (Baxter)	Yes	No	No
Novo Seven (Novo)	No	No	Yes

Footnotes: [1] identical to Helixate (Aventis); [2] although cells are grown in human albumin

of some products (see above). The current status of the various recombinant products is summarized in Table 2.

Concern has also been expressed that the use of highly purified factors might result in a greater incidence of inhibitory antibodies. Unfortunately, it is not possible to give a definitive answer to this important issue, as no prospective, double-blinded clinical studies have been conducted in which the incidence of inhibitor development has been compared in patients receiving recombinant products and those receiving conventional plasma-derived products. Approximately 5% of patients with haemophilia A in the UK are known to have developed inhibitory antibodies (or about 15% if severe patients with a baseline of <2% factor VIII are considered). The first two clinical trials of two different recombinant products in previously untreated patients (PUPs) reported an incidence of inhibitor development of around 20% [58, 59]. Inhibitors appeared after a mean of 9 exposure days in both clinical trials. A more recent study from France with a longer follow-up period reported an inhibitor incidence of 28% in patients receiving recombinant factor VIII, in contrast to an incidence of 9% in a historical control group which received only plasma-derived products [60]. Similar results have been observed in other groups. Most of the cases involved low titre and/or transient inhibitors that disappeared as treatment was continued. It is quite probable that many cases of transient or low-titre inhibitors amongst patients receiving conventional concentrates were simply not identified in the past, and most haematologists do not believe that the incidence of significant inhibitors in patients receiving recombinant products is truly elevated. The median number of exposure days until detection of the inhibitor was 9.5 days (range 5–14 days).

By contrast with recombinant factor VIII, there is no evidence of an increased risk of inhibitor development with the use of recombinant factor IX. In clinical trials, only one of 31 PUPs developed an inhibitor and only one of 56 previously treated patients (PTPs) developed a transient inhibitor. These findings are comparable with the incidence of inhibitors of approximately 1% of historical controls with haemophilia B. The formation of specific antibodies against recombinant factor VIIa has not been identified in subjects with either congenital or acquired haemophilia.

The ability to assay the activity of factor VIII both in actual coagulation factor concentrates and in the plasma of haemophiliac patients after infusion of products is vital for clinical care. Various methods have been developed for the assay of factor VIII, including the one-stage, two-stage and automated chromogenic methods. In general, clinical laboratories tend to prefer the one-stage method, which is both faster and easier to perform, for assay of factor VIII in both concentrates and patient plasma. By contrast, the potency of concentrates is now assigned by the chromogenic method, which is actually based on the two-stage method. Traditionally, human plasma is used as the standard for assays of plasma factor VIII. When plasma levels of factor VIII are assayed after infusion of recombinant factor VIII, recovery is significantly greater when using the chromogenic assay compared to the conventional one-stage assay. Pharmacokinetic evaluation also shows a 25% greater AUC (Area under curve (concentration × time) with the chromogenic method, but half-lives are identical on calculations using either assay method. It has recently been shown that these differences may be resolved by using recombinant concentrate diluted in haemophilic plasma as the laboratory standard. The recovery of recombinant factor IX in patients is slightly lower (on average by about 20%) than that observed with standard, plasma-derived products (see above). This means that a higher dose has to be given to patients to achieve a defined target plasma-level. Marked differences in laboratory assay results have been observed with "Refacto" (B-domainless factor VIII). The potency of this product should be assayed using the chromogenic substrate method, since conventional one-stage assays usually underestimate the real potency.

Summary and prospects

Recombinant factors VIII, IX and VIIa are now available for treatment of haemophilia A & B patients in countries where this newer form of "protein therapy" is affordable. They are safer than plasma-derived factors because they carry no, or minimal, risk of contamination by viruses. Unfortunately, at present, they are more expensive. In the future, gene therapy for haemophiliacs may become available. This subject has certainly been widely discussed as a potential cure for patients and there is considerable current interest in this topic [61]. Good progress has been made with adenoviral and adeno-associated viral vectors and clinical trials are in progress with adeno-associated viral vectors. Thus gene therapy is some way off and may not become available for haemophiliacs for some time.

Acknowledgments
G.G.B. thanks Dr. P. Handford, Dr. E.J. Boswell, Dr. R.J. Kaufman, Dr. J. Edwards, Dr. M. Mikaelsson and Prof. E.G.D. Tuddenham for critical comments.

References

1 Gailani D, Broze GJ (1991) Factor IX activation in a revised model of blood coagulation. *Science* 253: 909–912

2 Larsson SA (1985) Life expectancy of Swedish haemophiliacs 1831–1980. *Brit J Haematol* 59: 593–602

3 Giannelli F, Choo KH, Rees DJG, Boyd Y, Rizza CR, Brownlee GG (1983) Gene deletions in patients with haemophilia B and anti-factor IX antibodies. *Nature* 303: 181–182

4 Schwaab R, Brackmann HH, Meyer C, Seehafer J, Kirchgesser M, Haack A, Olek K, Tuddenham EGD, Oldenburg J (1995) Haemophilia A: mutation type determines risk of inhibitor formation. *Thromb Haemost* 74: 1402–1406

5 Antonarakis SE, Rossiter JP, Young M, Horst J, de Moerloose P, Sommer SS, Ketterling RP, Kazazian HH, Negrier C, Vinciguerra C et al (1995) Factor VIII gene inversions in severe hemophilia A: results of an international consortium study. *Blood* 86: 2206–2212

6 Green PM, Giannelli F, Sommer SS, Poon M-C, Ludwig M, Schwaab R, Reitsma PH, Goossens M, Yoshioka A, Figueiredo MS et al (2000) Haemophilia B: database of point mutations and short additions and deletions-v9.0, www.umds.ac.uk/molgen/haemBdatabase.html

7 Naylor JA, Green PM, Rizza CR, Giannelli F (1993) Analysis of factor VIII messenger RNA reveals defects in every one of 28 haemophilia A patients. *Hum Mol Genet* 2: 11–17

8 Rowley G, Saad S, Giannelli F, Green PM (1995) Ultrarapid mutation detection by multiplex, solid-phase chemical cleavage. *Genomics* 30: 574–582

9 Tuddenham EGD (1994) Flip tip inversion and haemophilia A. *Lancet* 342: 307–308

10 Kemball-Cook G, Tuddenham EGD, Wacey AI (1999) Haemophilia A mutation database, http://europium.mrc.rpms.ac.uk

11 Giannelli F, Green PM, Sommer SS, Poon M-C, Ludwig M, Schwaab R, Reitsma PH, Goossens M, Yoshioka A, Figueiredo MS et al (1998) Haemophilia B: database of point mutations and short additions and deletions: eighth edition. *Nucl Acid Res* 26: 265–268

12 Taylor SAM, Duffin J, Cameron C, Teitel J, Garvey B, Lillicrap DP (1992) Characterization of the original Christmas disease mutation (cysteine 206 → serine): from clinical recognition to molecular pathogenesis. *Thromb Haemost* 67: 63–65

13 Morgan GE, Rowley G, Green PM, Chisholm M, Giannelli F, Brownlee GG (1997) Further evidence for the importance of an androgen response element in the factor IX promoter. *Brit J Haematol* 98: 79–85

14 Biggs R (1967) Thirty years of haemophilia treatment in Oxford. *Brit J Haematol* 13: 452–463

15 Rosendaal FR, Varekamp I, Smit C, Brocker-Vriends AHJT, van Dijck H, Vandenbroucke JP, Hermans J, Suurmeijer TPBM, Briet E (1989) Mortality and causes of death in Dutch haemophiliacs 1972–86. *Brit J Haematol* 71: 71–76

16 Darby SC, Ewart DW, Giangrande PLF, Dolin PJ, Spooner RJD, Rizza CR on behalf of the UKHaemophilia Centre Directors' Organization (1995) Mortality before and after HIV infection in the complete UK population of haemophiliacs. *Nature* 377: 79–82

17 Darby SC, Ewart DW, Giangrande PLF, Spooner RJD, Rizza CR, Dusheiko GM, Lee CA, Ludlam CA, Preston FE, for the UK Haemophilia Centre Directors' Organization (1997) Mortality from liver cancer and liver disease in haemophilic men and boys in UK given blood products contaminated with hepatitis C. *Lancet* 350: 1425–1431

18 Lee CA, Ironside JW, Bell JE, Giangrande PLF, Ludlam CA, Esiri MM, McLaughlin JE (1998) Retrospective neuropathological review of prion disease in UK haemophilic patients. *Thromb Haemost* 80: 909–911

19 Katayama K, Ericsson LH, Enfield DL, Walsh KA, Neurath H, Davie EW, Titani K (1979) Comparison of amino acid sequence of bovine coagulation factor IX (Christmas factor) with that of other vitamin K-dependent plasma proteins. *Proc Natl Acad Sci USA* 76: 4990–4994

20 Proudfoot NJ, Brownlee GG (1974) Sequence at the 3' end of globin mRNA shows homology with immunoglobulin light chain mRNA. *Nature* 252: 359–362

21 Winter G, Fields S, Gait MJ, Brownlee GG (1981) The use of synthetic oligodeoxynucleotide primers in cloning and sequencing segment 8 of influenza virus A/PR/8/34. *Nucl Acid Res* 9: 237–245

22 Fields S, Winter G, Brownlee GG (1981) Structure of the neuraminidase gene in human influenza virus A/PR/8/34. *Nature* 290: 213–217

23 Choo KH, Gould KG, Rees DJG, Brownlee GG (1982) Molecular cloning of the gene for human antihaemophilic factor IX. *Nature* 299: 178–180

24 Wallace RB, Johnson MJ, Hirose T, Miyake T, Kawashima EH, Itakura K (1981) The use of synthetic oligonucleotides as hybridization probes: II. Hybridization of oligonucleotides of mixed sequence to rabbit β-globin DNA. *Nucl Acid Res* 9: 879–898

25 Kurachi K, Davie EW (1982) Isolation and characterization of a cDNA coding for human factor IX. *Proc Natl Acad Sci USA* 79: 6461–6464

26 Jaye M, de la Salle H, Schamber F, Balland A, Kohli V, Findeli A, Tolstoshev P, Lecocq J-P (1983) Isolation of a human anti-haemophilic factor IX cDNA clone using a unique 52-base synthetic oligonucleotide probe derived from the amino acid sequence of bovine factor IX. *Nucl Acid Res* 11: 2325–2335

27 Anson DS, Choo KH, Rees DJG, Giannelli F, Gould K, Huddleston JA, Brownlee GG (1984) Gene structure of human anti-haemophilic factor IX. *EMBO J* 3: 1053–1064

28 Yoshitake S, Schach BG, Foster DC, Davie EW, Kurachi K (1985) Nucleotide sequence of the gene for human factor IX (antihemophilic factor B). *Biochemistry* 24: 3736–3750

29 Bentley AK, Rees DJG, Rizza C, Brownlee GG (1986) Defective propeptide processing of blood clotting factor IX caused by mutation of arginine to glutamine at position-4. *Cell* 45: 343–348

30 Anson DS, Austen DEG, Brownlee GG (1985) Expression of active human clotting factor IX from recombinant DNA clones in mammalian cells. *Nature* 315: 683–685

31 Anson DS, Brownlee GG, Jones IM (1992) Factor IX preparations uncontaminated by plasma components or poxvirus. *US patent no.* 5,171,569

32 Busby S, Kumar A, Joseph M, Halfpap L, Insley M, Berkner K, Kurachi K, Woodbury R (1985) Expression of active human factor IX in transfected cells. *Nature* 316: 271–273

33 de la Salle H, Altenburger W, Elkaim R, Dott K, Dieterle A, Drillien R, Cazenave J-P, Tolstoshev P, Lecocq J-P (1985) Active γ-carboxylated human factor IX expressed using recombinant DNA techniques. *Nature* 316: 268–270

34 Kaufman RJ, Wasley LC, Furie BC, Furie B, Shoemaker CB (1986) Expression, purification and characterization of recombinant γ-carboxylated factor IX synthesized in chinese hamster ovary cells. *J Biol Chem* 261: 9622–9628

35 Rehemtulla A, Roth DA, Wasley LC, Kuliopulos A, Walsh CT, Furie B, Furie BC, Kaufman RJ (1993) *In vitro* and *in vivo* functional characterization of bovine vitamin K-dependent γ-carboxylase expressed in chinese hamster ovary cells. *Proc Natl Acad Sci USA* 90: 4611–4615

36 Wasley LC, Rehemtulla A, Bristol JA, Kaufman RJ (1993) PACE/furin can process the vitamin K-dependent pro-factor IX precursor within the secretory pathway. *J Biol Chem* 268: 8458–8465

37 White GC, Beebe A, Nielsen B (1997) Recombinant factor IX. *Thromb Haemost* 78: 261–265

38 Gillis S, Furie BC, Furie B, Patel H, Huberty MC, Switzer M, Foster WB, Scoble HA, Bond MD (1997) γ-Carboxyglutamic acids 36 and 40 do not contribute to human factor IX function. *Protein Sci* 6: 185–196

39 Brownlee GG, Rizza C (1984) Clotting factor VIII cloned. *Nature* 312: 307

40 Wood WI, Capon DJ, Simonsen CC, Eaton DL, Gitschier J, Keyt B, Seeburg PH, Smith DH, Hollingshead P, Wion KL et al (1984) Expression of active human factor VIII from recombinant DNA clones. *Nature* 312: 330–337

41 Toole JJ, Knopf JL, Wozney JM, Sultzman LA, Buecker JL, Pittman DD, Kaufman RJ, Brown E, Shoemaker C, Orr EC et al (1984) Molecular cloning of a cDNA encoding human antihaemophilic factor. *Nature* 312: 342–347

42 Pipe SW, Morris JA, Shah J, Kaufman R (1998) Differential interaction of coagulation factor VIII and factor V with protein chaperones calnexin and calreticulin. *Proc Natl Acad Sci USA* 273: 8537–8544

43 Kaufman RJ, Wasley LC, Dorner AJ (1988) Synthesis, processing and secretion of recombinant factor VIII expressed in mammalian cells. *J Biol Chem* 263: 6352–6362

44 Kaufman RJ, Wasley LC, Davies MV, Wise RJ, Israel DI, Dorner AJ (1989) Effect of von Willebrand factor coexpression on the synthesis and secretion of factor VIII in chinese hamster ovary cells. *Mol Cell Biol* 9: 1233–1242

45 Kaufman RJ (1992) Expression and structure-function properties of recombinant factor VIII. *Transfus Med Rev* 6: 235–246

46 Gomperts E, Lundblad R, Adamson R (1992) The manufacturing process of recombinant factor VIII, Recombinate. *Transfus Med Rev* 6: 247–251

47 Chan SY, Lembach KJ (1991) Genetic characterization of recombinbant BHK-21 cells expressing factor VIII. *Semin Hematol* 28: 10–16

48 Klein U (1991) Production and characterization of recombinant factor VIII. *Semin Hematol* 28: 17–21
49 Berntop E (1997) Second generation, B-domain deleted recombinant factor VIII. *Thromb Haemost* 78: 256–265
50 Toole JJ, Pittman DD, Orr EC, Murtha P, Wasley LC, Kaufman R (1986) A large region (c 95 kDa) of human factor VIII is dispensable for *in vitro* procoagulant activity. *Proc Natl Acad Sci USA* 83: 5939–5942
51 Andersson L-O, Forsman N, Huang K, Larsen K, Lundin A, Pavlu B, Sandberg H, Sewerin K, Smart J (1986) Isolation and characterization of human factor VIII: Molecular forms in commercial factor VIII concentrate, cryoprecipitate, and plasma. *Proc Natl Acad Sci USA* 83: 2979–2983
52 Eaton DL, Wood WI, Eaton D, Hass PE, Hollingshead P, Wion K, Mather J, Lawn RM, Wehar GA, Gorman C (1986) Construction and characterization of an active factor VIII variant lacking the central one-third of the molecule. *Biochemistry* 25: 8343–8347
53 Lind P, Larsson K, Spira J, Sydow-Backman M, Almstedt A, Gray E, Sandberg H (1995) Novel forms of B-domain-deleted recombinant factor VIII molecules. Construction and biochemical characterization. *Eur J Biochem* 232: 19–27
54 Lusher J, Ingerslev J, Roberts H, Hedner U (1998) Clinical experience with recombinant factor VIIa. *Blood Coagulat Fibrinolys* 9: 119–128
55 Warrier I, Ewenstein BM, Koerper MA, Shapiro A, Key N, Dimichele D, Miller RT, Pasi J, Rivard GE, Sommer SS et al (1996) Factor IX inhibitors and anaphylaxis in haemophilia B. *Haemophilia* 2: 239–260
56 Key NS, Aledort LM, Beardsley D, Cooper HA, Davignon G, Ewenstein BM, Gilchrist GS, Gill JC, Glader B, Hoots WK et al (1998) Home treatment of mild to moderate bleeding episodes using recombinant factor VIIa (Novoseven) in haemophiliacs with inhibitors. *Thromb Haemost* 80: 912–918
57 Shapiro AD, Gilchrist GS, Hoots WK, Cooper HA, Gastineau DA (1998) Prospective, randomised trial of two doses of rVIIa (NovoSeven) in haemophilia patients with inhibitors undergoing surgery. *Thromb Haemost* 80: 773–778
58 Lusher JM, Arkin S, Abildgaard CF, Schwartz RS (1993) Recombinant factor VIII for the treatment of previously untreated patients with haemophilia. *N Engl J Med* 328: 453–459
59 Bray GL, Gomperts ED, Courter S, Gordon EM, Manco-Johnson M, Shapiro A, Scheibel E, White G, Lee M (1994) A multicenter study of recombinant factor VIII (Recombinate): safety, efficacy, and inhibitor risk in previously untreated patients with haemophilia. *Blood* 83: 2428–2435
60 Rothschild C, Laurian Y, Satre EP, Borel Derlon A, Chambost H, Moreau P, Goudemand J (1998) French previously untreated patients with severe haemophilia A after exposure to recombinant factor VIII: incidence of inhibitor and evaluation of immune tolerance. *Thromb Haemost* 80: 779–783

Recombinant Protein Drugs
ed. by P. Buckel

Colony-stimulating factors: altering the practice of oncology

Karl Welte[1] and Erich Platzer[2]

[1] *Kinderklinik der Medizinischen Hochschule, Hannover, Germany*
[2] *Novuspharma, SpA, Monza, Italy*

Introduction

The process of haematopoiesis is regulated by a large number of glycoprotein cytokines which orchestrate the growth and development of haematopoietic cells, from the pluripotent self-renewing stem cell through committed lymphoid and myeloid progenitor and precursor cells to non-replicative, functionally mature blood cells. The control of haematopoiesis and the migration and functional activation of blood cells are closely controlled by stimulatory and inhibitory effects of at least 25 regulatory factors known as haematopoietic growth factors or cytokines.

Some cytokines have a broad spectrum of activity (e.g., interleukin-3), some mainly influence the survival and/or development of primitive, non-lineage-restricted multipotent progenitor cells (e.g., stem cell factor), while others principally promote the growth of cells with a more restricted developmental potential (e.g., granulocyte and granulocyte-macrophage colony-stimulating factors, G-CSF and GM-CSF). G-CSF is lineage-specific for granulocyte precursors, while GM-CSF is less restricted and influences the proliferation and differentiation of erythroid, megakaryocytic and myeloid lineage progenitor cells (Fig. 1).

The role of recombinant G-CSF and GM-CSF

Several glycoprotein cytokines have been isolated, biochemically characterized and are produced by recombinant DNA techniques in quantities sufficient for clinical use. Recombinant forms of G-CSF and GM-CSF are used in various clinical applications. The most commonly available recombinant G-CSFs are filgrastim and lenograstim. Filgrastim is expressed in *E. coli* and differs from the naturally occurring molecule by the addition of an N-terminal methionine and the absence of glycosylation. Lenograstim is expressed in mammalian (Chinese hamster ovary) cells and is glycosylated. GM-CSF is

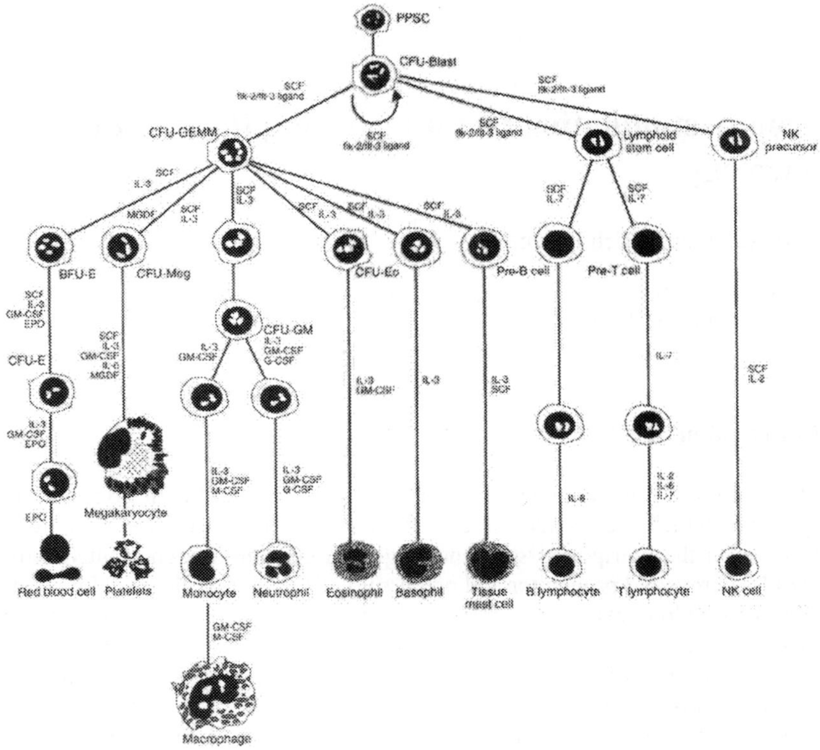

Figure 1. Haematopoiesis

available in Europe as molgramostim, a non-glycosylated product expressed in *E. coli*, and in the USA as sargramostim, a yeast-derived glycosylated protein that differs from the native molecule by a single amino acid substitution. The physiological and clinical relevance of different patterns of glycosylation and other minor differences between the recombinant proteins and their endogenous counterparts is unknown [1].

It is likely that G-CSF is involved in the response to neutropenia and bacterial infection. Normal plasma levels of G-CSF in healthy individuals are below the limit of detection (<10 pg/mL). An inverse relationship between G-CSF levels and neutrophil numbers has been demonstrated in patients with cyclic neutropenia, while levels are as high as 1000 to 100,000 pg/mL in patients with bacteraemia and febrile neutropenia. G-CSF knockout mice exhibited a 70–80% reduction in circulating neutrophil numbers, a major reduction in bone marrow neutrophils and an impaired ability to mobilize neutrophils. The ability to counter infection was impaired and was regained only with injection of recombinant G-CSF [2]. The knockout mice also showed decreased macrophage/monocyte progenitor cells and reduced circulating monocyte numbers, suggesting an influence of G-CSF on these cells as well.

Administration of recombinant G-CSF causes a transient leukopenia within minutes, followed by a sustained and dose-dependent increase in circulating neutrophils that is sustained during daily administration. There is an increased input of precursor cells into the myeloblast compartment, an increase in neutrophil production rate and a shortening of time required for neutrophil precursors to mature and appear in the circulation, from approximately 5 days to 1 day (Tab. 1). The increase in circulating neutrophils during treatment with recombinant G-CSF can be accounted for by the accelerated release from the bone marrow and extra amplification divisions in the post-progenitor compartments, thus placing little 'stress' in terms of increased proliferation of more primitive marrow cells [6].

Table 1. Effects *in vivo* of recombinant G-CSF and GM-CSF on neutrophil production [3–5]

	GM-CSF	G-CSF
Fold increase in neutrophil production rate	9.4	1.5
Emergence time of radiolabelled neutrophils		
In peripheral blood	1 day	normal (5 days)
Half-life in blood	normal (8 h)	48 h

GM-CSF is a multilineage factor that mainly induces proliferation of granulocyte, macrophage, and mixed granulocyte-macrophage colonies of bone marrow cells. GM-CSF is also involved in the proliferation of the megakaryocytic and erythroid progenitors, although other factors are required for maturation of these lineages [7]. GM-CSF-deficient mice have relatively normal levels of haematopoietic cells in marrow, spleen and blood, but develop pulmonary problems consistent with abnormally functioning alveolar macrophages [8]. GM-CSF increases neutrophil numbers in humans but the increase is less marked and slower than that observed with G-CSF [9]. GM-CSF, unlike G-CSF, does not reduce neutrophil maturation time and thus does not result in earlier release of mature neutrophils, but it does extend circulating neutrophil half-life [1].

GM-CSF is generally undetectable in the serum and appears under normal physiological conditions to act locally at inflammatory sites. GM-CSF increases neutrophil motility at low concentrations and inhibits neutrophil migration at high concentrations, possibly to immobilize these cells at sites of infection [10, 11]. Neutrophil respiratory burst, adherence, phagocytosis and bacterial killing are enhanced *in vivo* after therapy with either G-CSF or GM-CSF [5]. Neutrophils induced by G-CSF and GM-CSF treatment (in patients not suffering from primary defects in neutrophil function) show grossly normal functional abilities [5].

The broader activity of GM-CSF appears to confer an immunomodulatory role in enhancing antigen processing and presentation by monocytes. Administration of GM-CSF to patients with malignancies results in induction of MHC class II expression on monocytes, which is necessary for presentation of antigen to T-helper lymphocytes [12]. GM-CSF is involved in the development of dendritic cells from progenitor cells and from peripheral blood monocytes, although CD40 ligand rather than GM-CSF appears to be the most important factor in this process [13, 14]. Dendritic cells are the most efficient antigen-presenting cells and can promote antitumour immunity via the induction of a T-lymphocyte cytotoxic response. GM-CSF has a potential role as a vaccine adjuvant [15] and in the development of dendritic cell preparations for immunotherapy [16].

Both G-CSF and GM-CSF mobilize transplantable haematopoietic progenitor cells from the bone marrow to the bloodstream, an effect which was not expected from *in vitro* studies. Long-term reconstituting cells are present in the circulation but only at a low concentration. Levels increase in response to chemotherapy or G-CSF or GM-CSF therapy. Animal studies show that following transplantation, long-term regeneration occurs through proliferation and differentiation of donor stem cells rather than recovery of host stem cells [17]. Recombinant G-CSF is now used routinely to mobilize peripheral blood progenitor cells (PBPC) and to augment the mobilizing effects of chemotherapy. While it is not known with certainty if stem cells with significant long-term reconstituting potential are present in the mobilized PBPC product, the numbers of haematopoietic progenitor cells expressing the membrane antigen CD34 have been shown to correlate well with early neutrophil and platelet engraftment and with the incidence of CFC-GM in PBPC populations [18]. $CD34^+$ cell numbers are commonly used as a measure of the likelihood of successful engraftment. The mechanism for progenitor cell mobilization by G-CSF and GM-CSF is not established, but may involve interference with the activity of extracellular adhesion molecules and/or their receptors involved in the adhesion of $CD34^+$ cells to marrow stromal elements [6].

Clinical applications of G-CSF and GM-CSF

Chemotherapy support

Myelosuppression is one of the most common dose-limiting toxicities of cytotoxic drugs used at standard curative doses in the treatment of malignancies. While the resulting neutropenia may not in itself be life-threatening, the risk of infection is closely related to the depth and duration of neutropenia [19, 20]. Neutropenic infection requires hospitalization and treatment with broad-spectrum i.v. antibiotics and is associated with significant morbidity and mortality rates as high as 20%. Another important consequence of neutropenia is the need to reduce chemotherapy doses or to delay treatment until blood counts have recovered, leading to a decrease in dose intensity and a potential adverse effect on survival outcome [21].

The use of CSFs to reduce chemotherapy-induced toxicity can be divided into primary prophylaxis (given before the occurrence of neutropenia) and secondary prophylaxis (given in subsequent chemotherapy cycles after the occurrence of prolonged neutropenia or febrile neutropenia in an earlier cycle). They may also be used in the treatment of established febrile neutropenia, although efficacy appears to be less marked than with prophylactic use [22].

Given as primary prophylaxis, treatment with G-CSF after cycles of chemotherapy has been shown to shorten the incidence and duration of severe neutropenia, with improvements in associated clinical endpoints such as incidence of infection, duration of hospitalization and requirement for i.v. antibiotics in patients with solid tumours and haematological malignancies [23–26]. It allows chemotherapy to be delivered at or close to the planned dose intensity [24, 25]. In a study in children with acute lymphoblastic leukaemia, filgrastim reduced the incidence of febrile neutropenia and improved adherence to the tight time-frame of the curative chemotherapy protocol [27]. In one double-blind trial, filgrastim was given in an open-label fashion as secondary prophylaxis to placebo patients who had experienced febrile neutropenia. In these patients, the rate of febrile neutropenia decreased to 23% in cycle 2, and the duration of grade 4 neutropenia was reduced from 6 days to 3 days [23]. While the data supporting the use of secondary prophylaxis are limited, the approach appears to reduce toxicity while allowing the planned dose intensity of chemotherapy to be maintained [28, 29].

Thus far, studies have not been conducted with the aim of demonstrating that the use of G-CSF to support delivery of planned dose intensity translates into a long-term survival advantage, although small studies suggest a benefit [30–33].

In some patients, CSFs may not be needed, even with chemotherapy regimens that are associated with a moderately high incidence of febrile neutropenia [34, 35]. Conversely, certain patients may be at an intrinsically higher risk of neutropenic complications even with chemotherapy regimens associated with a lower incidence of complications and would benefit from G-CSF prophylaxis. A means to identify patients who are at highest risk of severe neutropenia and dose reduction or treatment delay would be a helpful clinical algorithm. One such model identified the first-cycle absolute neutrophil count (ANC) nadir as a significant predictor of the risk of dose reduction or treatment delay in patients with early breast cancer and calculated that using G-CSF support in the 50% of patients at highest risk of neutropenic complications would be an acceptably cost-effective way of sustaining chemotherapy dose intensity [36, 37].

The use of GM-CSF following myelosuppressive chemotherapy has also been reported to reduce neutropenia, infection and hospital stay [38, 39]. Comparative studies of the effect of G-CSF and GM-CSF on chemotherapy-induced neutropenia generally indicate superiority of G-CSF in terms of efficacy and safety [40–42]. For these reasons, G-CSF predominates as the

Table 2. Comparison of indications

	Filgrastim	Lenograstim	Sargramostim (USA)	Molgramostim (Europe)
Haematological support post-cytotoxic chemotherapy	Yes including AML (excludes CML, MDS)	Yes (excludes myeloid malignancies)	In AML patients aged >55 years	Yes (excludes myeloid malignancies
Post-BMT	Yes	Yes	AutoBMT in NHL, ALL, HD; alloBMT from HLA-matched donors	Autologous or syngeneic BMT
PBPC mobilization (autologous)	Yes	Yes	Yes	Not indicated
PBPC mobilization (allogeneic)	Pending	Yes	Not indicated	Not indicated
Severe congenital, cyclic or idiopathic neutropenia (long term)	Yes	Not indicated	Not indicated	Not indicated
BMT engraftment delay/failure	Not indicated	Not indicated	Yes	Not indicated
HIV/AIDS-related neutropenia	Some countries only	Not indicated	Not indicated	Ganciclovir-induced neutropenia in AIDS-related CMV retinitis

BMT bone marrow transplantation; PBPC peripheral blood progenitor cells. NHL non-Hodgkin's lymphoma; ALL acute lymphoblastic leukaemia; HD Hodgkin's disease.

haematopoietic growth factor used to reduce neutropenia-related complications associated with myelosuppressive chemotherapy.

Filgrastim (G-CSF) and sargramostim (GM-CSF) are also used after chemotherapy in patients with acute myeloid leukaemia (AML). In a large double-blind, placebo-controlled study of AML patients aged 55 or older, filgrastim accelerated neutrophil recovery following induction chemotherapy, and patients had significantly fewer days with fever or on antibiotics [43]. In another large study [26], filgrastim significantly reduced the duration of neutropenia and improved infection-related endpoints after induction and consolidation chemotherapy, as well as reducing the duration of hospitalization. In older patients, sargramostim produced a faster neutrophil recovery following induction chemotherapy, with reduced incidences of infections and fatal pneumonia and fewer induction therapy-related deaths [44]. Two studies of the use of molgramostim in elderly AML patients after induction chemotherapy found faster neutrophil recovery but no evidence of clinical benefit [45, 46]. Another study found no effect on neutropenia and a prolonged duration of thrombocytopenia [47]. Molgramostim is contraindicated in myeloid malignancies. Concerns that the use of growth factors will have an adverse effect on leukaemic cell proliferation due to stimulation of cytokine receptors on these cells appear generally unfounded [48] and there does not appear to be any adverse effect on response rates [26].

The growth factors are used extensively in the clinical evaluation of dose-escalated chemotherapy regimens in attempts to explore the upper reaches of the chemotherapy dose-response curve and improve survival, although none is formally approved for such use at present, and in some tumour types the benefits of dose-intensification have not been clearly established. The rationale for using growth factor support in this application was illustrated in a recent study of patients with advanced Hodgkin's disease, where the use of filgrastim enabled moderate dose escalation of the chemotherapy regimen without increasing the incidence of febrile neutropenia over that observed with the same regimen at baseline dosages [49].

Bone marrow transplantation (BMT)

The myeloablative, high-dose chemotherapy used in conjunction with BMT is followed inevitably by a period of bone marrow aplasia. The administration of G-CSF in the post-BMT period has been shown to accelerate neutrophil recovery and to improve associated clinical endpoints [50, 51]. A reduction in post-BMT morbidity has also been reported with the use of GM-CSF [52, 53].

In comparative terms, G-CSF may produce more rapid neutrophil and platelet engraftment post-BMT [54, 55], with associated improvements in fever and hospitalization [56]. The GM-CSF sargramostim is also approved in the setting of BMT graft failure or delay, which is defined in terms of low ANC with or without infection.

PBPC transplantation

Sheridan [57] was the first to report the superiority in terms of accelerated haematopoietic recovery when filgrastim-mobilized PBPC were reinfused with autologous bone marrow after high-dose chemotherapy, compared with the use of bone marrow alone. Schmitz [58] reported a randomized comparison of filgrastim-mobilized PBPC and autologous BMT in lymphoma patients treated with high-dose chemotherapy, and showed significant reductions in time to platelet recovery, requirement for platelet transfusions, neutrophil recovery, fewer red blood cell transfusions and less time in hospital. A subsequent economic analysis of this study showed significant cost savings [59], mostly due to lower costs of autograft collection, shorter hospital stay and less need for supportive care in patients receiving PBPC.

Comparative studies in healthy volunteers have shown G-CSF to be more effective than GM-CSF in numbers of $CD34^+$ cells mobilized [60, 61]. In women with breast cancer receiving high-dose chemotherapy and autologous PBPC, factors predictive of more rapid neutrophil engraftment included mobilization with G-CSF or cyclophosphamide/G-CSF (*versus* mobilization with GM-CSF or no mobilization) [62]. In a recent review of published studies, it was stated that haematological recovery following transplant of G-CSF-mobilized PBPC was faster than following GM-CSF mobilization, but that the difference disappeared when chemotherapy was included in the mobilization regimen [63]. A study comparing the two CSFs in a mobilization regimen in conjunction with chemotherapy found no differences in $CD34^+$ cell yield or in engraftment [64]. In a study comparing G-CSF and GM-CSF with high-dose cyclophosphamide for PBPC mobilization in multiple myeloma patients, both mobilization regimens were effective [65], although the use of GM-CSF resulted in delayed haematopoietic recovery and an increased complication rate. While GM-CSF is an effective mobilizing agent, moderate bone pain and low-grade fever mean that some patients are less likely to tolerate it in this setting [40].

Studies have also explored the potential synergy between CSFs. In one study, the addition of G-CSF to GM-CSF increased mobilization (CFU-GM, BFU-E) compared with either agent alone and with the reverse sequence [66]. The combination of G-CSF and GM-CSF *versus* G-CSF alone as part of a regimen containing low-dose cyclophosphamide has been reported to have advantages for $CD34^+$ cell mobilization over G-CSF plus chemotherapy [67]. However, Spitzer et al. [68] found no difference in mobilization (mononuclear cells, $CD34^+$ cells) and questionable clinical benefit with G-CSF + GM-CSF *versus* G-CSF alone.

Studies in patients comparing the mobilization efficacy of the two available forms of recombinant G-CSF, filgrastim and lenograstim, show no significant differences between the two forms [69, 70].

G-CSF may also be used for mobilizing PBPC in healthy donors for use in allogeneic transplantation, based on studies of mobilization efficacy in healthy volunteers [71]. In a multicentre EBMT study of allogeneic transplantation, filgrastim-mobilized PBPC provided comparable engraftment to BMT with earlier platelet recovery, while filgrastim administration and leukapheresis in normal donors were feasible and well tolerated [72].

Severe chronic neutropenia

Severe chronic neutropenia (SCN) describes a group of rare conditions, including congenital neutropenia, cyclic neutropenia and idiopathic neutropenia, characterized by an ANC of $<0.5 \times 10^9$/L. Patients suffer repeated episodes of fever, oropharyngeal inflammation, gastrointestinal symptoms, perirectal inflammation and cutaneous infections. Deep tissue infections and bacteraemias may occur. Since other host defence mechanisms remain intact in the absence of immunosuppressive drugs or prolonged antibiotics, chronic viral infections or infections with intracellular pathogens rarely occur.

Before the use of filgrastim (G-CSF) as a treatment for SCN, there was no reliably effective treatment for this condition. Filgrastim remains the only recombinant growth factor indicated for use in this condition (Tab. 2). Phase III studies showed restoration of ANC levels to $>1.5 \times 10^9$/L in most patients, along with a significant improvement in clinical endpoints (incidence of infection, fever, oropharyngeal ulcers and antibiotic use) with the daily filgrastim dose titrated to response [73]. Following approval of filgrastim for long-term therapy of SCN, the Severe Chronic Neutropenia International Registry was set up to monitor the clinical course, treatment and complications of patients with SCN, including those receiving filgrastim treatment. Registry data [74] show that the dose and schedule of filgrastim required to restore a normal ANC are variable, and the dose required is generally lower in idiopathic or cyclic neutropenia (median doses of 1.0 and 1.7 µg/kg/day, respectively) than in patients with congenital neutropenia (median 5.6 µg/kg/day). These doses can be used as starting doses, and titrated up or down at 1- or 2-week intervals according to response. With prolonged use, the benefits of filgrastim use appear to be sustained. The development of antibodies to filgrastim has not been observed. On beginning treatment, patients often experience bone pain, headache and musculoskeletal symptoms that are attributable to expansion of the haematopoietic tissues; these are usually controllable with mild analgesics and decline with continued therapy. Patients with congenital neutropenia (but not cyclic or idiopathic neutropenia) may develop myelodysplastic changes with chromosomal abnormalities (most frequently monosomy 7) and AML, although the association with filgrastim treatment is not well established. It is possible that in a subgroup of patients point mutations in the cytoplasmic region of the G-CSF receptor are involved in leukaemogenesis [75]. The overall risk is estimated to be less than 2% per year of observation on treatment. Patients showing such changes would be recommended for BMT.

Potential future indications

Some of the areas in which G-CSF and GM-CSF are being evaluated are described below. The list of possible applications will doubtless expand with continued research into areas in which their different activities can be exploited, either alone or in combination with other cytokines or therapies, e.g., the use of cytokine 'cocktails' for *ex vivo* expansion of haematopoietic progenitor cells [76]. In addition, new formulations of existing CSFs, for example with pegylation of filgrastim to produce a sustained duration of effect [77], may offer new therapeutic opportunities.

Neutropenia associated with HIV infection and AIDS

Anaemia, neutropenia and thrombocytopenia can present significant clinical problems in the treatment of HIV and AIDS. G-CSF and GM-CSF are effective in the treatment of AIDS-related neutropenia, which may occur as a result of the disease (defective neutrophil function) or the therapy (myelotoxic effects of antiretroviral agents and chemotherapy for secondary malignancies). Both agents have limited indications for HIV-infected patients. GM-CSF and G-CSF have been shown to increase neutrophil counts in patients with AIDS-related bone marrow failure and those receiving zidovudine, interferon α, or ganciclovir, and have been used to optimize the delivery of antiretroviral and prophylactic therapy [78].

G-CSF and GM-CSF have been reported to increase *in vitro* bactericidal activity of neutrophils from AIDS patients [79]. GM-CSF may have an additional activity in stimulating monocyte activity [80] but no reduction in incidence of opportunistic infections was observed in a study of patients with HIV-related leukopenia [81]. The CSFs may have a role in the treatment of HIV-associated neutropenia and defects in neutrophil function, while their use in the adjunctive treatment of specific HIV-related opportunistic infections continues to be explored [82]. G-CSF appears to be better tolerated than GM-CSF [83]. The effect of GM-CSF on viral activity is unclear. Human macrophages are the major target for HIV-1 and GM-CSF has been reported to increase HIV-1 entry and replication [84, 85], an effect which may not occur in the presence of retroviral therapy [83]. With no direct effect on monocytes/macrophages, G-CSF is unlikely to affect HIV replication.

Aplastic anaemia

Aplastic anaemia is characterized by bone marrow failure, possibly due to an intrinsic defect of haematopoietic stem cells. It does not appear to be related to defects in G-CSF or GM-CSF, since both these factors are present in elevated levels, though reduced levels of stem cell factor have been reported [86].

In vitro studies with a range of cytokines showed the strongest effect for G-CSF on clonogenic potential of $CD34^+$ cells [87]. The European Group for Blood and Marrow Transplantation (EBMT) Working Party on Severe Aplastic Anaemia conducted a pilot study of G-CSF with combined immunosuppressive therapy and observed trilineage haematopoietic reconstitution in 33 of 40 patients, and 92% survival at 2 years [88]. Mobilization of progenitor cells in some patients raises the possibility that transplantation will be a treatment option.

Severe autoimmune diseases

PBPC transplantation is also under exploration as a possible option for treating patients with severe autoimmune diseases, following the observation of coincidental improvements in the condition in patients undergoing transplantation for haematological malignancies. A joint committee of the EBMT/European League Against Rheumatism is assessing the feasibility of this approach in patients with systemic sclerosis, systemic lupus erythematosus, rheumatoid arthritis, juvenile chronic arthritis and multiple sclerosis. G-CSF with or without cyclophosphamide is usually used as the mobilizing regimen [89]. In a randomized study in patients with rheumatoid arthritis, G-CSF at a dose of 10 μg/kg/day permitted adequate PBPC mobilization in one leukapheresis without inducing an unacceptable incidence of flare-ups of underlying disease symptoms [90].

Cancer immunotherapy

The potential of GM-CSF as a vaccine adjuvant was explored in a phase I trial in 16 patients with dermal metastases. Significant inflammatory responses were seen at the skin and tumour injection sites, with increases in macrophages and dendritic cells. However, no elevation of T-cell activity was seen [91]. An immunotherapeutic role for GM-CSF was further illustrated by the observation that GM-CSF (but not G-CSF, IL-3 or stem cell factor) could enhance the cytotoxicity of peripheral blood mononuclear cells *in vitro* [92]. GM-CSF may have a synergistic effect with IL-2 in generating lymphokine-activated killer (LAK) cell activity [93]. *In vitro* incubation of PBPC with IL-2 and GM-CSF generated higher LAK cell activity than with IL-2 alone, and reinfusion of T-cell-derived LAK cells with *in vivo* administration of IL-2 and GM-CSF produced a dramatic increase in LAK activity in peripheral blood, suggesting a possible role in control of minimal residual disease [94].

Granulocyte transfusions

The use of granulocyte transfusions as an approach to the prevention and treatment of infections in neutropenic patients has attracted renewed interest with the availability of CSFs as a means to mobilize and collect adequate numbers of neutrophils. Filgrastim with or without a corticosteroid to improve pre-apheresis neutrophil levels has been found to provide high numbers of neutrophils with normal functional properties for transfusion therapy. Significant and sustained increases in ANC were observed when granulocytes were transfused to HLA-matched allogeneic BMT recipients [95–97]. Supplemental platelet support can arise as a result of platelet contamination of the apheresis product. Further studies of granulocyte transfusions in allogeneic and autologous transplant patients are under way.

Safety

G-CSF is well tolerated by the majority of patients; bone pain appears to be the most frequent adverse effect of therapy and is generally controlled with a mild analgesic. The broader functional activity of GM-CSF increases its potential to cause side-effects through release of pro-inflammatory cytokines [1, 98]. Although GM-CSF causes a number of adverse effects, including lethargy, myalgia, bone pain, anorexia, weight change, skin eruptions and flushing, these are generally tolerable. Erythematous lesions at the site of injection may occur. More problematical with GM-CSF are fever and chills which may be indistinguishable from fever due to infection, leading to potential overuse of i.v. antibiotics. With molgramostim, a 'first-dose' syndrome of flushing, tachycardia, hypotension, musculoskeletal pain, dyspnoea, nausea, rigours and leg spasms has been noted in 30–60% of patients, particularly with i.v. administration and in lung cancer patients [99]. Antibodies to recombinant GM-CSF have been reported occasionally, but not to G-CSF [100].

Summary and conclusions

The development of the colony-stimulating factors in the early 1990s altered the practice of oncology by permitting cytotoxic chemotherapy to be administered at doses and schedules that were previously limited by severe neutropenia and associated complications. The subsequent development of their use for the mobilization of PBPC for transplantation was an equally important therapeutic advance by providing an alternative to bone marrow as the source of stem cells for haematological support, conferring clinical benefits and savings in resources and costs. G-CSF (filgrastim) has also provided an effective treatment for the group of diseases of severe chronic neutropenia, for which no effective therapy was previously available. Their efficacy in surmounting neutropenia and mobilizing progenitor cells has also been exploited in different disease areas, for example HIV-associated neutropenia and PBPC transplantation for autoimmune diseases, while the immunomodulatory effects of GM-CSF continue to be elucidated for potential applications in disparate fields such as cancer vaccines and boosting influenza vaccinations. The colony-stimulating factors have also facilitated research into new areas such as *ex vivo* expansion of haematopoietic cells, where retroviral gene transfer studies will continue to advance our understanding of the processes of haematopoiesis and engraftment. The clinical roles for these useful agents will expand with the development of new formulations and the addition of recombinant forms of more haematopoietic growth factors and cytokines to provide further tools to manipulate the complex process of haematopoiesis.

References

1 Lieschke GJ, Burgess AW (1992) Granulocyte colony-stimulating factor and granulocyte-macrophage colony-stimulating factor. *N Engl J Med* 327: 28–35

2 Lieschke GJ, Grail D, Hodgson G, Metcalf D, Stanley E, Cheers C, Fowler KJ, Basu S, Zhan YF, Dunn AR (1994) Mice lacking granulocyte colony-stimulating factor have chronic neutropenia, granulocyte and macrophage progenitor cell deficiency, and impaired neutrophil mobilization. *Blood* 73: 117–122

3 Lord BI, Bronchud MH, Owens S, Chang J, howell A, Souza L, Dexter TM (1989) The kinetics of human granulopoiesis following treatment with granulocyte colony-stimulating factor *in vivo*. *Proc Natl Acad Sci USA* 86: 9499–9503

4 Lord BI, Gurney H, Chang J, Thatcher N, Crowther D, Dexter TM (1992) Haemopoietic cell kinetics in humans treated with rGM-CSF. *Int J Cancer* 50: 26–31

5 Spiekermann K, Roesler J, Emmendoerffer A, Elsner J, Welte K (1997) Functional features of neutrophils induced by G-CSF and GM-CSF treatment: differential effects and clinical implications. *Leukemia* 11: 466–478

6 Molineux G, Dexter TM (1998) Biology of G-CSF. *In*: G Morstyn, TM Dexter, M Foote (eds): *Filgrastim (r-metHuG-CSF) in clinical practice*. Marcel Dekker, New York, Basel, Hong Kong, 1–39

7 Metcalf D (1986) The molecular biology and functions of the granulocyte-macrophage colony-stimulating factors. *Blood* 67: 257–267

8 Stanley E, Lieschke GJ, Grail D, Metcalf D, Hodgson G, Gall JA, Maher DW, Cebon J, Sinickas V, Dunn AR (1994) Granulocyte/macrophage colony-stimulating factor-deficient mice show no major perturbation of hematopoiesis but develop a characteristic pulmonary pathology. *Proc Natl Acad Sci USA* 91: 5592–5596

9 Morstyn G, Lieschke GJ, Sheridan W, Layton J, Cebon J (1989) Pharmacology of the colony-stimulating factors. *Trends Pharmacol* 10: 154–159

10 Weisbart RH, Kwan L, Goldie DW, Gasson JC (1987) Human GM-CSF primes neutrophils for enhanced oxidative metabolism in response to the major physiological chemoattractants. *Blood* 69: 18–21

11 Wang JM, Colella S, Allavena P, Mantovani A (1987) Chemotactic activity of human recombinant granulocyte-macrophage colony-stimulating factor. *Immunology* 138: 439–444

12 Aman MJ, Stockdreher K, Thews A, Kienast K, Aulitzky WE, Farber L, Haus U, Koci B, Huber C, Peschel C (1996) Regulation of immunomodulatory functions by granulocyte-macrophage colony-stimulating factor and granulocyte colony-stimulating factor *in vivo*. *Ann Hematol* 73: 231–238

13 Brossart P, Grünebach F, Stuhler G, Reichardt VL, Mohle R, Kanz L, Brugger W (1998) Generation of functional human dendritic cells from adherent peripheral blood monocytes by CD40 ligation in the absence of granulocyte-macrophage colony-stimulating factor. *Blood* 11: 4238–4247

14 Labeur MS, Roters B, Pers B, Mehling A, Luger TA, Schwarz T, Grabbe S (1999) Generation of tumor immunity by bone marrow-derived dendritic cells correlates with dendritic cell maturation stage. *J Immunol* 162: 168–175

15 Dunussi-Joannopoulos K, Dranoff G, Weinstein HJ, Ferrara JLM, Bierer BE, Croop JM (1998) Gene immunotherapy in murine acute myeloid leukemia: granulocyte-macrophage colony-stimulating factor tumor cell vaccines elicit more potent antitumor immunity compared with B7 family and other cytokine vaccines. *Blood* 91: 222–230

16 Nestle FO, Alijagic S, Gilliet M, Sun Y, Grabbe S, Dummer R, Burg G, Schadendorf D (1998) Vaccination of melanoma patients with peptide- or tumor lysate-pulsed dendritic cells. *Nat Med* 4: 328–332

17 Molineux G, Pojda Z, Hampson IN, Lord BI, Dexter TM (1990) Transplantation potential of peripheral blood stem cells induced by granulocyte colony-stimulating factor. *Blood* 76: 2153–2158

18 Kiss JE, Rybka WB, Winklestein A, de Magalhoes Silverman M, Lister J, D'Andrea P, Ball ED (1997) Relationship of CD34+ cell dose to early and late hematopoiesis following autologous peripheral blood stem cell transplantation. *Bone Marrow Transplant* 19: 303–310

19 Bodey GP, Buckley M, Sathe YS, Freireich EJ (1966) Quantitative relationships between circulating leukocytes and infection in patients with acute leukemia. *Ann Intern Med* 64: 328–340

20 Pizzo PA (1993) Management of fever in patients with cancer and treatement-induced neutropenia. *N Engl J Med* 328: 1323–1332

21 DeVita VT Jr, (1997) Principles of cancer management: chemotherapy. *In*: VT Devita Jr, S Hellman, SA Rosenberg (eds): *Cancer: principles and practice of oncology.* Lippincott-Raven, Philadelphia 333–347

22 ASCO (1994) Recommendations for the use of hematopoietic colony-stimulating factors: evidence-based, clinical practice guidelines. *J Clin Oncol* 12: 2471–2508

23 Crawford J, Ozer H, Stoller R, Johnson D, Lyman G, Tabbara I, Kris M, Grous J, Picozzi V, Rausch G et al (1991) Reduction by granulocyte colony-stimulating factor of fever and neutropenia induced by chemotherapy in patients with small-cell lung cancer. *N Engl J Med* 325: 164–170

24 Trillet-Lenoir V, Green J, Manegold C, Von Pawel J, Gatzemeier U, Lebeau B, Depierre A, Johnson P, Decoster G, Tomita D et al (1993) Recombinant granulocyte colony stimulating factor reduces the infectious complications of cytotoxic chemotherapy. *Eur J Cancer* 29A: 319–324

25 Pettengell R, Gurney H, Radford JA, Deakin DP, James R, Wilkinson PM, Kane K, Bentley J, Crowther D (1992) Granulocyte colony-stimulating factor to prevent dose-limiting neutropenia in non-Hodgkin's lymphoma: a randomized controlled trial. *Blood* 80: 1430–1436

26 Heil G, Hoelzer D, Sanz MA, Lechner K, Liu Yin JA, Papa G, Noens L, Szer J, Ganser A, O'Brien C et al (1997) A randomized, double-blind, placebo-controlled, phase III study of filgrastim in remission induction and consolidation therapy for adults with *de novo* acute myeloid leukemia. *Blood* 90: 4710–4718

27 Welte K, Reiter A, Mempel K, Pfetsch M, Schwab G, Schrappe M, Riehm H (1996) A randomized phase-III study of the efficacy of granulocyte colony-stimulating factor in children with high-risk acute lymphoblastic leukemia. *Blood* 87: 3143–3150

28 de Graaf H, Willemse PHB, Bong SB (1996) Dose intensity of standard adjuvant CMF with granulocyte colony-stimulating factor for premenopausal patients with node-positive breast cancer. *Oncology* 53: 289–294

29 Ribas A, Albanell J, Bellmunt J, Solé-Calvo L-A, Bermejo B, Gallardo E, Vidal R, Vera R, Eres N, Carulla J et al (1996) Five-day course of granulocyte colony-stimulating factor in patients with prolonged neutropenia after adjuvant chemotherapy for breast cancer is a safe and cost-effective schedule to maintain dose-intensity. *J Clin Oncol* 14: 1573–1580

30 Michon JM, Hartmann O, Bouffet E, Meresse V, Coze C, Rubie H, Bordigoni P, Cattiaux E, Ward N, Bernard JL et al (1998) An open-label, multicentre, randomised phase 2 study of recombinant human granulocyte colony-stimulating factor (filgrastim) as an adjunct to combination chemotherapy in paediatric patients with metastatic neuroblastoma. *Eur J Cancer* 34: 1063–1069

31 Fukuoka M, Masuda N, Negoro S (1997) CODE chemotherapy with and without granulocyte colony-stimulating factor in small-cell lung cancer. *Brit J Cancer* 75: 307–309

32 Splinter TA, Kranse R (1996) Randomized trial of chemotherapy +/– G-CSF without dose-intensification in small cell lung cancer (SCLC): improved survival in the G-CSF arm. *Proc Am Soc Clin Oncol* 15: A993

33 Woll P, Hodgetts JLomax L, Bildet F, Cour-Chabernaud V, Thatcher N (1995) Can cytotoxic dose-

intensity be increased by using granulocyte colony-stimulating factor? A randomized controlled trial of lenograstim in small cell lung cancer. *J Clin Oncol* 13: 652–659

34 Hartmann LC, Tschetter LK, Habermann TM, Ebbert LP, Johnson PS, Mailliard JA, Levitt R, Suman VJ, Witzig TE, Wieand HS et al ([redacted]) Granulocyte colony-stimulating factor in severe chemotherapy-induced afebrile neutropenia. *N Engl J Med* 336: 1776–1780

35 Hoelzer D (1997) Hematopoietic growth factors – not whether, but when and where. *N Engl J Med* 336: 1822–1824

36 Silber JH, Fridman M, DiPaola RS, Haim Erder M, Pauly MV, Fox KR (1998) First cycle blood counts and subsequent neutropenia, dose reduction or delay in early stage breast cancer therapy. *J Clin Oncol* 16: 2392–2400

37 Silber JH, Fridman M, Shpilsky A, Even-Shoshan O, Smink DS, Jayaraman J, Fox KR, Pauly MV (1998) Modelling the cost effectiveness of granulocyte colony-stimulating factor use in early stage breast cancer. *J Clin Oncol* 16: 2435–2444

38 Gerhartz HH, Engelhard M, Meusers P, Brittinger G, Wilmanns W, Schlimok G, Mueller P, Huhn D, Musch R, Siegert W et al (1993) Randomized, double-blind, placebo-controlled, phase III study of recombinant human granulocyte-macrophage colony-stimulating factor as adjunct to induction treatment of high-grade malignant non-Hodgkin's lymphomas. *Blood* 82: 2329–2339

39 Yau JC, Neidhart JA, Triozzi P, Verma S, Nemunaitis J, Quick DP, Mayernik DG, Oette DH, Haynes FA, Holcenberg J (1996) Randomized placebo-controlled trial of granulocyte-macrophage colony-stimulating-factor support for dose-intensive cyclophosphamide, etoposide, and cisplatin. *Amer J Hematol* 51: 289–295

40 Nemunaitis J (1997) A comparative review of colony-stimulating factors. *Drugs* 54: 709–729

41 Lydaki E, Bolonaki E, Stiakaki E, Dimitriou H, Kalmantis T, Kalmanti M (1995) Efficacy of recombinant human granulocyte colony-stimulating factor and recombinant human granulocyte-macrophage colony-stimulating factor in neutropenic children with malignancies. *Pediatr Hematol Oncol* 12: 551–558

42 Mamounas EP, Anderson S, Wickerham DL, Clark R, Stoller R, Hamm JT, Stewart J, Bear HD, Glass AG, Bornstein R et al (1994) The efficacy of recombinant human granulocyte colony-stimulating factor and recombinant human granulocyte macrophage colony-stimulating factor in permitting the administration of higher doses of cyclophosphamide in a doxorubicin-cyclophosphamide combination. An NSABP pilot study in patients with metastatic or high-risk primary breast cancer. National Surgical Adjuvant Breast and Bowel Project. *Amer J Clin Oncol* 17: 374–381

43 Godwin JE, Kopecky KJ, Head DR, Willman CL, Leith CP, Hynes HE, Balcerzak SP, Appelbaum FR (1998) A double-blind placebo-controlled trial of granulocyte colony-stimulating factor in elderly patients with previously untreated acute myeloid leukemia: a Southwest oncology group study (9031). *Blood* 91: 3607–3615

44 Rowe JM, Andersen JW, Mazza JJ, Bennett JM, Paietta E, Hayes FA, Oette D, Cassileth PA, Stadtmauer EA, Wiernik PH et al (1995) A randomized placebo-controlled phase III study of granulocyte-macrophage colony-stimulating factor in adult patients (>55 to 70 years of age) with acute myelogenous leukemia: a study of the Eastern Cooperative Oncology Group (E1490). *Blood* 86: 457–462

45 Stone RM, Berg DT, George SL, Dodge RK, Paciucci PA, Schulman P, Lee EJ, Moore JO, Powell BL, Schiffer CA (1995) Granulocyte-macrophage colony-stimulating factor after initial chemotherapy for elderly patients with primary acute myelogenous leukemia. *N Engl J Med* 332: 1671–1677

46 Löwenberg B, Suciu S, Archimbaud E, Ossenkoppele G, Verhoef GE, Vellenga E, Wijermans P, Berneman Z, Dekker AW, Stryckmans P et al (1997) Use of recombinant granulocyte-macrophage colony-stimulating factor during and after remission induction chemotherapy in patients aged 61 years and older with acute myeloid leukemia (AML): final report of AML-11, a phase III randomized study of the Leukemia Cooperative Group of European Organisation for the Research and Treatment of Cancer (EORTC-LCG) and the Dutch Belgian Hemato-Oncology Cooperative Group (HOVON). *Blood* 90: 2952–2961

47 Heil G, Chadid L, Hoelzer D, Seipelt S, Mitrou P, Huber C, Kolbe K, Mertelsmann R, Lindemann A, Frisch J et al (1995) GM-CSF in a double-blind randomized, placebo controlled trial in therapy of adult patients with *de novo* acute myeloid leukemia (AML). *Leukemia* 9: 3–9

48 Rowe JM, Liesveld JL (1997) Hematopoietic growth factors in acute leukemia. *Leukemia* 11: 328–341

49 Diehl V, Franklin J, Hasenclever D, Tesch H, Pfreundschuh M, Lathan B, Paulus U, Sieber M,

Rueffer JU, Sextro M et al (1998) BEACOPP, a new dose-escalated and accelerated regimen, is at least as effective as COPP/ABVD in patients with advanced stage Hodgkin's lymphoma: interim report from a trial of the German Hodgkin's Lymphoma Study Group. *J Clin Oncol* 16: 3810–3821

50 Stahel J, Jost LM, Cerny T, Pichert G, Honegger H, Tobler A, Jacky E, Fey M, Platzer E (1994) Randomized study of recombinant human granulocyte colony-stimulating factor after high-dose chemotherapy and autologous bone marrow transplantation for high-risk lymphoid malignancies. *J Clin Oncol* 12: 1931–1938

51 Gisselbrecht G, Prentice H, Bacigalupo A, Biron P, Milpied N, Rubie H, Cunningham D, Legros M, Pico JL, Linch DC et al (1994) Placebo-controlled phase III trial of lenograstim in bone-marrow transplantation. *Lancet* 343: 696–700

52 Nemunaitis J, Rabinowe SN, Singer JW, Bierman DJ, Vose JM, Freedman AS, Onetto N, Gillis S, Oette D, Gold M et al (1991) Recombinant granulocyte-macrophage colony-stimulating factor after autologous bone marrow transplantation for lymphoid cancer. *N Engl J Med* 324: 1773–1778

53 Nemunaitis J, Rosenfeld CS, Ash R, Freedman MH, Deeg HJ, Appelbaum F, Singer JW, Flomenberg N, Dalton W, Elfenbein GJ et al (1995) Phase III randomized, double-blind placebo-controlled trial of rhGM-CSF following allogeneic bone marrow transplantation. *Bone Marrow Transplant* 15: 949–954

54 Bolwell BJ, Goormastic M, Yanssens T, Dannley R, Baucco P, Fishleder A (1994) Comparison of G-CSF with GM-CSF for mobilizing peripheral blood progenitor cells and for enhancing marrow recovery after autologous bone marrow transplant. *Bone Marrow Transplant* 14: 913–918

55 Schriber JR, Negrin RS, Chao NJ, Long GD, Horning SJ, Blume KG (1993) The efficacy of granulocyte colony-stimulating factor following autologous bone marrow transplantation for non-Hodgkin's lymphoma with monoclonal antibody purged bone marrow. *Leukemia* 7: 1491–1495

56 Miggiano MC, Gherlinzoni F, Visani G, Belardinelli A, Ricci P, Rosti G, Mazza P, Motta MR, Rizzi S, Lemoli RM (1994) Hematological recovery after autologous bone marrow transplantation for high-grade non Hodgkin's lymphomas: a single center experience. *Haematologica* 79: 225–232

57 Sheridan WP, Begley CG, Juttner CA, Szer J, To LB, Maher D, MaGrath KM, Morstyn G, Fox RM (1992) Effect of peripheral-blood progenitor cells mobilised by filgrastim (G-CSF) on platelet recovery after high-dose chemotherapy. *Lancet* 339: 640–644

58 Schmitz N, Linch DC, Dreger P, Goldstone AH, Boogaerts MA, Ferrant A, Demuynck HMS, Link H, Zander A, Barge A et al (1996) Randomised trial of filgrastim-mobilised peripheral blood progenitor cell transplantation *versus* autologous bone-marrow transplantation in lymphoma patients. *Lancet* 347: 353–357

59 Smith TJ, Hillner BE, Schmitz N, Linch DC, Dreger P, Goldstone AH, Boogaerts MA, Ferrant A, Link H, Zander A et al (1997) Economic analysis of a randomized clinical trial to compare filgrastim-mobilized peripheral-blood progenitor-cell transplantation and autologous bone marrow transplantation in patients with Hodgkin's and non-Hodgkin's lymphoma. *J Clin Oncol* 15: 5–10

60 Ho AD, Young D, Maruyama M, Corringham RE, Mason JR, Thompson P, Grenier K, Law P, Terstappen LW, Lane T (1996) Pluripotent and lineage-committed CD34+ subsets in leukapheresis products mobilized by G-CSF, GM-CSF vs a combination of both. *Exp Hematol* 14: 1460–1468

61 Lane TA, Law P, Maruyama M, Young D, Burgess J, Mullen M, Mealiffe M, Terstappen LW, Hardwick A, Moubayed M et al (1995) Harvesting and enrichment of hematopoietic progenitor cells mobilized into the peripheral blood of normal donors by granulocyte-macrophage colony-stimulating factor (GM-CSF) or G-CSF: potential role in allogeneic bone marrow transplantation. *Blood* 85: 275–282

62 Klumpp TR, Goldberg SL, Magdalinski AJ, Mangan KF (1997) Phase II study of high-dose cyclophosphamide, etoposide, and carboplatin (CEC) followed by autologous hematopoietic stem cell rescue in women with metastatic or high-risk non-metastatic breast cancer: multivariate analysis of factors affecting survival and engraftment. *Bone Marrow Transplant* 20: 273–281

63 Van Hoef MEHM (1998) Haematological recovery after high-dose consolidation chemotherapy with peripheral blood progenitor cell rescue: the effects of the mobilization regimen and post-transplant growth factors. *Neth J Med* 52: 30–39

64 Hohaus S, Martin H, Wassmann B, Egerer G, Haus U, Farber L, Burger KJ, Goldschmidt H, Hoelzer D, Haas R (1998) Recombinant human granulocyte and granulocyte-macrophage colony-stimulating factor (G-CSF and GM-CSF) administered following cytotoxic chemotherapy have a

similar ability to mobilize peripheral blood stem cells. *Bone Marrow Transplant* 22: 625–630
65 Demuynck H, Delforge M, Verhoef G, Zachée P, Vandenberghe P Boogaerts M (1995) A comparative study of peripheral blood progenitor cell collection in patients with multiple myeloma after single-dose cyclophosphamide combined with rhGM-CSF or rhG-CSF. *Brit J Haematol* 90: 384–392
66 Winter JN, Lazarus HM, Rademaker A, Villa M, Mangan C, Tallman M, Jahnke L, Gordon L, Newman S, Byrd K et al (1996) Phase I/II study of combined granulocyte colony-stimulating factor and granulocyte-macrophage colony-stimulating factor administration for the mobilization of hematopoietic progenitor cells. *J Clin Oncol* 14: 277–286
67 Meisenberg B, Brehm T, Schmeckel A, Miller W, McMillan R (1998) A combination of low-dose cyclophosphamide and colony-stimulating factors is more cost-effective than granulocyte-colony-stimulating factors alone in mobilizing peripheral blood stem and progenitor cells. *Transfusion* 38: 209–215
68 Spitzer G, Adkins D, Mathews M, Velasquez W, Bowers C, Dunphy F, Kronmueller N, Niemeyer R, McIntyre W, Petruska P (1997) Randomized comparison of G-CSF + GM-CSF vs G-CSF alone for mobilization of peripheral blood stem cells: effects on hematopoietic recovery after high-dose chemotherapy. *Bone Marrow Transplant* 20: 921–930
69 Schiodt I, Knudsen L, Jensen L, Nikolajsen K, Gaarsdal E, Johnsen HE (1998) Flow cytometry comparison of CD34+ subsets in bone marrow and peripheral blood after priming with glycosylated or non-glycosylated G-CSF. *Bone Marrow Transplant* 21: 1167–1170
70 Watts M, Sullivan AM, Jamieson E, Pearce R, Fielding A, Devereux S, Goldstone AH, Linch DC (1997) Progenitor-cell mobilization after low-dose cyclophosphamide and granulocyte colony-stimulating factor: An analysis of progenitor-cell quantity and quality and factor predicting for these parameters in 101 pretreated patients with malignant lymphoma. *J Clin Oncol* 15: 535–546
71 Höglund M, Smedmyr B, Bengtsson M, Tötterman TH, Cour-Chabernaud V, Yver A, Simonsson B (1997) Mobilization of CD34+ cells by glycosylated and non-glycosylated G-CSF in healthy volunteers – a comparative study. *Eur J Haematol* 59: 177–183
72 Schmitz N, Bacigalupo A, Hasenclever D, Nagler A, Gluckman E, Clark P, Bourquelot P, Greinix H, Frickhofen N, Ringdén O et al (1998) Allogeneic bone marrow transplantation vs filgrastim-mobilised peripheral blood progenitor cell transplantation in patients with early leukaemia: first results of a randomised multicentre trial of the European Group for Blood and Marrow Transplantation. *Bone Marrow Transplant* 21: 995–1003
73 Dale DC, Bonilla MA, Davis MW, Nakanishi AM, Hammond WP, Hurtzberg J, Wang W, Jakubowski A, Winton E, Lalezari P et al (1993) A randomized controlled phase III trial of recombinant human G-CSF for treatment of severe chronic neutropenia. *Blood* 81: 2496–2502
74 Welte K, Boxer LA (1997) Severe chronic neutropenia: Pathophysiology and Therapy. *Semin Hematol* 34: 267–278
75 Tidow N, Welte K (1997) Advances in understanding postreceptor signalling in response to granulocyte colony-stimulating factor. *Curr Opin Hematol* 4: 171–175
76 Reiffers J, Cailliot C, Dazey B, Duchez I, Pigneux A, Cousin T, Bussière Boiron JM (1998) Infusion of expanded CD34+ selected cells can abrogate post myeloablative chemotherapy neutropenia in patients with hematologic malignancies. *Blood* 92: 126a
77 Johnston E, Crawford J, Lockbaum P, Shoemaker D, Bjurstrom A, Mallon K, Miller-Messana M, Schwab G (1998) Single-dose, subcutaneous (SC), sustained-duration filgrastim (SD) *versus* daily filgrastim in non-small cell lung cancer patients (NSCLC): A randomized, controlled, dose-escalation study. *Proc Amer Soc Oncol* 17: 73a
78 Miles S (1995) The use of hematopoietic growth factors in treating HIV infection. *Curr Opin Hematol* 2: 227–233
79 Newman GW, Guarnaccia JR, Remold HG, Kazanjian PH Jr, (1997) Cytokines enhance neutrophils from human immunodeficiency virus-negative donors and AIDS patients to inhibit the growth of *Mycobacterium avium in vitro*. *J Infect Dis* 175: 891–900
80 Kemper CA, Bermudez LE, Deresinski SC (1998) Immunomodulatory treatment of *Mycobacterium avium* complex bacteremia in patients with AIDS by use of recombinant granulocyte-macrophage colony-stimulating factor. *J Infect Dis* 177: 914–920
81 Barbaro G, Di Lorenzo G, Grisorio B, Soldini M, Barbarini G (1997) Effect of recombinant human granulocyte-macrophage colony-stimulating factor on HIV-related leukopenia: a randomized, controlled clinical study. *AIDS* 11: 1453–1461
82 Frumkin-L-R (1997) Role of granulocyte colony-stimulating factor and granulocyte-macrophage

colony-stimulating factor in the treatment of patients with HIV infection. *Curr Opin Hematol* 4: 200–206
83 Hermans P (1995) Haematopoietic growth factors as supportive therapy in HIV-infected patients. *AIDS* 9: S9–S14
84 Crowe SM, Lopez A (1997) GM-CSF and its effects on replication of HIV-1 in cells of macrophage lineage. *J Leukocyte Biol* 62: 41–48
85 Wang J, Roderiquez G, Oravecz T, Norcross MA (1998) Cytokine regulation of human immunodeficiency virus type 1 entry and replication in human monocytes/macrophages through modulation of CCR5 expression. *J Virol* 9: 7642–7647
86 Nimer SD, Leung DH, Wolin MJ, Golde DW (1994) Serum stem cell factor levels in patients with aplastic anemia. *Int JHematol* 60: 185–189
87 Scopes J, Daly S, Atkinson R, Ball SE, Gordon-Smith Ecm Gibson FM (1996) Aplastic anemia: evidence for dysfunctional bone marrow progenitor cells and the corrective effect of granulocyte colony stimulating factor *in vitro*. *Blood* 87: 3179–3185
88 Bacigalupo A, Broccia G, Corda G, Arcese W, Carotenuto M, Gallamini A, Loctelli F, Mori PG, Sarcacco P, Todeschini G et al (1995) Antilymphocyte globulin, cyclosporin, and granulocyte colony-stimulating factor in patients with acquired severe aplastic anemia (SAA): a pilot study of the EBMT SAA Working Party. *Blood* 85: 1348–1353
89 Passweg JR, Tyndall A (1999) Autologous stem cell transplantation for autoimmune disease. *Bone Marrow Transplant* 23: S35
90 Snowden JA, Biggs JC, Milliken ST, Fuller A, Staniforth D, Passuello F, Renwick J, Brooks PM (1998) A randomised, blinded, placebo-controlled, dose escalation study of the tolerability and efficacy of filgrastim for haemopoietic stem cell mobilisation in patients with severe active rheumatoid arthritis. *Bone Marrow Transplant* 22: 1035–1041
91 Nasi ML, Lieberman PH, Lewis J, Prieto VG, Busam K, Williams L, Dantis L, Reyes S, Meyers ML, Livingston PO et al (1998) Intradermal (ID) injection of granulocyte-macrophage colony stimulating factor (GM-CSF) in patients with metastatic melanoma. *Proc Am Soc Clin Oncol* 17: 429a
92 Durek C, Schäfer I, Braasch H, Ulmer AJ, Ernst M, Flad HD, Jocham D, Böhle A (1997) Effects of colony-stimulating factors on cellular cytotoxicity. *Cancer Immunol Immunother* 44: 35–40
93 Baxevanis CN, Dedoussis GVZ, Papadopoulos NG, Missitzis I, Beroukas C, Stathopoulos GP, Papamichail M (1995) Enhanced human lymphokine-activated killer cell function after brief exposure to granulocyte-macrophage-colony stimulating factor. *Cancer* 76: 1253–1260
94 Herrera C, García Pérez MJ, Ramirez R, Martín C, Alvarez MA, Martinez F, Gómez P, García Castellano JM, Torres A (1997) Lymphokine-activated killer (LAK) cell generation from peripheral blood stem cells by *in vitro* incubation with low-dose interleukin-2 plus granulocyte-macrophage colony-stimulating factor. *Bone Marrow Transplant* 19: 545–551
95 Dale DC, Liles WC, Llewellyn C, Rodger E, Price TH (1998) Neutrophil transfusions: kinetics and functions of neutrophils mobilized with granulocyte-colony-stimulating factor and dexamethasone. *Transfusion* 38: 713–721
96 Adkins DR, Spitzer G, Johnston M, Velasquez W, Dunphy F, Petruska P (1997) Transfusions of granulocyte-colony-stimulating factor-mobilized granulocyte components to allogeneic transplant recipients: analysis of kinetics and factors determining posttransfusion neutrophil and platelet counts. *Transfusion* 37: 737–748
97 Adkins DR, Brown RA, Goodnough LT, DiPersio JF (1998) Use of filgrastim (r-metHuG-CSF) in neutrophil transfusions. *In*: Morstyn G, Dexter TM, Foote M (eds):. *Filgrastim (r-metHuG-CSF) In clinical practice*. New York, Basel, Hong Kong: Marcel Dekker, Inc., 149–164
98 Groopman JE, Molina J-M, Scadden DT (1989) Hematopoietic growth factors. *N Engl J Med* 321: 1449–1459
99 Lieschke GJ, Cebon J, Morstyn G (1989) Characterization of the clinical effects after the first dose of bacterially synthesized recombinant human granulocyte-macrophage colony-stimulating factor. *Blood* 74: 2634–2643
100 Vial T, Descotes J (1995) Clinical toxicity of cytokines used as haemopoietic growth factors. *Drug Safety* 13: 371–406

Recombinant Protein Drugs
ed. by P. Buckel

Tissue-type plasminogen activator: helping patients with acute myocardial infarction

Désiré Collen[1] and H. Roger Lijnen[2]

[1] *Center for Transgene Technology and Gene Therapy, Flanders Interuniversity Institute for Biotechnology, Leuven, Belgium*
[2] *Center for Molecular and Vascular Biology, Katholieke Universiteit Leuven, Leuven, Belgium*

Introduction

The blood fibrinolytic system comprises an inactive proenzyme, plasminogen, that can be converted to the active enzyme, plasmin, that in turn degrades fibrin into soluble fibrin degradation products (Fig. 1). Two immunologically distinct physiological plasminogen activators (PA) have been identified: the tissue-type PA (t-PA) and the urokinase-type PA (u-PA). Inhibition of the fibrinolytic system may occur either at the level of the PA, by specific plasminogen activator inhibitors (PAI), or at the level of plasmin, mainly by α_2-antiplasmin. t-PA-mediated plasminogen activation is mainly involved in the dissolu-

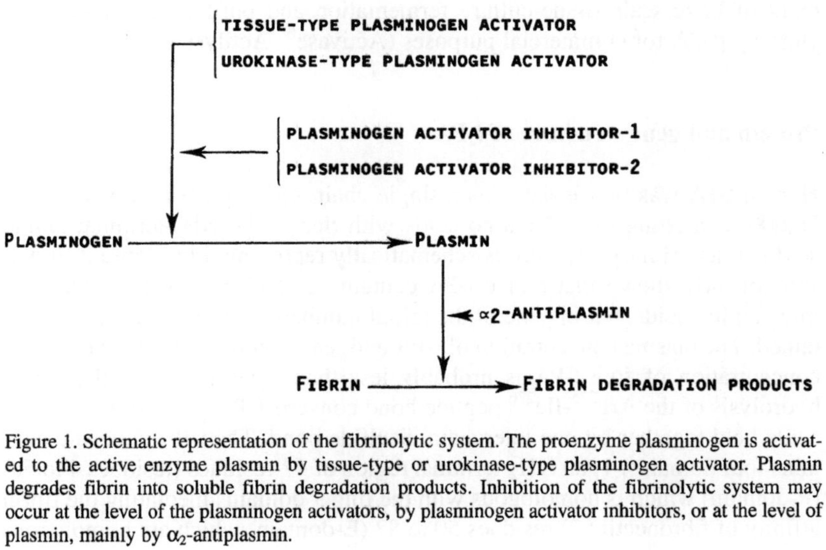

Figure 1. Schematic representation of the fibrinolytic system. The proenzyme plasminogen is activated to the active enzyme plasmin by tissue-type or urokinase-type plasminogen activator. Plasmin degrades fibrin into soluble fibrin degradation products. Inhibition of the fibrinolytic system may occur at the level of the plasminogen activators, by plasminogen activator inhibitors, or at the level of plasmin, mainly by α_2-antiplasmin.

tion of fibrin in the circulation [1]. u-PA binds to a specific cellular receptor (u-PAR) and plays a role in the induction of pericellular proteolysis [2]. Physiological fibrinolysis is regulated by specific molecular interactions between its main components as well as by controlled synthesis and release of PAs and PAIs [1].

Already in 1947 it was reported that animal tissues contain an agent that can activate plasminogen; this factor was originally called fibrinokinase [3]. Many studies have since reported on the purification and characterization of tissue PAs from various sources, including pig heart, hog ovaries, post-mortem vascular perfusates and post-exercise blood. The first highly purified form of human t-PA has been obtained from uterine tissue [4]. Using an antiserum raised against uterine PA, it was shown that tissue PA, vascular PA, and blood PA are immunologically identical, but different from urokinase [5]. The PA found in blood represents vascular PA which is released primarily from endothelial cells.

t-PA has been purified from the culture fluid of a stable human melanoma cell line (Bowes, RPMI-7272) in sufficient amounts to study its biochemical and biological properties [6]. Purification methods include immunoadsorption and chromatography on zinc-chelate, lysine-Sepharose or fibrin-Sepharose. t-PA has subsequently been produced by recombinant DNA technology (rt-PA). The cDNA of human t-PA has been cloned and expressed in *E. coli* and in mammalian cell systems [7]. rt-PA expressed in mammalian cells, yielding a properly processed and glycosylated molecule, was shown to be indistinguishable from the natural activator isolated from human melanoma cell cultures with respect to biochemical properties, turnover *in vivo* and specific thrombolytic activity [8]. The generation of CHO (Chinese hamster ovary) cells capable of producing single-chain human t-PA has allowed the development of large-scale tissue-culture fermentation and purification procedures, yielding rt-PA for commercial purposes (Activase®; Actilyse®).

Protein and gene structure of t-PA

Human t-PA was first isolated as a single-chain serine proteinase with $\underline{M}_r$ of 70,000, consisting of 527 amino acids with Ser as the NH_2-terminal amino acid [7]; its primary structure is schematically represented in Figure 2. It was subsequently shown that native t-PA contains an NH_2-terminal extension of three amino acids, but in general the initial numbering system has been maintained. The plasma concentration of t-PA antigen is about 5 ng/ml, whereas the concentration of free t-PA is probably less than 1 ng/ml. Limited plasmic hydrolysis of the Arg^{275}-Ile^{276} peptide bond converts t-PA to a two-chain molecule held together by one interchain disulfide bond. The t-PA molecule contains four domains: 1) an NH_2-terminal region of 47-residues (residues 4 to 50) (F-domain) which is homologous with the finger domains mediating the fibrin affinity of fibronectin; 2) residues 50 to 87 (E-domain) which are homologous

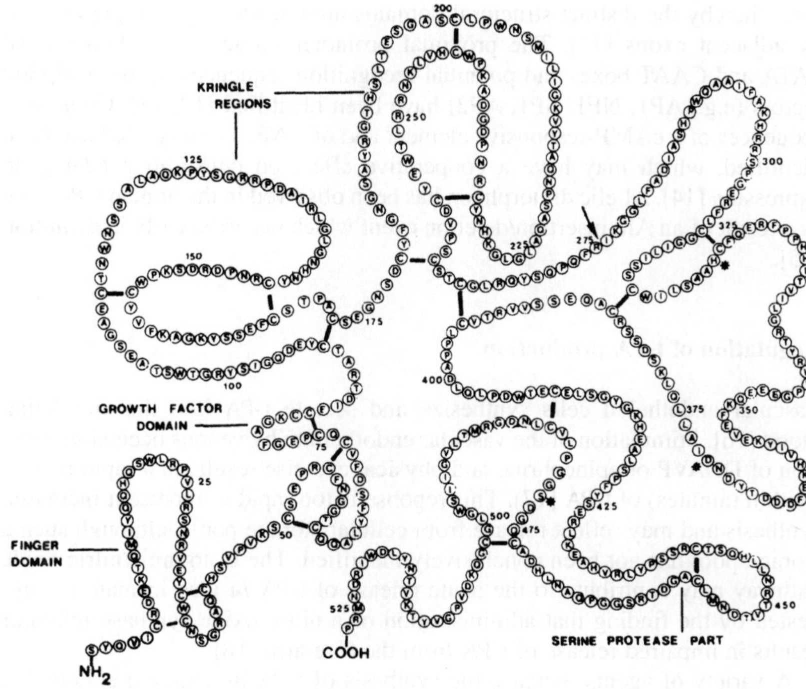

Figure 2. Schematic representation of the primary structure of t-PA. The amino acids are represented by their single letter symbols and black bars indicate disulphide bonds. The active site residues His^{322}, Asp^{371} and Ser^{478} are indicated with an asterisk. The arrow indicates the plasmin cleavage site for conversion of single-chain t-PA to two-chain t-PA (adapted from ref. [21]).

with epidermal growth factor; 3) two kringle regions comprising residues 87 to 176 and 176 to 262 (K_1 and K_2 domains) which share a high degree of homology with the five kringles of plasminogen and 4) a serine proteinase domain (P, residues 276 to 527) with the active site residues His^{322}, Asp^{371} and Ser^{478} [7]. There are three potential N-glycosylation sites, at Asn^{117} (K_1), Asn^{184} (K_2) and Asn^{448} (P). t-PA preparations may contain a mixture of variant I (with all three glycosylation sites) and variant II (lacking carbohydrate at Asn^{184}) [7]. In contrast to the single-chain precursor form of most serine proteinases, single-chain t-PA is enzymatically active. Amino acid Lys^{156} was shown to contribute directly to the enzymatic activity of single-chain t-PA, by forming a salt bridge with Asp^{194} that selectively stabilizes the active conformation [9].

The human *t-PA* gene is localized on chromosome 8 (bands 8.p.12 $\rightarrow$ q.11.2) [10] and more than 36 kb of its sequence have been determined. The *t-PA* gene consists of 14 exons and the intron-exon organization suggests that the assembly occurred according to the "exon shuffling" principle, whereby the distinct structural domains are encoded by a single exon or by adjacent exons [11]. The proximal promoter sequences contain typical TATA and CAAT boxes and potential recognition sequences for transcription factors (e.g., AP1, NF1, SP1, AP2) have been identified [12, 13]. Consensus sequences of a cAMP-responsive element and of a AP2 binding site have been identified, which may have a cooperative effect on constitutive *t-PA* gene expression [14]. Allelic dimorphism has been observed in the human *t-PA* gene as a result of an Alu insertion/deletion event which occurred early in evolution [15].

Regulation of t-PA production

Vascular endothelial cells synthesize and secrete t-PA into the circulating blood [16]. Stimulation of the vascular endothelium by venous occlusion, infusion of DDAVP or epinephrine and physical exercise results in a rapid release (within minutes) of t-PA [17]. This reponse is too rapid to represent increased synthesis and may reflect release from cellular storage pools, although such a storage pool has not been conclusively identified. The L-arginine/nitric oxide pathway may contribute to the acute release of t-PA *in vivo* in man, as suggested by the finding that administration of a nitric oxide synthase inhibitor results in impaired release of t-PA from the fore-arm [18].

A variety of agents increase the synthesis of t-PA by cultured endothelial cells, including thrombin [19, 20], histamine [20], dexamethasone [21], butyrate [22], phorbol myristate acetate (PMA) [23], basic fibroblast growth factor [24], activated protein C [25], butanol and alcohol derivatives [26] and retinoids [27, 28]. Agents, such as thrombin, that stimulate the release of t-PA from endothelial cells, also stimulate the secretion of PAI-1 [19, 20]. Dexamethasone increases t-PA antigen levels in hepatoma cells moderately but increases PAI-1 antigen levels to a greater extent, resulting in inhibition of t-PA activity [29].

The mechanisms involved in the stimulatory effect of these various agents on t-PA synthesis appear to be different and are now being gradually elucidated. Vitamin A, retinoic acid (RA) and some of its analogues induce t-PA-related antigen secretion by human umbilical vein endothelial cells *in vitro*, but also in the plasma and specific tissues of vitamin A-deficient rats [27], suggesting that circulating RA may regulate t-PA expression in the vessel wall. The receptors for these agents are members of the nuclear receptor superfamily, a class of transcription factors that specifically bind to *cis*-elements in the gene regulatory region. Recently, a functional RA response element (RARE), which consists of a direct repeat of the GGTCA motif spaced by 5 nucleotides (DR5), has been localized 7.3 kb upstream from the transcription start site of the human *t-PA* gene. This element mediates the direct regulation by RA in human fibrosarcoma, endothelial and neuroblastoma cells [30]. This t-PA/DR5-RARE is part of a multihormone responsive enhancer covering an upstream fragment, which contains a complex glucocorticoid responsive unit composed of 4 binding sites for the receptor [31]. Induction of t-PA by RA in human umbilical vein endothelial cells involves a two-step mechanism, requiring induction of RA receptor β_2(RARβ_2) via RARα_1, followed by induction of t-PA synthesis via RARβ_2 [32].

Vasoactive substances, such as histamine and thrombin, bind to specific receptors and activate phospholipase C which acts on phosphatidyl-inositol biphosphate to produce diacylglycerol. Diacylglycerol activates membrane-bound protein kinase C, which plays an important role in the regulation of t-PA synthesis. This is suggested by the findings that direct activation of protein kinase C by phorbol esters induces t-PA synthesis, whereas suppression of protein kinase C impairs the increase in t-PA synthesis by histamine and by PMA [33]. The increase of t-PA induced by histamine, thrombin and PMA in endothelial cells is paralleled by increased levels of mRNA, as a result of enhanced transcription of the *t-PA* gene [34]. Very little is known, however, about the regulation of human *t-PA* gene transcription. Two *cis*-elements (a cAMP response element (CRE) in the proximal promoter and an activator protein-2 (AP-2) binding site in exon 1) have been identified which are involved in basal expression and induction of human *t-PA* gene transcription by cAMP and phorbolesters [14]. *In vivo* footprinting analysis revealed that specificity protein 1 (Sp1) binds the t-PA promoter at two proximal sites, of which one overlaps with the AP-2 site in exon 1 [35].

Overexpression of t-PA in endothelial cells *in vitro* using a retroviral expression vector has been achieved without altering the morphology, attachment, proliferation, migration or invasion. Potentially such *t-PA* transduced cells could increase local fibrinolysis and may be useful for *in vivo* therapeutic interventions [36]. Interestingly, plasmin inhibits the biosynthesis of t-PA antigen by human umbilical vein endothelial cells in a dose-dependent manner, possibly through the signal transduction pathway involving one or more protein kinases [37].

Mechanism of plasminogen activation by t-PA

t-PA, as all other known PAs, converts the zymogen plasminogen into the active serine proteinase plasmin by cleavage of a single Arg^{561}-Val^{562} peptide bond. The NH_2-terminal polypeptide chain of plasmin contains 5 kringle structures, some of which have lysine-binding sites, and the active site is comprised within the COOH-terminal polypeptide chain. The lysine-binding sites are required for the binding of plasmin(ogen) to fibrin and for the rapid inhibition of plasmin by α_2-antiplasmin [39].

t-PA is a poor enzyme in the absence of fibrin, but the presence of fibrin strikingly enhances the activation rate of plasminogen [38]. Plasmin formed at the fibrin surface has both its lysine binding sites and active site occupied and is thus only slowly inactivated by α_2-antiplasmin (half-life of about 10–100 s);

in contrast, free plasmin, when formed, is rapidly inhibited by α_2-antiplasmin (half-life of about 0.1 s) [39, 40].

During fibrinolysis, fibrinogen and fibrin itself are continuously modified by cleavage with thrombin or plasmin, yielding a diversity of reaction products. Thrombin-catalyzed formation of desA-fibrin monomer, and a certain degree of desA-fibrin polymerization are essential for stimulation of plasminogen activation by t-PA. Optimal stimulation is only obtained after early plasmin-cleavage in the COOH-terminal Aα-chain and the NH_2-terminal Bβ-chain of fibrin, yielding fragment X-polymer [41]. Kinetic data [38] support a mechanism in which fibrin provides a surface to which t-PA and plasminogen adsorb in a sequential and ordered way, yielding a cyclic ternary complex. Formation of this complex results in an enhanced affinity of t-PA for plasminogen, yielding up to three orders of magnitude higher efficiencies for plasminogen activation. In agreement with this mechanism, the increase in fibrin stimulation after formation of fibrin X-polymers is associated with an enhanced binding of t-PA and plasminogen. This increased and altered binding of both enzyme and substrate to fibrin is mediated in part by COOH-terminal lysine residues generated by plasmin-cleavage. Interaction of these COOH-terminal lysines with lysine binding sites on t-PA and plasminogen may allow an improved alignment as well as allosteric changes of the t-PA and plasminogen moieties, thus enhancing the rate of plasminogen activation [41]. During fibrin clot lysis, single-chain t-PA is converted to two-chain t-PA at the fibrin surface. This conversion is probably of little physiological relevance, since the activity of single-chain t-PA and two-chain t-PA is enhanced to the same extent in the presence of fibrin or fragment X-polymer [42].

Proteins that compete with plasminogen for binding to fibrin may have an antifibrinolytic action. Thus, Lp(a), a protein with multiple copies of a plasminogen kringle 4-like domain, a single copy of a kringle 5-like domain and an inactive proteinase domain [43], binds to fibrin via its lysine-binding domains. As for plasminogen, binding of Lp(a) to fibrin is enhanced by partial proteolytic degradation of the fibrin surface [44]. The fibrin-dependent enhancement of plasminogen activation by t-PA is thereby reduced [45–47], although kinetic studies indicate that the effect of Lp(a) on plasminogen activation by t-PA is only very limited [48].

Alternatively, proteins that remove lysine residues from the fibrin surface, such as the Thrombin Activatable Fibrinolysis Inhibitor (TAFI), may have an antifibrinolytic action. TAFI is a $\underline{M}_r$ 60,000 single-chain protein, identical to plasma procarboxypeptidase B, occurring at a concentration of 75 nM [49, 50]. Thrombin, trypsin or plasmin convert the protein to an active carboxypeptidase B. Activated TAFI suppresses fibrinolysis, most likely by removing COOH-terminal lysine residues from (partially degraded) fibrin, thereby preventing additional binding of plasminogen and/or t-PA to fibrin [51].

Inhibition of t-PA

Multiple mechanisms are involved in the rapid inhibition of t-PA in human plasma. The main mechanism of removal of t-PA from the blood is by clearance via the liver. In healthy volunteers and in patients with acute myocardial infarction, the initial half-life of t-PA is 4 to 6 min [52, 53]. In addition, t-PA is inhibited slowly by α_2-antiplasmin, α_1-antitrypsin and C1-inhibitor [54]. PAI-1 is a specific rapid-reacting inhibitor of t-PA, which is present at a low concentration in normal plasma, but at higher concentrations in many clinical conditions [55].

PAI-1 is a single-chain glycoprotein with $\underline{M}_r$ of about 52,000 consisting of 379 amino acids. The cDNA sequence revealed that PAI-1 is a member of the serpin family with reactive site peptide bond Arg^{346}-Met^{347} [56, 57]. PAI-1 is stabilized by binding to a PAI binding protein identified as S-protein or vitronectin [58].

PAI-1 reacts very rapidly with single-chain and two-chain t-PA, with second-order inhibition rate constants of the order of $10^7\ M^{-1}\cdot s^{-1}$ [59, 60]. Like other serpins, PAI-1 inhibits its target proteinases by formation of a 1:1 stoichiometric reversible complex, followed by covalent binding between the hydroxyl group of the active site serine residue of the proteinase and the carboxyl group of the P1 residue at the reactive center ("bait region") of the serpin. The rapid inhibition of t-PA by PAI-1 involves a reversible high-affinity second-site interaction between the sequence 350–355 of PAI-1, which contains three negatively charged amino acids, with highly positively charged regions in t-PA (residues 296–304) [61]. In the presence of fibrin, single-chain t-PA is protected from rapid inhibition by PAI-1 [62]. It has, however, also been reported that PAI-1 binds to fibrin and that fibrin-bound PAI-1 may inhibit t-PA-mediated clot lysis [63, 64].

PAI-2 is a serpin of 393 amino acids with reactive site peptide bond Arg^{358}-Thr^{359}. It inhibits two-chain t-PA and less efficiently single-chain t-PA [59]. PAI-2 levels in plasma are very low, but are drastically elevated during pregnancy [65].

Thrombolytic therapy

Thrombolysis consists of the pharmacological dissolution of a blood clot by intravenous infusion of PAs that activate the fibrinolytic system. The fibrin-specificity of t-PA, as described above, has triggered great interest in its use for thrombolytic therapy, mainly in patients with acute myocardial infarction. Recently, rt-PA was also approved for treatment of ischemic stroke. The beneficial effects of thrombolytic therapy in acute myocardial infarction have been well established in controlled clinical trials and it has become routine treatment; it is given to more than 500,000 patients per year worldwide, while at least three times that number could benefit from this treatment [66].

However, all available thrombolytic agents still suffer significant shortcomings, including large therapeutic doses, limited efficacy, reocclusion and bleeding complications. Thus rt-PA, the most effective agent presently available, will produce functional recanalization of the occluded coronary artery in approximately 55% of patients, recanalization requiring 45 minutes or more, whereas reocclusion occurs in 5 to 10% and cerebral bleeding in 0.5 to 1.0% of patients [66].

Wild-type t-PA

Wild-type t-PA has a short half-life in man. The initial and terminal half-lives of single-chain rt-PA, following infusion of 8.3 µg/kg/min over 30 minutes in healthy volunteers, were 3.3 and 26 minutes, respectively [67]. In patients with acute myocardial infarction, clearance of single-chain rt-PA was found to be 30 to 40% more rapid than two-chain rt-PA [53]. Clearance is the result of interaction with several receptor systems. Liver endothelial cells have a mannose receptor which recognizes the high mannose-type carbohydrate side-chain at Asn^{117} in the K_1 domain, whereas liver parenchymal cells contain a calcium-dependent receptor which interacts mainly with the growth factor domain of t-PA. In addition, the low-density lipoprotein receptor-related protein (LRP), expressed in high copy number on hepatocytes, binds free t-PA and complexes with PAI-1 (for references, cf.68].

The recommended dose of rt-PA (alteplase, Activase®, Actilyse®) for the treatment of acute myocardial infarction was 100 mg, administered as 60 mg in the first hour (of which 6 to 10 mg is administered as a bolus over the first 1 to 2 minutes), 20 mg over the second hour and 20 mg over the third hour [69]. More recently it was proposed to give the same total dose of 100 mg but "front-loaded", starting with a bolus of 15 mg followed by 50 mg in the next 30 minutes and the remaining 35 mg in the following hour [70]. In the GUSTO trial, a dose of 15 mg intravenous bolus of alteplase followed by 0.75 mg/kg over 30 minutes (not to exceed 50 mg) and then 0.50 mg/kg over 60 minutes (not to exceed 35 mg) was utilized [71]. This study conclusively demonstrated that fibrin-selective rt-PA combined with intravenous heparin is superior to non-fibrin-selective streptokinase for early mortality reduction [71]. A recent meta-analysis of all megatrials concluded differently [72], but wrongly pooled the rt-PA and the rt-PA plus streptokinase groups of GUSTO, which constitute fibrin-selective and non-fibrin-selective thrombolytic strategies with different mortality reductions. *Post-hoc* analysis of GUSTO results indicated that the difference in mortality persisted after 1 year [73] and that patients who were at higher risk derived a greater absolute benefit from treatment with rt-PA with intravenous heparin than with streptokinase [74]. In the COBALT trial, accelerated infusion of rt-PA over 90 minutes was found to be superior to double bolus administration (50 mg given 30 minutes apart) in patients with myocardial infarction [75].

Large-scale placebo-controlled randomized studies with i.v. streptokinase in the treatment of acute ischemic stroke were disappointing because of high hemorrhage-related mortality [76]. Similar observations were made initially with rt-PA in the ECASS study (1.1 mg rt-PA/kg given over 60 minutes with a maximum dose of 100 mg); 30-day mortality and clinical outcome in treated patients and in controls were comparable and hemorrhage-related mortality was 6.3% in the treated group [76, 77]. Subsequently, in the NINDS study, treatment with rt-PA (0.9 mg/kg with a maximum of 90 mg, 10% given as a bolus and the rest infused over 60 minutes) was initiated within 3 hours of symptom onset. Mortality rates were not different, but there was evidence of functional improvement within 3 months in a greater proportion of t-PA treated patients. Intracerebral hemorrhage, however, occurred more frequently with thrombolytic therapy (6.4% *versus* 0.6% in controls) [78]. Optimal patient selection and treatment regimen for stroke will thus require further clinical studies.

Mutants and variants of t-PA

By deletion or substitution of functional domains, by site-specific point mutations and/or by altering the carbohydrate composition, mutants of rt-PA have been produced with higher fibrin-specificity, more zymogenicity, slower clearance from the circulation and resistance to plasma proteinase inhibitors [79]. During thrombolytic therapy there is a vast excess of t-PA over PAI-1 in the circulation, but critical lysis occurs at the surface of an arterial thrombus where the local PAI-1 concentration can be very high [80]. Therefore, mutants with resistance to PAI-1 may be useful to reduce reocclusion. In addition, mutants with a prolonged half-life may allow efficient thrombolysis by bolus administration at a reduced dose. Several mutants and variants of t-PA are presently being evaluated at the preclinical level in animal models of venous and arterial thrombosis and in pilot studies, mainly in patients with acute myocardial infarction. These agents include reteplase (Rapilysin® or Ecokinase®), TNK-rt-PA and the vampire bat (*Desmodus rotundus*) salivary PA.

Reteplase (BM 06.022) is a single-chain non-glycosylated deletion variant consisting only of the kringle 2 and the proteinase domain of human t-PA; it contains amino acids 1–3 and 176–527 of rt-PA (deletion of Val^{4}-Glu^{175}; cf. Figure 2). The Arg^{275}-Ile^{276} plasmin cleavage site is maintained [81]. The plasminogenolytic activity of reteplase and of t-PA in the absence of a stimulator does not differ, but the activity of reteplase in the presence of cyanogen bromide (CNBr) fragments of fibrinogen as a stimulator was 4-fold lower as compared to t-PA, and its binding to fibrin was 5-fold lower [81, 82]. These differences might possibly be due to the missing finger domain in reteplase. It is indeed known that fibrin binding is mediated through both the finger domain and the lysine-binding site in the kringle 2 domain of t-PA. Reteplase and t-PA are inhibited by PAI-1 to a similar degree. The affinity of reteplase for binding to endothelial cells and monocytes is reduced as compared to t-PA, probably as a consequence of deletion of the finger and epidermal growth factor domains in reteplase, which seem to be involved in the interaction with endothelial cell receptors [83]. Pharmacokinetic analysis in the rabbit revealed a half-life of 19 min for reteplase as compared to 2 min for rt-PA, associated with a 4.3-fold slower plasma clearance [84]. In healthy human volunteers [85] and in patients with acute myocardial infarction [86], an intitial half-life of 14–18 min was observed for reteplase. Different doses of reteplase in patients with acute myocardial infarction were evaluated in two open non-randomized pilot trials [87, 88]. The randomized RAPID I trial showed that reteplase, when given as a double bolus of 10 plus 10 MU 30 minutes apart, achieves more rapid, complete and sustained thrombolysis than standard dose alteplase (100 mg over 3 hours) [89]. In the RAPID II trial, the same reteplase dose regimen appeared to achieve higher rates of early reperfusion than front-loaded alteplase [90]. In the INJECT study, a double-blind randomized trial in patients with acute myocardial infarction, administration of two boluses of 10 MU reteplase given 30 min apart was compared with streptokinase (1.5 MU i.v. over 60 minutes) [91]. In the definitive GUSTO-III trial, however, no clinical benefit of reteplase over alteplase could be demonstrated, leading to the conclusion that both agents are equivalent [92].

In TNK-rt-PA, replacement of Asn^{117} with Gln (N117Q) deletes the glycosylation site in K_1 whereas substitution of Thr^{103} by Asn(T103N) reintroduces a glycosylation site in K_1, but at a different locus; these modifications substantially decrease the plasma clearance rate. In addition, the amino acids Lys^{296}-His^{297}-Arg^{298}-Arg^{299} were each replaced with Ala, which confers resistance to inhibition by PAI-1 (cf. Fig. 2) [93, 94]. TNK-rt-PA has a similar ability as wild-type rt-PA to bind to fibrin and lyses fibrin clots in a plasma milieu with enhanced fibrin-specificity. TNK-rt-PA has an increased thrombolytic potency on platelet-rich clots in rabbits, it conserves fibrinogen and is effective upon bolus administration at half the dose of rt-PA [93, 95]. Similar results were obtained in a combined arterial and venous thrombosis model in the dog [96] and in a rabbit carotid artery thrombosis model [97]. In patients with acute myocardial infarction, TNK-rt-PA has a plasma clearance of 151 ± 55 ml/min and a half-life of 17 ± 7 min, as compared to 572 ± 132 ml/min and 3.5 ± 1.4 min for wild-type rt-PA [98]. In the Thrombolysis in Myocardial Infarction (TIMI) 10A trial, a phase 1 dose-ranging pilot study, single bolus TNK-rt-PA was administered over 5 to 10 seconds with doses ranging from 5 to 50 mg [98]. The agent was fibrin-specific with initial patency and safety profile at the 30 to 50 mg doses which appeared encouraging. In the TIMI-10B trial, a larger phase 2 efficacy trial, a single bolus of 40 mg TNK-t-PA yielded similar TIMI-3 flow rates at 90 minutes as accelerated rt-PA, with faster and more complete reperfusion [99]. In the ASSENT-1 phase 2 safety trial, an intracranial hemorrhage rate of 0.76% was observed with the 40 mg dose, which is acceptable considering the fact that nearly 15% of the patients were above 75 years [100].

Different molecular forms of the *Desmodus* salivary PA (DSPA) have been purified, characterized, cloned and expressed. Two high molecular weight forms, DSPAα1 (43 kDa) and DSPAα2 (39 kDa), exhibit about 85% homology to human t-PA, but contain neither a kringle 2 domain nor a plasmin-sensitive cleavage site. DSPAβ lacks the finger-domain and DSPAγ lacks the finger and epidermal growth factor domains [101–103]. DSPAα1 and DSPAα2 exhibit a specific activity *in vitro* that is equal to or higher than that of rt-PA, a relative PAI-1 resistance and a greatly enhanced fibrin-specificity with a strict requirement for polymeric fibrin as a cofactor [101–103]. In several animal models of thrombolysis, DSPAα1 has a 2.5 times higher potency and four- to eight-fold slower clearance than rt-PA [104–108].

Lanoteplase is a deletion mutant of rt-PA (without the finger and growth factor domains) in which glycosylation at Asn^{117} is lacking [109]. Given as a single bolus of 120 U/kg in the "Intravenous n-PA for Treating Infarcting Myocardium Early (InTIME-1)" trial, higher infarct-related vessel patency rates were obtained than with alteplase [110].

Other fibrin-specific plasminogen activators

The physiological single-chain urokinase-type PA (scu-PA, saruplase) and the bacterial PA staphylokinase are also under investigation as fibrin-specific thrombolytic agents.

Single-chain urokinase-type PA

scu-PA is a serine proteinase of 411 amino acids in a single polypeptide chain, with active site triad His^{204}, Asp^{255} and Ser^{356}. The molecule contains an NH_2-terminal growth factor domain and one kringle structure homologous to the five kringles found in plasminogen and the two kringles in t-PA. Conversion of scu-PA to tcu-PA occurs after proteolytic cleavage at position Lys^{158}–Ile^{159}; a fully active tcu-PA derivative is obtained after additional proteolysis by plasmin at position Lys^{135}–Lys^{136}. A low molecular weight form of scu-PA (32 kDa) can be obtained by selective cleavage at position Glu^{143}–Leu^{144} [1].

scu-PA appears to have some intrinsic plasminogen-activating potential, which represents ≤ 0.5% of the catalytic efficiency of tcu-PA [111, 112]. It is not an efficient activator of plasminogen bound to internal lysine residues on intact fibrin, but it develops a higher activity toward plasminogen bound to newly generated COOH-terminal lysine residues on partially degraded fibrin [113]. The fibrin-specificity of scu-PA does not require its conversion to tcu-PA, but appears to be mediated by enhanced binding of plasminogen to partially digested fibrin [114]. In plasma, in the absence of fibrin, scu-PA is stable and does not activate plasminogen; in the presence of a fibrin clot, scu-PA, but not tcu-PA, induces fibrin-specific clot lysis [111]. The intrinsic activity of scu-PA towards fibrin-bound plasminogen may contribute to its fibrin-specificity. Furthermore, α_2-antiplasmin in plasma prevents conversion of scu-PA to tcu-PA outside the clot and thus preserves fibrin-specificity [115].

Following intravenous infusion of natural or recombinant scu-PA in patients with acute myocardial infarction, a biphasic disappearance is observed with initial half-lives in plasma of 4 minutes or 8 minutes, respectively [116, 117]. With a preparation containing 160,000 IU/mg, the dose of saruplase (full-length unglycosylated human recombinant scu-PA obtained from *Escherichia coli*) used successfully in patients with acute myocardial infarction (PRIMI Study) was 20 mg given as a bolus and 60 mg over the next 60 min, immediately followed by an intravenous heparin infusion (20 IU/kg per h) for 72 h [118]. In the LIMITS Study in patients with acute myocardial infarction, the same dose regimen of saruplase was used, but with a prethrombolytic heparin bolus of 5000 IU and an i.v. heparin infusion for 5 days starting 30 min after completion of thrombolysis [119].

Staphylokinase

Staphylokinase, a PA produced by certain strains of *Staphylococcus aureus*, was shown to have profibrinolytic properties about 5 decades ago [120]. Mature staphylokinase consists of 136 amino acids in a single polypeptide chain without disulfide bridges.

Staphylokinase forms a 1:1 stoichiometric complex with plasmin(ogen). It is not an enzyme, and generation of an active site in its equimolar complex with plasminogen requires conversion of plasminogen to plasmin [121, 122]. In plasma, in the absence of fibrin, no significant amounts of plasmin·staphylokinase complex are generated because traces of plasmin are inhibited by α_2-antiplasmin. In the presence of fibrin, generation of the active complex is facilitated because traces of fibrin-bound plasmin are protected from α_2-antiplasmin and inhibition of the complex by α_2-antiplasmin at the clot surface is delayed more than 100-fold [123]. Furthermore, staphylokinase does not bind to a significant extent to plasminogen in circulating plasma, but binds with high affinity to plasmin and to plasminogen which is bound to partially degraded fibrin [124].

Recently, biochemical studies with highly purified recombinant staphylokinase, initial experiments in animal models of thrombosis and pilot studies in patients with acute myocardial infarction or peripheral arterial occlusion have revealed that staphylokinase is an efficient and highly fibrin-specific PA [125, 126].

In patients with acute myocardial infarction treated with an intravenous infusion of 10 mg staphylokinase over 30 min, staphylokinase-related antigen disappeared from plasma in a biphasic manner with a $t1/2\alpha$ of 6.3 min and a $t1/2\beta$ of 37 min, corresponding to a plasma clearance of 270 ml/min [127]. The vast majority of patients with either myocardial infarction [127, 128] or peripheral arterial occlusion [129] developed neutralizing antibodies to staphylokinase, albeit after a long lag phase of 7 to 12 days, that remained elevated well above pretreatment levels for several months after administration [130]. Variants of recombinant staphylokinase with reduced immunogenicity obtained by site-directed mutagenesis have recently been investigated in patients with peripheral arterial occlusion [126].

In the first pilot recanalization studies, patients with acute myocardial infarction were given 10 mg i.v. staphylokinase as a 1 mg bolus followed by infusion of 9 mg over 30 min [127]. In the STAR trial, patients randomized to i.v. staphylokinase were given 10 mg over 30 min in the first half of the study and, following a prospectively planned interim analysis, 20 mg over 30 min in the second half, always with an initial 10% bolus [128]. In a multicenter randomized trial in patients with evolving myocardial infarction, accelerated rt-PA was compared with a double bolus of 15 mg staphylokinase given 30 min apart [126]. In a pilot study in patients with peripheral arterial occlusion, intra-arterial catheter-directed staphylokinase was given as a bolus of 1 mg, followed by a continuous infusion of 0.5 mg per hour, or as a 2 mg bolus followed by an infusion of 1 mg per hour, together with heparin. Complete recanalization was obtained in 83% of the patients after 7.0 ± 0.7 mg staphylokinase infused over 8.7 ± 1.0 hours [129].

From these studies it was concluded that i.v. staphylokinase, combined with heparin and aspirin, is a potent, rapidly acting and complete fibrin-specific thrombolytic agent. Its safety and efficacy for coronary thrombolysis appear to compare well with those of accelerated rt-PA [126].

Summary

Tissue-type PA (t-PA) activates the fibrinolytic system by conversion of the zymogen plasminogen into the active serine proteinase plasmin. It is a 70 kDa single chain serine proteinase which is composed of several structural domains that are involved in different functional properties, including binding to fibrin, rapid *in vivo* clearance and rapid inhibition by plasminogen activator inhibitor-1 (PAI-1). t-PA preferentially activates plasminogen at the fibrin surface and less in the circulation. Plasmin associated with the fibrin surface is protected from inhibition and may efficiently degrade the fibrin of a thrombus without causing significant systemic fibrinolytic activation. This fibrin-specific mechanism of action has triggered great interest in its use for thrombolytic therapy. Recombinant t-PA (Activase®; Actilyse®) is used worldwide mainly in the treatment of patients with acute myocardial infarction and has recently also been approved for treatment of acute ischemic stroke. Several mutants and variants of t-PA with prolonged half-life and resistance to PAI-1 are presently under clinical investigation. In addition, other fibrin-specific recombinant PAs, including single-chain urokinase-type plasminogen activator (scu-PA, saruplase) and staphylokinase, are becoming available for thrombolytic therapy.

References

1 Collen D, Lijnen HR (1991) Basic and clinical aspects of fibrinolysis and thrombolysis. *Blood* 78: 3114–3124

2 Blasi F (1993) Urokinase and urokinase receptor: A paracrine/autocrine system regulating cell migration and invasiveness. *BioEssays* 15: 105–111

3 Astrup T, Permin PM (1947) Fibrinolysis in animal organism. *Nature* 159: 681–682

4 Rijken DC, Wijngaards G, Zaal-de Jong M, Welbergen J (1979) Purification and partial characterization of plasminogen activator from human uterine tissue. *Biochim Biophys Acta* 580: 140–153

5 Rijken DC, Wijngaards G, Welbergen J (1980) Relationship between tissue plasminogen activator and the activators in blood and vascular wall. *Thromb Res* 18: 815–830

6 Rijken DC, Collen D (1981) Purification and characterization of the plasminogen activator secreted by human melanoma cells in culture. *J Biol Chem* 256: 7035–7041

7 Pennica D, Holmes WE, Kohr WJ, Harkins RN, Vehar GA, Ward CA, Bennett WF, Yelverton E, Seeburg PH, Heyneker HL et al (1983) Cloning and expression of human tissue-type plasminogen activator cDNA in *E. coli*. *Nature* 301: 214–221

8 Collen D, Stassen JM, Marafino BJ, Builder S, De Cock F, Ogez J, Tajiri D, Pennica D, Bennett WF, Salwa J (1984) Biological properties of human tissue-type plasminogen activator obtained by expression of recombinant DNA in mammalian cells. *J Pharmacol Exp Ther* 231: 146–152

9 Tachias K, Madison EL (1997) Converting tissue type plasminogen activator into a zymogen. *J Biol Chem* 272: 28–31

10 Rajput B, Degen SF, Reich E, Waller EK, Axelrod J, Eddy RL, Shows TB (1985) Chromosomal locations of human tissue plasminogen activator and urokinase genes. *Science* 230: 672–674

11 Patthy L (1985) Evolution of the proteases of blood coagulation and fibrinolysis by assembly from modules. *Cell* 41: 657–663

12 Feng P, Ohlsson M, Ny T (1990) The structure of the TATA-less rat tissue-type plasminogen activator gene. Species-specific sequence divergences in the promoter predict differences in regulation of gene expression. *J Biol Chem* 265: 2022–2027

13 Kooistra T, Bosma PJ, Toet K, Cohen LH, Griffioen M, van den Berg E, le Clercq L (1991) Role of protein kinase C and cyclic adenosine monophosphate in the regulation of tissue-type plasminogen activator, plasminogen activator inhibitor-1, and platelet-derived growth factor mRNA levels in human endothelial cells. Possible involvement of proto-oncogenes c-jun and c-fos. *Arterioscler Thromb* 11: 1042–1052

14 Medcalf RL, Rueegg M, Schleuning WD (1990) A DNA motif related to the cAMP-responsive element and an exon-located activator protein-2 binding site in the human tissue-type plasminogen activator gene promoter cooperate in basal expression and convey activation by phorbol ester and cAMP. *J Biol Chem* 265: 14 618–14 626

15 Ludwig M, Wohn KD, Schleuning WD, Olek K (1992) Allelic dimorphism in the human tissue-type plasminogen activator (tPA) gene as a result of an Alu insertion/deletion event. *Hum Genet* 88: 388–392

16 Van Hinsbergh VWM, Kooistra T, Emeis JJ, Koolwijk P (1991) Regulation of plasminogen activator production by endothelial cells: role in fibrinolysis and local proteolysis. *Int J Radiat Biol* 60: 261–272

17 Smith D, Gilbert M, Owen WG (1985) Tissue plasminogen activator release *in vivo* in response to vasoactive agents. *Blood* 66: 835–839

18 Newby DE, Wright RA, Dawson P, Ludlam CA, Boon NA, Fox KAA, Webb DJ (1998) The L-arginine/nitric oxide pathway contributes to the acute release of tissue plasminogen activator *in vivo* in man. *Cardiovasc Res* 38: 485–492

19 Gelehrter TD, Sznycer-Laszuk R (1986) Thrombin induction of plasminogen activator-inhibitor in cultured human endothelial cells. *J Clin Invest* 77: 165–169

20 Hanss M, Collen D (1987) Secretion of tissue-type plasminogen activator and plasminogen activator inhibitor by cultured human endothelial cells: modulation by thrombin, endotoxin and histamine. *J Lab Clin Med* 109: 97–104

21 Medcalf RL, Van den Berg E, Schleuning WD (1988) Glucocorticoid-modulated gene expression of tissue- and urinary-type plasminogen activator and plasminogen activator inhibitor 1 and 2. *J Cell Biol* 106: 971–978

22 Kooistra T, Van den Berg J, Töns A, Platenburg G, Rijken DC, van den Berg E (1987) Butyrate

stimulates tissue-type plasminogen activator synthesis in cultured human endothelial cells. *Biochem J* 247: 605–612
23 Moscatelli D (1986) Urokinase-type and tissue-type plasminogen activators have different distributions in cultured bovine capillary endothelial cells. *J Cell Biochem* 30: 19–29
24 Montesano R, Vassalli JD, Baird A, Guillemin R, Orci L (1986) Basic fibroblast growth factor induces angiogenesis *in vitro*. *Proc Natl Acad Sci USA* 83: 7297–7301
25 Sakata Y, Curriden S, Lawrence D, Griffin JH, Loskutoff DJ (1985) Activated protein C stimulates the fibrinolytic activity of cultured endothelial cells and decreases antiactivator activity. *Proc Natl Acad Sci USA* 82: 1121–1125
26 Laug WE (1983) Ethyl alcohol enhances plasminogen activator secretion by endothelial cells. *JAMA* 250: 772–776
27 Kooistra T, Opdenberg JP, Toet K, Hendriks HF, van den Hoogen RM, Emeis JJ (1991) Stimulation of tissue-type plasminogen activator synthesis by retinoids in cultured human endothelial cells and rat tissues *in vivo*. *Thromb Haemost* 65: 565–572
28 Thompson EA, Nelles L, Collen D (1991) Effect of retinoic acid on the synthesis of tissue-type plasminogen activator and plasminogen activator inhibitor-1 in human endothelial cells. *Eur J Biochem* 201: 627–632
29 Gelehrter TD, Sznycer-Laszuk R, Zeheb R, Cwikel BJ (1987) Dexamethasone inhibition of tissue-type plasminogen activator (t-PA) activity: paradoxical induction of both t-PA antigen and plasminogen activator inhibitor. *Mol Endocrinol* 1: 97–101
30 Bulens F, Ibanez-Tallon I, Van Acker P, De Vriese A, Nelles L, Belayew A, Collen D (1995) Retinoic acid induction of human tissue-type plasminogen activator (t-PA) gene expression via a direct repeat element (DR5) located at -7 kilobases. *J Biol Chem* 270: 7167–7175
31 Bulens F, Merchiers P, Ibanes-Tallon I, De Vriese A, Nelles L, Claessens F, Belayew A, Collen D (1997) Identification of a multihormone responsive enhancer far upstream from the human tissue-type plasminogen activator gene. *J Biol Chem* 272: 663–671
32 Lansink M, Kooistra T (1996) Stimulation of tissue-type plasminogen activator expression by retinoic acid in human endothelial cells requires retinoic acid receptor β_2 induction. *Blood* 88: 531–541
33 Levin EG, Santell L (1988) Stimulation and desensitization of tissue plasminogen activator release from human endothelial cells. *J Biol Chem* 263: 9360–9365
34 Levin EG, Marotti KR, Santell L (1989) Protein kinase C and the stimulation of tissue plasminogen activator release from human endothelial cells. Dependence on the elevation of messenger RNA. *J Biol Chem* 264: 16 030–16 036
35 Arts J, Herr I, Lansink M, Angel P, Kooistra T (1997) Cell-type specific DNA-protein interactions at the tissue-type plasminogen activator promoter in human endothelial and HeLa cells *in vivo* and *in vitro*. *Nucl Acid Res* 25: 311–317
36 Jaklitsch MT, Biro S, Casscells W, Dichek DA (1993) Transduced endothelial cells expressing high levels of tissue plasminogen activator have an unaltered phenotype *in vitro*. *J Cell Physiol* 154: 207–216
37 Shi GY, Hau JS, Wang SJ, Wu IS, Chang BI, Lin MT, Chow YH, Chang WC, Wing LY, Jen CY et al (1992) Plasmin and the regulation of tissue-type plasminogen activator biosynthesis in human endothelial cells. *J Biol Chem* 267: 19 363–19 368
38 Hoylaerts M, Rijken DC, Lijnen HR, Collen D (1982) Kinetics of the activation of plasminogen by human tissue plasminogen activator. Role of fibrin. *J Biol Chem* 257: 2912–2919
39 Wiman B, Collen D (1978) Molecular mechanism of physiological fibrinolysis. *Nature* 272: 549–550
40 Wiman B, Collen D (1978) On the kinetics of the reaction between human antiplasmin and plasmin. *Eur J Biochem* 84: 573–578
41 Thorsen S (1992) The mechanism of plasminogen activation and the variability of the fibrin effector during tissue-type plasminogen activator-mediated fibrinolysis. *Ann N Y Acad Sci* 667: 52–63
42 Andreasen PA, Petersen LC, Danø K (1991) Diversity in catalytic properties of single-chain and two-chain tissue-type plasminogen activator. *Fibrinolysis* 5: 207–215
43 McLean JW, Tomlinson JE, Kuang WJ, Eaton DL, Chen EY, Fless GM, Scanu AM, Lawn RM (1987) cDNA sequence of human apolipoprotein(a) is homologous to plasminogen. *Nature* 330: 132–137
44 Harpel PC, Gordon BR, Parker TS (1989) Plasmin catalyzes binding of lipoprotein (a) to immobilized fibrinogen and fibrin. *Proc Natl Acad Sci USA* 86: 3847–3851

45 Fleury V, Anglès-Cano (1991) Characterization of the binding of plasminogen to fibrin surfaces: the role of carboxy-terminal lysines. *Biochemistry* 30: 7630–7638
46 Loscalzo J, Weinfeld M, Fless GM, Scanu AM (1990) Lipoprotein(a), fibrin binding and plasminogen activation. *Arteriosclerosis* 10: 240–245
47 Edelberg JM, Gonzales-Gronow M, Pizzo SV (1990) Lipoprotein(a) inhibition of plasminogen activation by tissue-type plasminogen activator. *Thromb Res* 57: 155–162
48 Liu JN, Harpel PC, Pannell R, Gurewich V (1993) Lipoprotein(a): A kinetic study of its influence on fibrin-dependent plasminogen activation by prourokinase or tissue plasminogen activator. *Biochemistry* 32: 9694–9700
49 Bajzar L, Manuel R, Nesheim ME (1995) Purification and characterization of TAFI, a thrombin-activable fibrinolysis inhibitor. *J Biol Chem* 270: 14 477–14 484
50 Eaton DL, Malloy BE, Tsai SP, Henzel W, Drayna D (1991) Isolation, molecular cloning, and partial characterization of a novel carboxypeptidase B from human plasma. *J Biol Chem* 266: 21 833–21 838
51 Nesheim M, Wang W, Boffa M, Nagashima M, Morser J, Bajza L (1997) Thrombin, thrombomodulin and TAFI in the molecular link between coagulation and fibrinolysis. *Thromb Haemost* 78: 386–391
52 Verstraete M, Su CAPF, Tanswell P, Feuerer W, Collen D (1986) Pharmacokinetics and effects of fibrinolytic and coagulation parameters of two doses of recombinant tissue-type plasminogen activator in healthy volunteers. *Thromb Haemost* 56: 1–5
53 Garabedian HD, Gold HK, Leinbach RC, Johns JA, Yasuda T, Kanke M, Collen D (1987) Comparative properties of two clinical preparations of recombinant human tissue-type plasminogen activator in patients with acute myocardial infarction. *J Amer Coll Cardiol* 9: 599–607
54 Collen D, Lijnen HR (1986) The fibrinolytic system in man. *CRC. Crit Rev Haemat Oncol* 4: 249–301
55 Sprengers ED, Kluft C (1987) Plasminogen activator inhibitors. *Blood* 69: 381–387
56 Ny T, Sawdey M, Lawrence D, Millan JL, Loskutoff DJ (1986) Cloning and sequence of a cDNA coding for the human β-migrating endothelial-cell-type plasminogen activator inhibitor. *Proc Natl Acad Sci USA* 83: 6776–6780
57 Pannekoek H, Veerman H, Lambers H, Diergaarde P, Verweij CL, van Zonneveld AJ, van Mourik JA (1986) Endothelial plasminogen activator inhibitor (PAI): a new member of the serpin gene family. *EMBO J* 5: 2539–2544
58 Declerck PJ, De Mol M, Alessi MC, Baudner S, Pâques EP, Preissner KT, Müller-Berghaus G, Collen D (1988) Purification and characterization of a plasminogen activator inhibitor-1 binding protein from human plasma. Identification as a multimeric form of S protein (Vitronectin). *J Biol Chem* 263: 15 454–15 461
59 Kruithof EKO (1988) Plasminogen activator inhibitors – a review. *Enzyme* 40: 113–121
60 Thorsen S, Philips M, Selmer J, Lecander I, Astedt B (1988) Kinetics of inhibition of tissue-type and urokinase-type plasminogen activator by plasminogen-activator inhibitor type 1 and type 2. *Eur J Biochem* 175: 33–39
61 Madison EL, Goldsmith EJ, Gerard RD, Gething MJ, Sambrook JF (1989) Serpin-resistant mutants of human tissue-type plasminogen activator. *Nature* 339: 721–724
62 Chmielewska J, Ranby M, Wiman B (1988) Kinetics of the inhibition of plasminogen activators by the plasminogen-activator inhibitor. Evidence for 'second site' interactions. *Biochem J* 251: 327–332
63 Wagner OF, de Vries C, Hohmann C, Veerman H, Pannekoek H (1989) Interaction between plasminogen activator inhibitor type 1 (PAI-1) bound to fibrin and either tissue-type plasminogen activator (t-PA) or urokinase-type plasminogen activator (u-PA). *J Clin Invest* 84: 647–655
64 Reilly CF, Hutzelmann JE (1992) Plasminogen activator inhibitor-1 binds to fibrin and inhibits tissue-type plasminogen activator-mediated fibrin dissolution. *J Biol Chem* 267: 17 128–17 135
65 Kruithof EKO, Gudinchet A, Bachmann F (1988) Plasminogen activator inhibitor 1 and plasminogen activator inhibitor 2 in various disease states. *Thromb Haemost* 59: 7–12
66 Schlandt RC (Chairman) (1994) Reperfusion in acute myocardial infarction. *Circulation* 90: 2091–2102
67 Seifried E, Tanswell P, Rijken DC, Barrett-Bergshoeff MM, Su CA, Kluft C (1988) Pharmacokinetics of antigen and activity of recombinant tissue-type plasminogen activator after infusion in healthy volunteers. *Arzneim-Forsch* 38: 418–422
68 Lijnen HR, Bachmann F, Collen D, Ellis V, Pannekoek H, Rijken DC, Thorsen S (1994)

Mechanisms of plasminogen activation. *J Int Med* 236: 415–424
69 Van de Werf F, Arnold AER, for the European Cooperative Study Group (1988) Effect of intravenous tissue plasminogen activator on infarct size, left ventricular function and survival in patients with acute myocardial infarction. *Brit Med J* 297: 1374–1379
70 Neuhaus KL, Feuerer W, Jeep-Tebbe S, Niederer W, Vogt A, Tebbe U (1989) Improved thrombolysis with a modified dose regimen of recombinant tissue-type plasminogen activator. *J Amer Coll Cardiol* 14: 1566–1569
71 The GUSTOInvestigators (1993) An international randomized trial comparing four thrombolytic strategies for acute myocardial infarction. *N Engl J Med* 329: 673–682
72 Collins R, Peto R, Baigent C, Sleight P (1997) Aspirin, heparin, and fibrinolytic therapy in suspected acute myocardial infarction. *N Engl J Med* 336: 847–860
73 Califf RM, White HD, Van de Werf F, Sadowski A, Armstrong PW, Vahanian A, Simoons ML, Simes RJ, Lee KL, Topol EJ (1996) One-year results from the Global Utilization of Streptokinase and TPA for Occluded Coronary Arteries (GUSTO-I) Trial. *Circulation* 4: 1233–1238
74 Califf RM, Woodlief LH, Harrell FE Jr, Lee KL, White HD, Guerci A, Barbash GI, Simes RJ, Weaver WD, Simoons ML et al (1997) Selection of thrombolytic therapy for individual patients: development of a clinical model. *Amer Heart J* 133: 630–639
75 Van de Werf F, on behalf of the COBALTInvestigators (1997) A comparison of continuous infusion of alteplase with double-bolus administration for acute myocardial infarction. The Continuous Infusion *versus* Double-Bolus Administration of Alteplase (COBALT). *N Engl J Med* 337: 1124–1130
76 Becker RC (1997) Editorial. *Stroke* 28: 1657–1659
77 Hacke W, Kaste M, Fieschi C, Toni D, Lesaffre E, von Kummer R, Boysen G, Bluhmki E, Hixter G, Mahagne MH et al, for the ECASSStudy Group (1995) Intravenous thrombolysis with recombinant tissue plasminogen activator for acute hemispheric stroke. The European Cooperative Acute Stroke Study (ECASS). *JAMA* 274: 1017–1025
78 The National Institute for Neurological Disorders, Stroke rt-PAStroke Study Group (1995) Tissue plasminogen activator for acute ischemic stroke. *N Engl J Med* 333: 1581–1587
79 Lijnen HR, Collen D (1991) Strategies for the improvement of thrombolytic agents. *Thromb Haemost* 66: 88–110
80 Fay WP, Eitzman DT, Shapiro AD, Madison EL, Ginsburg D (1994) Platelets inhibit fibrinolysis *in vitro* by both plasminogen activator inhibitor-1-dependent and -independent mechanisms. *Blood* 83: 351–361
81 Kohnert U, Rudolph R, Verheijen JH, Weening-Verhoeff EJ, Stern A, Opitz U, Martin U, Lill H, Prinz H, Lechner M et al (1992) Biochemical properties of the kringle 2 and protease domains are maintained in the refolded t-PA deletion variant BM 06.022. *Protein Eng* 5: 93–100
82 Stürzebecher J, Neumann U, Kohnert U, Kresse GB, Fischer S (1992) Mapping of the catalytic site of CHO-t-PA and the t-PA variant BM 06.022 by synthetic inhibitors and substrates. *Protein Sci* 1: 1007–1013
83 Hajjar KA (1991) The endothelial cell tissue plasminogen activator receptor. Specific interaction with plasminogen. *J Biol Chem* 266: 21 962–21 970
84 Martin U, Fischer S, Kohnert U, Opitz U, Rudolph R, Sponer G, Stern A, Strein K (1991) Thrombolysis with an *Escherichia coli*-produced recombinant plasminogen activator (BM 06.022) in the rabbit model of jugular vein thrombosis. *Thromb Haemost* 65: 560–564
85 Martin U, van Möllendorf E, Akpan W, Kientsch Engel R, Kaufmann B, Neugebauer G (1991) Dose-ranging study of the novel recombinant plasminogen activator BM 06.022 in healthy volunteers. *Clin Pharmacol Ther* 50: 429–436
86 Müller M, Haerer W, Ellbrück D, for the GRECOStudy Group (1992) Pharmacokinetics and effects on the hemostatic system of bolus application of a novel recombinant plasminogen activator in AMI patients. *Fibrinolysis* 6 (Suppl 2): 26 (Abstract 63), 1992
87 Neuhaus KL, von Essen R, Vogt A, Tebbe U, Rustige J, Wagner HJ, Appel KF, Stienen U, Konig R, Meyer Sabellek W (1994) Dose finding with a novel recombinant plasminogen activator (BM 06.022) in patients with acute myocardial infarction: results of the German Recombinant Plasminogen Activator Study. *J Amer Coll Cardiol* 24: 55–60
88 Tebbe U, von Essen R, Smolarz A, Limbourg P, Rox J, Rustige J, Vogt A, Wagner J, Meyer Sabellek W, Neuhaus KL (1993) Open, noncontrolled dose-finding study with a novel recombinant plasminogen activator (BM 06.022) given as a double bolus in patients with acute myocardial infarction. *Amer J Cardiol* 72: 518–524

89 Smalling RW, Bode C, Kalbfleisch J, Sen S, Limbourg P, Forycki F, Habib G, Feldman R, Hohnloser S, Seals A (1995) More rapid, complete, and stable coronary thrombolysis with bolus administration of reteplase compared with alteplase infusion in acute myocardial infarction. RAPID Investigators. *Circulation* 91: 2725–2732
90 Bode C, Smalling RW, Berg G, Burnett C, Lorch G, Kalbfleisch JM, Chernoff R, Christie LG, Feldman RL, Seals AA et al (1996) Randomized comparison of coronary thrombolysis achieved with double-bolus reteplase (recombinant plasminogen activator) and front-loaded, accelerated alteplase (recombinant tissue plasminogen activator) in patients with acute myocardial infarction. The RAPID II Investigators. *Circulation* 94: 891–898
91 International Joint Efficacy Comparison of Thrombolytics (1995) Randomised, double-blind comparison to reteplase double-bolus administration with streptokinase in acute myocardial infarction (INJECT): trial to investigate equivalence. *Lancet* 346: 329–336
92 The GUSTO-III investigators (1997) A comparison of reteplase with alteplase for acute myocardial infarction. *N Engl J Med* 337: 1118–1123
93 Keyt BA, Paoni NF, Refino CJ, Berleau L, Nguyen H, Chow A, Lai J, Pena L, Pater C, Ogez J (1994) A faster-acting and more potent form of tissue plasminogen activator. *Proc Natl Acad Sci USA* 91: 3670–3674
94 Paoni NF, Keyt BA, Refino CJ, Chow AM, Nguyen HV, Berleau LT, Badillo J, Pena LC, Brady K, Wurm FM et al (1993) A slow clearing, fibrin-specific, PAI-1 resistant variant of t-PA (T103N,KHRR296-299AAAA). *Thromb Haemost* 70: 307–312
95 Refino CJ, Paoni NF, Keyt BA, Pater CS, Badillo JM, Wurm FM, Ogez J, Bennett WF (1993) A variant of t-PA (T103N, KHRR 296-299 AAAA) that, by bolus, has increased potency and decreased systemic activation of plasminogen. *Thromb Haemost* 70: 313–319
96 Collen D, Stassen JM, Yasuda T, Refino CJ, Paoni N, Keyt B, Roskams T, Guerrero JL, Lijnen HR, Gold HK et al (1994) Comparative thrombolytic properties of tissue-type plasminogen activator and of a plasminogen activator inhibitor-1-resistant glycosylation variant, in a combined arterial and venous thrombosis model in the dog. *Thromb Haemost* 72: 98–104
97 Benedict CR, Refino CJ, Keyt BA, Pakala R, Paoni NF, Thomas GR, Bennett WF (1995) New variant of tissue plasminogen activator (t-PA) with enhanced efficacy and lower incidence of bleeding compared with recombinant human t-PA. *Circulation* 92: 3032–3040
98 Cannon CP, McCabe CH, Gibson CM, Ghali M, Sequeira RF, McKendall GR, Breed J, Modi NB, Fox NL, Tracy RP et al (1997) TNK-tissue plasminogen activator in acute myocardial infarction: results of the Thrombolysis in Myocardial Infarction (TIMI) 10A dose-ranging trial. *Circulation* 95: 351–356
99 Cannon CP, McCabe CH, Gibson MC, Adgey JA, Sweiger MJ, Sequeira RF, Muller HS, McCluskey ER, Fox NL, Van de Werf F et al (1997) TNK-tissue plasminogen activator compared with front-loaded tissue plasminogen activator in acute myocardial infarction: primary results of the TIMI-10B trial. *Circulation* 96 (Suppl I): 206
100 Van de Werf F, for the ASSENT-1 investigators (1997) The preliminary results of the ASSENT-1 trial. Presented at the XIXth Congress of the European Society of Cardiology, Stockholm, August 24–28, 1997
101 Gardell SJ, Hare TR, Bergum PW, Cuca GC, O'Neill-Palladino L, Zavodny SM (1990) Vampire bat salivary plasminogen activator is quiescent in human plasma in the absence of fibrin unlike human tissue plasminogen activator. *Blood* 76: 2560–2564
102 Kratzschmar J, Haendler B, Langer G, Boidol W, Bringmann P, Alagon A, Donner P, Schleuning WD (1991) The plasminogen activator family from the salivary gland of the vampire bat *Desmodus rotundus*: cloning and expression. *Gene* 105: 229–237
103 Bergum PW, Gardell SJ (1992) Vampire bat salivary plasminogen activator exhibits a strict and fastidious requirement for polymeric fibrin as its cofactor, unlike human tissue-type plasminogen activator. A kinetic analysis. *J Biol Chem* 267: 17 726–17 731
104 Gardell SJ, Ramjit DR, Stabilito II, Fujita T, Lynch JJ, Cuca GC, Jain D, Wang SP, Tung JS, Mark GE et al (1991) Effective thrombolysis without marked plasminemia after bolus intravenous administration of vampire bat salivary plasminogen activator in rabbits. *Circulation* 84: 244–253
105 Mellot MJ, Stabilito II, Holahan MA, Cuca GC, Wang S, Li P, Barrett JS, Lynch JJ, Gardell SJ (1992) Vampire bat salivary plasminogen activator promotes rapid and sustained reperfusion without concomitant systemic plasminogen activation in a canine model of arterial thrombosis. *Arterioscler Thromb* 12: 212–221
106 Mellot MJ, Ramjit DR, Stabilito II, Hare TR, Senderak ET, Lynch JJ Jr, Gardell SJ (1995)

Vampire bat salivary plasminogen activator evokes minimal bleeding relative to tissue-type plasminogen activator as assessed by a rabbit cuticle bleeding time model. *Thromb Haemost* 73: 478–483
107 Witt W, Baldus B, Bringmann P, Cashion L, Donner P, Schleuning WD (1992) Thrombolytic properties of *Desmodus rotundus* (vampire bat) salivary plasminogen activator in experimental pulmonary embolism in rats. *Blood* 79: 1213–1217
108 Witt W, Maass B, Baldus B, Hildebrand M, Donner P, Schleuning WD (1994) Coronary thrombolysis with *Desmodus* salivary plasminogen activator in dogs. Fast and persistent recanalization by intravenous bolus administration. *Circulation* 90: 421–426
109 Larsen GR, Timony GA, Horgan PG, Barone KM, Henson KS, Argus LB, Stoudemire JB (1991) Protein engineering of novel plasminogen activators with increased thrombolytic potency in rabbits relative to activase. *J Biol Chem* 266: 8156–8161
110 Thadani U. INTIME trial. Presented at the Tenth Annual Myocardial Reperfusion Symposium, American College of Cardiology, Anaheim, CA, March 15, 1997
111 Gurewich V, Pannell R, Louie S, Kelley P, Suddith RL, Greenlee R (1984) Effective and fibrin-specific clot lysis by a zymogen precursor form of urokinase (pro-urokinase). A study *in vitro* and in two animal species. *J Clin Invest* 73: 1731–1739
112 Lijnen HR, Van Hoef B, Nelles L, Collen D (1990) Plasminogen activation with single-chain urokinase-type plasminogen activator (scu-PA). Studies with active site mutagenized plasminogen ($Ser^{740} \rightarrow Ala$) and plasmin resistant scu-PA ($Lys^{158} \rightarrow Glu$). *J Biol Chem* 265: 5232–5236
113 Fleury V, Gurewich V, Anglés-Cano E (1993) A study of the activation of fibrin-bound plasminogen by tissue-type plasminogen activator, single chain urokinase and sequential combinations of the activators. *Fibrinolysis* 7: 87–96
114 Fleury V, Lijnen HR, Anglés-Cano E (1993) Mechanism of the enhanced intrinsic activity of single-chain urokinase-type plasminogen activator during ongoing fibrinolysis. *J Biol Chem* 268: 18 554–18 559
115 Declerck PJ, Lijnen HR, Verstreken M, Collen D (1991) Role of α_2-antiplasmin in fibrin-specific clot lysis with single-chain urokinase-type plasminogen activator in human plasma. *Thromb Haemost* 65: 394–398
116 Van de Werf F, Nobuhara M, Collen D (1986) Coronary thrombolysis with human single chain urokinase-type plasminogen activator (scu-PA) in patients with acute myocardial infarction. *Ann Intern Med* 104: 345–348
117 Van de Werf F, Vanhaecke J, De Geest H, Verstraete M, Collen D (1986) Coronary thrombolysis with recombinant single-chain urokinase-type plasminogen activator (rscu-PA) in patients with acute myocardial infarction. *Circulation* 74: 1066–1070
118 PRIMITrial Study Group (1989) Randomised double-blind trial of recombinant pro-urokinase against streptokinase in acute myocardial infarction. *Lancet* 1: 863–868
119 Tebbe U, Windeler J, Boesl I, Hoffmann H, Wojcikj, Ashmawy M, Rudiger-Schwarz E, von Loewis P, Rosemeyer P, Hopkins G et al, behalf of the LIMITSStudy Group (1995) Thrombolysis with recombinant unglycosylated single-chain urokinase-type plasminogen activator (Saruplase) in acute myocardial infarction: influence on early patency rate (LIMITS Study). *J Amer Coll Cardiol* 26: 365–373
120 Lack CH (1948) Staphylokinase: an activator of plasma protease. *Nature* 161: 559–560
121 Lijnen HR, Van Hoef B, De Cock F, Okada K, Ueshima S, Matsuo O, Collen D (1991) On the mechanism of fibrin-specific plasminogen activation by staphylokinase. *J Biol Chem* 266: 11 826–11 832
122 Collen D, Schlott B, Engelborghs Y, Van Hoef B, Hartmann M, Lijnen HR, Behnke D (1993) On the mechanism of the activation of human plasminogen by recombinant staphylokinase. *J Biol Chem* 268: 8284–8289
123 Silence K, Collen D, Lijnen HR (1993) Regulation by alpha 2-antiplasmin and fibrin of the activation of plasminogen with recombinant staphylokinase in plasma. *Blood* 82: 1175–1183
124 Sakharov DV, Lijnen HR, Rijken DC (1996) Interactions between staphylokinase, plasmin(ogen) and fibr*In*: staphylokinase discriminates between free plasminogen and plasminogen bound to partially degraded fibrin. *J Biol Chem* 271: 27 912–27 918
125 Lijnen HR, Collen D (1996) Staphylokinase, a fibrin-specific bacterial plasminogen activator. *Fibrinolysis* 10: 119–126
126 Collen D (1998) Staphylokinase: a potent, uniquely fibrin-selective thrombolytic agent. *Nat Med* 4: 279–284

127 Collen D, Van de Werf F (1993) Coronary thrombolysis with recombinant staphylokinase in patients with evolving myocardial infarction. *Circulation* 87: 1850–1853
128 Vanderschueren S, Barrios L, Kerdsinchai P, Van den Heuvel P, Hermans L, Vrolix M, De Man F, Benit E, Muyldermans L, Collen D et al (1995) A randomized trial of recombinant staphylokinase *versus* alteplase for coronary artery patency in acute myocardial infarction. *Circulation* 92: 2044–2049
129 Vanderschueren S, Stockx L, Wilms G, Lacroix H, Verhaeghe R, Vermylen J, Collen D (1995) Thrombolytic therapy of peripheral arterial occlusion with recombinant staphylokinase. *Circulation* 92: 2050–2057
130 Vanderschueren SMF, Stassen JM, Collen D (1994) On the immunogenicity of recombinant staphylokinase in patients and in animal models. *Thromb Haemost* 72: 297–301

Proteins with new functions: protein engineering

Recombinant Protein Drugs
ed. by P. Buckel

Designing immunocytokines: genetically engineered fusion proteins for targeted immune therapy

Stephen D. Gillies

Lexigen Pharmaceuticals Corp., Lexington, MA, USA

Introduction

The use of antibodies and antibody-based therapeutic agents has accelerated in the last ten years through the combined technological advances in hybridoma technology and genetic engineering. In fact, molecular biological approaches have now been applied to the antibody engineering field in ways that both enhance the hybridoma approach, e.g., through the generation of transgenic mice capable of expressing human immunoglobulins and, in some cases, by replacing the use of animals altogether. The latter approaches involve the use of phage display or *in vitro* molecular evolution technologies that use antigen binding selection coupled with linked gene sequence identification to isolate binding proteins and their coding sequences from enormously complex mixtures of randomly generated molecules.

Along with the development of the binding components of antibody molecules, the directed evolution of the antibody "payload" has progressed from the original "magic bullet" concept of Paul Ehrlich [1], proposed at the early part of this century, to virtually any kind of agent capable of being attached chemically or genetically to an immunoglobulin molecule. As more sophisticated genetic methods have been developed to break down antibodies into their component parts, the trend toward molecular minimalism has resulted in proteins of the smallest possible size that contain the desired biological components. Thus, the complete variable region binding component of a 150 kD antibody can be compressed into a single polypeptide of 25 kD called a single-chain FV (scFV) molecule. Such antigen-binding units can be linked genetically to any type of polypeptide to form a fusion protein with both antibody targeting activity and the activity of the second protein. In the context of the magic bullet approach, the second protein would logically be a type of toxin. Examples might include Diptheria toxin and the *Pseudomonas* exotoxin.

While many of these molecular biological techniques can prove useful in the laboratory and, in many cases, in animal models of human disease, the quantum leap to the treatment of human disease is, more often than not, problematic. This concept could not be more true than for the subject matter of this chapter. The targeted delivery of cytokines to disease sites through systemic administration attempts to achieve what has been a major stumbling block in the clinical use of most cytokines: the fact that these molecules maintain their selectivity of response through their highly localized release by effector cells at disease sites. Systemic administration of cytokines, on the other hand, generally achieve high concentrations in the circulation but often fail to achieve optimal concentration at the intended target sites, e.g., in the tumor microenvironment during anti-tumor therapy.

Thus, the simple combination of a targeting component and a cytokine, genetically fused into a single recombinant molecule, addresses the basic principles of the desired biological features that can be demonstrated in the laboratory setting. How this translates into a useful biopharmaceutical drug is a far more complex issue and relates to the overall composition of the specific fusion protein, its resultant pharmacological and pharmacokinetic properties and especially the nature of the cytokine itself. Important considerations include the fusion protein's circulating half-life, the degree of targeting to the intended disease site, the extent of systemic *versus* local cytokine response and the mechanism and route of clearance of the drug.

This overview will describe the brief history of what we have termed "immunocytokines", including the various approaches that have been taken for their molecular construction. It will also focus on pre-clinical animal studies designed not only to demonstrate efficacy in rodents but also to optimize their design for eventual human clinical use.

Construction of immunocytokines

The first reports of genetically engineered antibody-cytokine fusion proteins involved fusions with lymphotoxin (now called TNF-β), TNF-α and IL-2 [2–4]. In these first three articles, several different approaches were used to optimize biological activity and several points shed light on how antibody structure might play a role in the activity of the fused cytokine.

In the studies with lymphotoxin, two constructs were compared in which the cytokine was genetically fused to the end of either the CH2 or CH3 domains of the H chain (see Fig. 1 for a diagram of the various forms of immunocytokines). In other words, lymphotoxin replaced the CH3 domain in the first construct and was added as an extra domain at the carboxyl terminus of the CH3 domain in the second. The function of the CH3 domain in the immunoglobulin molecule is to provide structural interactions leading to dimerization of the two H chains, so the replacement of this domain with another unrelated protein domain would have unpredictable consequences. Since it was known that lymphotoxin (and TNF-α, as well) forms trimers in solution [5], it was thought that this function could lead to a similar trimeric structure in the constructs fused to the CH2 domain and provide the structural requirements for lymphotoxin bioactivity. Fusion to the CH3 domain, on the

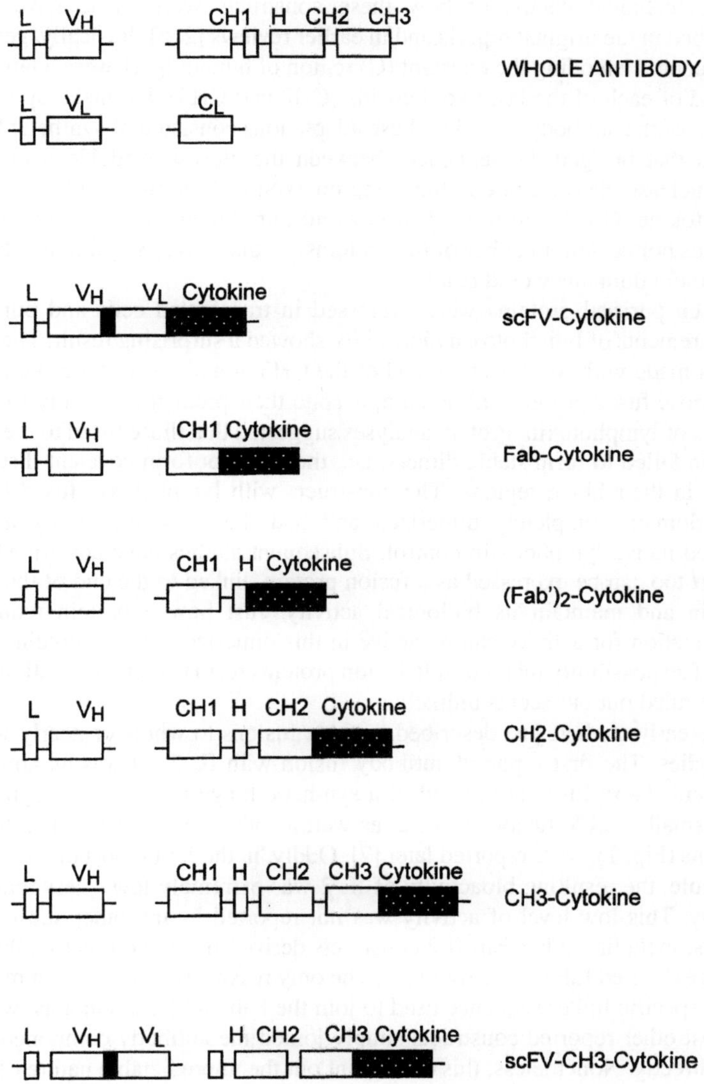

Figure 1. Genetic constructs encoding different forms of antibody-cytokine fusion proteins. Open boxes represent antibody domain coding regions. Dotted boxes represent cytokine cDNA coding regions. The light chain coding regions are shown for the whole antibody only, but would be co-expressed together with other constructs containing VH and CH1 exons. The separate light chain is not needed for expression of the scFV-based constructs.

other hand, might limit the chain association to only dimers of the fused H chains and reduce the activity accordingly.

The technical details of how these constructs were made have been described in the original reports and in earlier reviews [2, 6]. Basically, genomic sequences encoding the constant (C) region of human IgG1 were adapted at the end of each of the last two domains (CH2 and CH3) that make up the Fc portion of the antibody (Fig. 1). These adaptations consisted of synthetic DNA linkers that bridged the sequences between the closest available restriction endonuclease cleavage site in the C region exon and the first available site in the cytokine. Great care was taken to avoid introducing any new amino acid residues not present in either of the proteins, so that a precise joining between the protein domains would result.

When purified proteins were expressed in transfected cells and purified, measurements of lymphotoxin bioactivity showed a surprising result. The constructs made with fusions at the end of the CH3 domain were far more active than those fused at the CH2 domain, despite their predicted inability to form trimers of lymphotoxin. Protein analyses suggested that those fused to the CH2 domain failed to form stable dimers, i.e., they did not form covalent disulfide bonds in their hinge regions. The constructs with lymphotoxin fused to the CH3 domain completely dimerized and had the same bioactivity as the unfused native lymphotoxin control. Subsequent studies have confirmed that TNF-α too can be expressed as a fusion protein, linked to the end of the CH3 domain and maintain its biological activity. Just how a protein requiring trimerization for activity can be active in this dimerized fusion protein is not clear. The possibility that multiple fusion proteins form trimers in solution cannot be ruled out but seems unlikely.

The early studies, just described, involve fusions to whole or nearly whole antibodies. The first reported antibody fusion with IL-2 [4] was an antibody fragment (Fab), fused at the end of a synthetic hinge region to the cytokine. Even smaller scFV fusions to IL-2, as well as other forms of Fab-IL2 fusion proteins (Fig. 1), were reported later [7]. Oddly, in the first report of a Fab-IL2 molecule, the resulting bioactivity of IL-2 was extremely low – less than 1% activity. This low level of activity was not reported in any other subsequent studies, including other Fab-IL2 constructs derived from two other antibodies which exhibited full IL-2 activity [8]. The only reasonable explanation may lie in the specific linker sequence used to join the Fab and IL-2 domains, whereas most other reported constructs simply joined the antibody component and IL-2 directly. Nonetheless, this does point out the unpredictable nature of protein engineering and the possible consequences of fusing domains of unrelated proteins together into one molecule.

A comparison of three different forms of antibody-IL2 fusions, attached without synthetic linker sequences at the carboxyl termini of either the CH1, CH2 or CH3 domains, had full IL-2 activity as measured by the ability to stimulate the proliferation of either the mouse CTLL-2 cell line, or a human tumor-infiltrating lymphocyte (TIL) line [8]. What varied among the different constructs was the ability of the fused H chains to form the typical dimeric antibody structure. The construct in which IL-2 was attached to the CH1 domain constitutes a Fab-IL2 and thus was expected to be monomeric. The fusion of IL-2 to the carboxyl terminus of the CH2 domain, on the other hand, could possibly result in dimers through the hinge region and be stabilized through the interchain cysteine disulfide bond. However, as was seen earlier with lymphotoxin fusion proteins, constructs made by fusion to the CH2 domain did not dimerize, whereas the fusions of IL-2 to the CH3 domain were completely assembled into intact antibody molecules. Most of the subsequent studies to date from my laboratory and those of my collaborators have focused on the latter type of fusion protein in which the cytokine is added to the normal carboxyl terminus of an intact antibody rather than replacing one or more of the antibody's domains. The reasons for this include more uniform product, ease of purification on protein A Sepharose, increased circulating half-life and preservation of antibody effector functions.

Additional fusion proteins made with other cytokines have also been reported including those with GM-CSF [9–11], TNF-α [3, 9], IFN-γ [12, 13] and IL-12 [14]. Most of these constructs followed the approach of fusing the cytokine to the end of the CH3 domain and all reported normal or nearly normal cytokine activities, at least those with GM-CSF and TNF-α. The latter two cytokines represent a bigger challenge to protein engineering due to their more complex structures. For example, IFN-γ normally exists in solution as an anti-parallel homodimer and this structure is critical for activity. Therefore, it is hard to imagine how dimeric antibody fusion proteins with IFN-γ could maintain the cytokine activity when the adjacent chains are expressed and assembled in a parallel orientation. Monomeric forms may be able to complex in an anti-parallel orientation (through the protein-protein interactions between IFN-γ components) and exhibit sufficient receptor binding for activity, but such structures would be expected to be unstable. Nonetheless, Xiang et al. [12, 13] have reported on the expression of scFV-IFN-γ and $(Fab')_2$-IFN-γ proteins in bacteria and mammalian cells, respectively, and have provided evidence of biological activity at high concentrations. It was unclear from these studies, however, what the specific activity was since only high concentrations of the fusion proteins were tested in vast excess of the affinity constants for receptor binding. Furthermore, there was no analysis of the structure of the $(Fab')_2$-IFN-γ molecule showing that it formed dimers, or whether purified proteins, exposed to acid conditions during processing, retained biological activity. It is well known that certain cytokines, including IFN-γ and lymphotoxin, are very sensitive to acid pH and can quickly lose their biological activity even after brief exposures to such conditions. In fact, the lymphotoxin activity of antibody fusion proteins was reported to be highly sensitive to pH and alternative purification procedures were needed to produce fully active proteins [2].

An even more complex expression problem presents itself with IL-12. This unique cytokine is composed of two different protein subunits that form a heterodimeric structure that is stabilized by an interchain disulfide bond. Nonetheless, it has been possible to engineer antibody fusion proteins either with an scFV or a whole antibody structure fused to one subunit, and co-expressing the second subunit in the same cell to form an antibody-IL12 heterodimer structure [14]. In these studies it was shown that by fusing the p35 subunit to the antibody component, the fusion protein could not be exported out of the cell without first associating with the co-expressed p40 subunit. This is due to the inherent property of the p35 subunit which is degraded inside the cell in the absence of the complexed p40 subunit [15]. By expressing the fusion protein this way, the antibody-IL12 protein is ensured of being fully assembled with the stoichiometric amount of each subunit, in the same manner that H and L chains are required for secretion of an intact antibody [16]. In fact, the whole antibody-IL12 fusion protein consists of a pair of each of three separate proteins which assemble into a 6-chain, fully assembled molecule [14].

Despite this rather complex requirement for protein assembly, we have been able to express whole-antibody IL-12 immunocytokines in transfected mouse myeloma cells at high levels. Two different approaches were used. In both approaches, two separate expression plasmid vectors were constructed: one encoding the antibody L chain, the antibody H chain fused to the p35 subunit of IL-12 and the drug selection marker, dihydrofolate reductase (dhfr). The second vector encodes the p40 subunit of IL-12 and a second (Neo®) drug selection marker conferring resistance to the antibiotic, G-418.

For the first expression approach, the two vectors are mixed together and introduced into the myeloma target cells by electroporation. After recovering from this process, the cells are cultured in the presence of methotrexate which kills all cells except those expressing the transfected dhfr gene product. Once the drug-resistant cells have grown into colonies, they are tested for the secretion of antibody using typical ELISA methods. Only those cells expressing proteins from both of the vectors were found to secrete antibody determinants into their culture media. In other words, the antibody-p35 complex could not leave the cell unless p40 was expressed by the same cell and formed the complete antibody-p35/p40 structure.

In the second approach, the vector expressing only the p40 subunit and the Neo® gene was introduced into myeloma cells and drug selection was achieved using G-418. Surviving cell clones were tested for p40 subunit expression and secretion using an ELISA, since this protein can be secreted in the absence of the p35 subunit. Clones with the highest p40 expression rates were used as recipients in a second round of transfection with the antibody-p35 expression vector and, in this case, drug selection utilized the dhfr/methotrexate system. While both of these methods produced lines expressing intact IL-12 immunocytokines, the second method generated the clones with the highest expression rates. This is likely to be due to the fact that p40 expression can be rate-limiting for secretion of the intact complex and so if all transfectants already express a high-level of p40, the chance of getting a high-level expressing clone is dependent on the fortuitous integration of only the antibody-p35 vector, and not each separate vector, in the same cell.

Further development of immunocytokines will require additional engineering strategies for optimization of protein expression as well as biological properties and these are discussed in detail below. As far as initial construction strategies for new cytokines are concerned, alternative approaches, not already discussed, include the following situations.

Some cytokines may be more active as fusion proteins if their amino termini are free to interact with their receptor. This may be the case for the chemokine family of cytokines [17]. Recently, a fusion protein between the RANTES chemokine and an intact anti-tumor antibody was reported in which the cytokine was genetically fused to the amino terminus, rather than the carboxyl terminus of the H chain [18]. The fusion protein maintained both chemokine and antigen binding activities. In still another study, IL-2 was fused to the amino terminus of a scFV, which in turn was fused to the C region of the κ L chain [19]. Both of these studies demonstrate the numerous possibilities for constructing immunocytokines, but the utility of such proteins still awaits their testing in pre-clinical animal models and eventually in the clinic.

Biological activities

As discussed above, the type of fusion between the antibody and cytokine, as well as the multimeric nature of the fusion protein, can greatly influence its biological activity. These effects are likely to reflect the ability of the fused cytokine to interact with its receptor and can be measured both by receptor binding assays, as well as biological responses of the cells bearing the receptors. The vast majority of studies to date have been with IL-2 immunocytokines and their ability to induce the proliferation of resting or activated cell lines or freshly isolated lymphocytes. The first report, with very low specific activity Fab-IL2, showed that despite poor activity in a standard CTLL activity, the fusion protein bound to cells could induce a reasonable level of proliferation [4]. When fully active fusion proteins were used in another study [8], the ability of immunocytokine-coated cells to stimulate TIL destruction of target cells was found to exceed that of free rIL-2. The same immunocytokines, in this case whole antibody-IL2 constructs, were shown to have full activity in proliferation assays with both the CTLL-2 mouse line and a human TIL cell line. Later studies showed that IL-2 immunocytokines can also stimulate the proliferation of cells expressing only the intermediate (β) receptor as well as free IL-2, including a transfected cell line and resting peripheral blood mononuclear cells (PBMC) [20]. It was also shown that IL-2 immunocytokine bound to cells, could mediate the stimulation of the same cells. This suggests that targeted IL-2, still bound to cells, can activate resting immune cells in the tumor microenvironment and not just pre-activated cells. Such an effect seems to be borne out by successful treatment of established tumors in mice (see below).

Biological activities of other cytokines, expressed as antibody fusion proteins, have generally been found to be equivalent to those of the free cytokines (with the possible exception of INF-γ, noted above). For example, GM-CSF activity of human antibody-GM-CSF was reported to be 20% as active as the control GM-CSF produced in bacteria [9]. This degree of activity is typical of the glycosylated form produced in mammalian cells, at least in measurements based on cell proliferation. Assays based on granulocyte-macrophage colony formation, on the other hand, show comparable activity for the immunocytokine and the GM-CSF standard produced in bacteria.

Two different activities of IL-12 were also tested with immunocytokine forms specific for human effector cells and a hybrid mouse/human construct with activity on both cell types [14]. For the human-specific construct, the ability to induce proliferation of mitogen-activated cells was nearly the same as the IL-12 standard, while the ability to induce IFN-γ production (arguably the most important immune function of IL-12) from the same cells was reduced approximately 4-fold. The hybrid form had a greatly reduced level of activity in both assays when tested on pre-activated mouse spleen cells. Later studies using a completely mouse-specific IL-12 immunocytokine showed somewhat improved activities but not to the level of the human-specific form. The reason for reduced bioactivities is probably due to steric hindrance of the bulky antibody component, closely juxtaposed to two very large cytokine components (one at the carboxyl terminus of each H chain). This still does not explain the differences seen in activity between the proliferation of mitogen-activated cells and INF-γ induction with the human-specific IL-12 immunocytokine. In this case, such differences could reflect altered affinity for one or more forms of the IL-12 receptor [21] expressed on either NK or T-cells. Thus, the bulk of the proliferation could be due to T-cells responding through one receptor form, while the bulk of the IFN-γ induction could be derived from NK cells and be mediated through a different IL-12 receptor complex.

The other potentially important biological activities of whole antibody-based immunocytokines include the standard antibody effector function of complement fixation (and eventual target cell lysis or complement-dependent cytotoxicity (CDC)) and antibody-dependent cellular cytotoxicity (ADCC). What, if any, role these activities might play *in vivo* still remains to be demonstrated, but intuitively they would seem to add further immune activation potential for the destruction of target cells such as cancer or virus-infected cells. In general, both CDC and ADCC activities are maintained following fusions of cytokines to the carboxyl termini of IgG1 [8, 11, 14] and IgG3 antibodies [22]. Immunocytokines produced with fragments of antibodies or specific deletion mutants would, of course, not have these activities. Neither would whole antibody-based immunocytokines using antibody isotypes that do not normally have these activities mediated by sequence-specific binding of either complement components (for CDC) or one or more Fc receptors (FcR). The effects of such changes of the immunocytokine antibody component on anti-tumor efficacy will be discussed below.

Pharmacokinetic studies

In addition to specific targeting, one goal of immunocytokines is to increase the circulating half-life of the cytokine. Typical circulating $T_{1/2}$ for most cytokines range from 10 to 60 minutes, with the exception of IL-12. In this case, the much larger size of this heterodimeric molecule may be related to its $T_{1/2}$ of more than three hours [23]. The pharmacokinetics of immunocytokines vary greatly with different cytokines and not just as a function of the size of the fusion protein.

The first study of immunocytokine pharmacokinetics compared IL-2 and GM-CSF fusion proteins made with the same V regions, specific for the ganglioside GD2 [9]. In this study, the immunocytokines were administered by i.v. injection and the clearance properties were followed by quantitative ELISA of serial blood samples. This is a typical way of measuring the clearance of injected drugs but is different from the techniques used by other laboratories [22, 25] who have compared their results with this study. In these other cases, radiolabeled immunocytokines were injected into the peritoneal cavity and the clearance was followed by measuring whole-body radioactivity. With i.v. administration of the IL-2 immunocytokine, a rapid redistribution out of the circulation was observed that removed about 90% of the protein from the circulation in the first 2 hours. This was followed by a much longer catabolic (β) phase with a $T_{1/2}$ of approximately 30 hr. It should be pointed out that this early study did not discriminate between intact fusion protein and antibody that may circulate free of the cytokine after proteolytic cleavage of the cytokine from the whole molecule. In fact, later studies [24] have shown that this is the case and that the $T_{1/2}$ β of intact fusion protein (~6 h) is significantly shorter than first thought.

In marked contrast to the IL-2 immunocytokine, another fusion protein made with the same antibody and GM-CSF had very different pharmacokinetic properties. In this case, the redistribution (α) phase $T_{1/2}$ was 1.4 hr (*versus* 0.3 for the IL-2 fusion protein) and the catabolic phase was 28 hr. The result was that far more immunocytokine remained in the circulation for extended periods of time. It was also shown that the GM-CSF fusion protein was not susceptible to proteolytic cleavage [9] so, unlike the IL-2 case, the material in the blood at the later times represented fusion protein and not cleaved antibody.

Other laboratories [22, 25] have measured the pharmacokinetics of IL-2 immunocytokines using intraperitoneal (i.p.) injection of radiolabeled protein and followed the half-life by elimination of radioactivity. This technique eliminates the distribution phase seen following i.v. injection by placing the protein in a body cavity from which it redistributes in a very different manner. Using such a method, the $T_{1/2}$ was reported to be 7 hr, or almost exactly the same as the $T_{1/2}$ β found after i.v. injection and analyzed for intact fusion protein components by ELISA (see above). Thus, different groups find very similar results for the catabolism phase of IL-2 immunocytokine clearance when the route of administration is taken into consideration.

Why IL-2 but not GM-CSF immunocytokines exhibit this unusual distribution phenomenon in the circulation was not determined in the early studies, but some other interesting properties of the two proteins suggested that structural alterations of the antibody itself may be responsible. Both fusion proteins were made using the same antibody recognizing GD2 ganglioside. When purified immunocytokines were tested for binding to plate-bound antigen, significantly higher binding was observed with the IL-2 fusion protein than with either the antibody alone or the antibody-GM-CSF fusion protein. This suggests that fusion of IL-2 to each H chain alters the overall structure of the antibody to the extent that even antigen binding at the extreme opposite end of the molecule is affected. Earlier work had shown that proteolytic cleavage of IL-2 from the fusion protein resulted in normal antigen-binding activity [8]. These results support the idea that the IL-2 domains actively alter the antibody structure, rather than affecting the assembly of the molecule during the initial folding of the independent protein domains.

How this effect is transmitted from one end of the molecule to the other is not clear, but it is likely to be mediated through interactions with the CH2 domain. It was suggested that IL-2 interactions with the CH2 domain might disrupt interactions with the Fab arm, thus increasing antibody flexibility and antigen binding. Such an effect had already been noted with deletion mutants of the same antibody lacking the CH2 domain [26]. Further evidence that IL-2 alters the structure of the CH2 domain will be discussed below.

The effect of IL-12 fusion on the pharmacokinetic properties of another antibody (in this case, recognizing the epithelial antigen EpCAM) was studied and found to be more similar to that seen with GM-CSF, although some proteolytic cleavage of IL-12 from the antibody was noted [14]. When the antibody and intact fusion protein components were independently measured using specific ELISA reagents, the intact fusion protein $T_{1/2}\,\beta$ was shorter than that of the released antibody (21 hr *versus* 30 hr). This compares to values of 6 hr and 28 hr for IL-2 and GM-CSF immunocytokines, respectively. Thus, there is no correlation between the size of the immunocytokine and its half-life but rather with how the cytokine affects the antibody structure. The important question that remains to be determined is what is the optimal half-life of a given immunocytokine and whether a longer circulation time translates into increased targeting *in vivo*.

Preclinical animal models

IL-2 Immunocytokines

The majority of pre-clinical anti-tumor efficacy studies of immunocytokines have involved those made with IL-2. The first set of studies utilized human neuroblastoma tumor cells expressing the appropriate antigen target of the ch14.18 antibody from which the IL-2 immunocytokine was derived, in this case the GD2 ganglioside. These human tumors are highly immunogenic in immune competent mice and are spontaneously rejected after implantation. They do grow in immunodeficient SCID mice both as solid tumors and as pulmonary or hepatic metastases. Since the rationale was to activate the local immune system by specifically targeting the tumor microenvironment, human lymphokine-activated killer (LAK) cells were provided as effectors that could respond to the immune stimulation. The first studies by Sabzevari et al. [27] and later extended by Pancook et al. [28], showed that established neuroblastoma metastases could be eradicated by a short course of treatment with the ch14.18-IL2 immunocytokine. Control mice transplanted with LAK cells and then treated with the same dose of antibody and IL-2, did not have such dramatic anti-tumor responses. A similar type of anti-tumor response was reported in a melanoma model [29] for both hepatic and pulmonary metastases, even those established for as long as 8 days prior to initiation of treatment.

The mechanism by which the IL-2 immunocytokines eradicate tumor cells is best studied in models that do not require the addition of exogenous immune cell xenografts. Since mouse tumor cells do not generally express human tumor antigens, it was necessary to induce the expression of the antigens recognized by the anti-human tumor antibodies under development. In one case, the genes encoding the enzymes required for the synthesis of the GD2 ganglioside from precursors, already present in the B16 melanoma, were transfected in order to generate a GD2-expressing mouse melanoma called B78-D14 [30]. This cell line forms solid tumors and metastases in immune competent C57Bl/6 mice and can be targeted with the ch14.18-IL2 immunocytokine.

Studies in this syngeneic tumor model demonstrated several important points. It was shown that a 7-day course of treatment with low doses of ch14.18-IL2 completely eradicated established pulmonary or hepatic metastases in most mice [31]. Control mice treated with antibody and IL-2 (not fused) or an IL-2 immunocytokine not reactive with these tumor cells showed no such anti-tumor activity. Life-span studies also demonstrated long-term survival of the ch14.18-IL2-treated mice exceeding double the median survival time of the controls.

Another important finding was that mixtures of antigen-positive and antigen-negative tumor cells growing in the same mice could both be eradicated by treatment with the antigen-specific ch14.18-IL2 antibody [32]. At first glance this appears to contradict the finding, stated above, that antigen specificity of the immunocytokine is essential for anti-tumor activity. However, the following proposed mechanism of action can explain this potential discrepancy. Binding of tumor cells by a specific IL-2 immunocytokine elicits an immune reaction at the tumor site (and/or in draining lymph nodes) and leads to the presentation of tumor antigens to T-cells, coupled with the IL-2 co-stimulatory signal. Expanded T-cells recognizing these tumor antigens are activated to kill any tumor displaying them, whether or not they also express the GD2 ganglioside. Unlike MHC-restricted peptide antigens recognized by the T-cells, the GD2 antigen serves only as a means of localizing the IL-2 immunocytokine to the tumor microenvironment and thus does not have to be present on all cells to achieve this task.

Data supporting this proposed mechanism include the demonstration that $CD8^+$ T-cells are necessary for the anti-tumor activity in the B78-D14 model (by antibody depletion of T-cell subsets), while $CD4^+$ cells improve activity but are not essential [31]. Furthermore, cytotoxic lymphocyte (CTL) activity was detected in spleen cell preparations from ch14.18-IL2-treated mice but not from control mice treated with non-specific IL-2 immunocytokine or other control reagents. This activity could also be blocked *in vitro* using antibodies specific for MHC class I molecules. Lastly, spleen cells or purified $CD8^+$ cells from ch14.18-IL2-treated mice could be adoptively transferred to SCID mice (lacking functional T and B cells) and protect them from B78-D14 metastases [33]. Taken together these data support the T-cell-mediated mechanism of anti-tumor activity and suggest that antigens other than those related to the antibody-targeted antigen (GD2, in this case) are the target of effector cell recognition. This is a very important point since many antibody-based therapies have encountered problems when antigen modulation by tumors led to the emergence of escape variants.

Formal proof that T-cell reactivities induced by IL-2 immunocytokines are unrelated to the antibody-targeted antigen was demonstrated in another model. In this case, a humanized antibody (huKS) recognizing the human epithelial antigen EpCAM (also called KS antigen or KSA) was transfected into a mouse colon carcinoma line, CT26, syngeneic with Balb/c mice [14]. Established pulmonary and hepatic metastases were treated with huKS-IL2 for 7 days resulting in eradication of the disease, as shown by histological examination and a sensitive RT-PCR analysis of human KSA expression in liver tissues [34]. When CTL responses were tested in this system, it was shown that freshly isolated splenocytes killed the CT26 transfectants expressing KSA and non-transfected CT26 cells to exactly the same extent. Again, this killing was MHC class I restricted and could be adoptively transferred to naive mice to confer protection from the same tumor [35].

While both the melanoma and colon carcinoma models have shown an important role for $CD8^+$ T-cells in anti-tumor activity, no such role could be demonstrated in a syngeneic neuroblastoma model [36]. In this case, the ch14.18-IL2 immunocytokine could eradicate spontaneous or experimental metastases in immune competent A/J mice; the primary effector was shown to be NK cells. Since NK cells do not have immunological memory, long-term survival in treated animals following a single course of treatment was observed in a smaller proportion of mice (3/8) than was seen in the melanoma and colon carcinoma models (usually >80%).

The reason for this predominance of an NK-mediated response over that of a T-cell response is not known; however, it was shown later in this model that a T-cell response against the same syngeneic neuroblastoma tumor could be induced if the tumor cells secreted IL-12 [37]. In this case, a protective vaccine effect was generated against parental tumor cell challenge but this protection was short-lived. Nonetheless, the important point is that IL-2 based immunocytokines can generate potent anti-tumor activity in many pre-clinical models through the activation of multiple immune cell types. A more recent study in a xenograft model of metastatic prostate cancer has even demonstrated that macrophage can be important effectors of anti-tumor activity mediated by IL-2 immunocytokines [38]. Thus, one can consider IL-2 immunocytokine therapy in clinical situations where patients are unlikely to have healthy T-cell responses, such as shortly after chemotherapy or bone marrow transplant.

Finally, two other groups have reported on pre-clinical studies of IL-2 immunocytokines targeted against a mouse B lymphoma line, 38C13. In one study [39], an anti-tumor antibody-IL2 immunocytokine was constructed using human IgG3 instead of IgG1 and used to test different dosing strategies. Both methods produced anti-tumor effects, but a single i.p. dose resulted in a 50% response rate and evidence of a immune memory response when the tumor cells were implanted i.p., while a 5-day course of treatment of tumor cells implanted s.c. resulted in a far better response rate (87%) but no evidence of immune memory. Thus, it is likely that one route stimulated a T-cell response and the other was dominated by an NK-mediated effector reaction.

Another group [40] reported that an IgG1-based IL-2 immunocytokine could effectively treat 38C13 tumors if administered 24 hr after tumor inoculation. An important finding in this study was that the Fc portion of the antibody was important to its anti-tumor activity, since an scFV-IL2 fusion protein prepared with the same V regions had no anti-tumor activity in this model. The authors speculated that the requirement for the Fc was most likely related to the immunocytokine's longer half-life and its associated CDC and ADCC effector functions.

TNF-β based immunocytokines

Far less data are available for immunocytokines based on molecules other than IL-2. Several groups have reported on the construction and expression of antibody fusion proteins with TNF-α and TNF-β (lymphotoxin, or LT), but very little pre-clinical animal testing has been reported. In one study using a melanoma xenograft model and ch14.18-LT, anti-tumor activity could be demonstrated in nude mice but not in SCID mice, and that functional B cells were essential for this activity [41]. This was a particularly interesting result because the tumor line used was very sensitive to LT-mediated apoptosis and yet could only be eradicated in the presence of B cells. Histological analyses showed a marked accumulation of B cells in the perivascular space around the tumors.

These results suggest that additional signals for tumor cell destruction were required but it is still unclear whether they are immune-based or simply a cytotoxic reaction mediated, for example, through membrane-bound adhesion molecules expressed on the B cells. The perivascular localization of B cells outside of the tumor sites seem to support an immune type of reaction, probably in the form of a secreted molecule(s) capable of stimulating the infiltration of tumors with leukocytes [41]. Unfortunately, these studies were done before a syngeneic mouse model was available for this immunocytokine and further studies have not been performed in order to clarify the mechanism of this anti-tumor activity. An interesting question is what role anti-angiogenic factors might play and how B cells might be related to this process. Epstein-Barr virus (EBV)-transformed B-cells expressing both IL-12 and IP-10, two potent inhibitors of angiogenesis, have been shown to cause the regression of other co-injected tumors through an anti-angiogenic mechanism [42].

Another study reported the construction of a TNF-α-based immunocytokine fused at its carboxyl terminus with a scFV specific for the LeY antigen found on several tumor cells [43]. The scFV domain was deliberately joined through the C-terminus of the cytokine to reduce its TNF-receptor binding and "detoxify" the fusion protein. The rationale was that accumulation on antigen-presenting cells would lead to the selective killing of antigen-expressing cells but spare antigen-negative, TNFR-positive ones. The authors reported that this detoxified protein could cause significant regression of human breast cancer xenografts in immune-deficient mice at concentrations that were not toxic.

Il-12 immunocytokines

Pre-clinical tumor models for testing IL-12 immunocytokines are far more complicated due to the highly species-specific nature of the cytokine. Not only is human IL-12 itself inactive on mouse responder cells, but so too is IFN-γ, the primary cytokine that is induced by IL-12 [44]. Some systems can be designed to test the human proteins in mice, although the data need to be qualified with respect to their potential mechanisms of action. For example, we reported that a human anti-EpCAM antibody-based IL-12 immunocytokine (KS-IL12) showed significant activity against established human prostate carcinoma metastases in SCID mice transplanted with human LAK cells [14]. This activity required specific antibody targeting because another IL-12 immunocytokine made with an irrelevant antibody was not active. The mechanism of anti-tumor activity in this model would necessarily be mediated through the human immune effector cells since they alone would respond to human IL-12. Furthermore, any response to the human IFN-γ, induced from these cells by IL-12, would be mediated by the transplanted human effectors, not endogenous mouse cells. Thus, any of the proposed anti-angiogenic activities of IL-12 [45] are unlikely to be operating in this model. Likewise, mechanisms based on the activation of macrophage by induced IFN-γ are unlikely to be operating in this model since the transplanted human LAK cells consist primarily of activated NK cells and some T-cells, not macrophage or granulocytes.

Despite the limitations, noted above, the KS-IL12 immunocytokines showed significant enough anti-tumor activity to justify further studies in a more appropriate model. In order to cross the species barrier, we engineered a hybrid IL-12 immunocytokine comprising the human antibody, the human IL-12 p40 subunit and the mouse IL-12 p35 subunit. The resulting fusion protein had IL-12 activity when tested on either human or mouse cells, although far less than the IL-12 standards [14]. Despite this relatively low activity, the hybrid IL-12 immunocytokine had potent anti-tumor activity in a SCID mouse colon carcinoma model, in the absence of exogenously administered LAK cells. The dramatic increase in activity is likely due to the ability to activate several of the potential anti-tumor activities of this cytokine, and not just those mediated by LAK cells.

Engineering for optimal biological activity

The overall activity of immunocytokines *in vivo* depends on several independent functional properties including: (1) antigen binding (e.g., target cell binding); (2) cytokine activity and (3) pharmacokinetics. In general, the first two properties are maintained after the fusion of the antibody and cytokine, with a few exceptions noted above. Thus, the area needing more protein engineering for the design of optimal therapeutic immunocytokines is related to their *in vivo* clearance properties.

One of the surprising results of the studies with immunocytokines is the unpredictable nature of the pharmacokinetic properties of a given antibody-cytokine combination. This was first shown in the earliest studies comparing the circulating half lives of a set of IL-2 and GM-CSF immunocytokines made with the same antibody (described in detail above). While the GM-CSF immunocytokine had a long half-life, similar to the original antibody, a large portion of the IL-2 immunocytokine was rapidly cleared from the circulation in the first 2 hr, followed by a slower rate of clearance thereafter. What made these findings so interesting was the fact that these changes in pharmacokinetic properties were directly related to alterations in antigen binding of the antibody, in this case to the ganglioside GD2 [9].

More recently we have re-addressed the potential source of this clearance phenomenon in an attempt to increase the circulating half-life and, potentially, improve the therapeutic efficacy. Using the findings of the earlier studies as a clue, we reasoned that if the carboxyl terminal IL-2 could affect antigen binding at the amino terminus of the molecule, the alteration in structure might also be realized somewhere in the middle of the molecule. In fact, we proposed that the IL-2 domains at the end of each H chain could fold back over the CH3 domain and make contact with the CH2 domain in the middle of the antibody. This interaction could distort CH2 and disrupt its interactions with the Fab arms, that otherwise restrict the CH2's flexibility and ability to bind [6]. In this model, the distortion of CH2 could also change the affinity to other molecules that normally bind in this region of the antibody, such as FcR and complement component C1q.

To test this hypothesis, we recently constructed a set of IL-2 fusion proteins based on both the 14.18 anti-ganglioside antibody and the anti-EpCAM antibody KS1/4 [46]. The rationale was to use different H chain isotypes known to have reduced binding affinities for FcR and/or C1q, and test whether these changes had an impact on their clearance from the circulation. The results indicated that the fusion of IL-2 to these humanized antibodies increased their binding to a mouse macrophage cell line expressing FcgRI and that these increases in binding were decreased nearly to the original levels if the Cγ4 H chain replaced the original Cγ1 H chain in the immunocytokine.

The reduction in FcR binding was correlated with improved pharmacokinetic properties, especially during the first 2-hr period after injection, when >90% of the Cγ1-IL-2 immunocytokine is normally cleared from the circulation. Furthermore, the same effects could be achieved using specific mutations in the known FcR binding site in the Cγ1 H chain, indicating that some of the other sequence differences between Cγ1 and Cγ4, e.g., those related to C1q binding, were not playing a major role in this phenomenon. Both antibody systems showed the same improvement in pharmacokinetic behavior with these modifications, indicating that this effect is not related to a particular set of antibody V regions. This is important in the context of the earlier results with the 14.18 antibody, in which we observed increased antigen binding that could be falsely attributed to causing the rapid clearance in mice [9].

The improved pharmacokinetic properties, just described, required modifications that resulted in dramatic changes in antibody effector functions ADCC and CDC. These activities are generally measured with purified tumor target cells and immune effector cells (generally enriched NK cells) *in vitro,* and indeed, these properties were lost in the Cγ4-based IL-2 immunocytokines. The testing of these modified molecules in pre-clinical efficacy models might help address the relative importance of these functions *in vivo.*

Our preliminary findings showed different results for different models [46]. In immuno-deficient SCID mice, transplanted with human LAK cells, anti-tumor efficacy was virtually the same as that of the original 14.18-IL2 (Cγ1) immunocytokine. Thus, improved half-life in the circulation did not improve the anti-tumor activity. On the other hand, reduced ADCC and CDC functions did not reduce the anti-tumor activity. Perhaps this suggests that these effector functions play a role in the anti-tumor activity but that the improved levels of immunocytokine compensated for the less efficient effector activities. Alternatively, the Cγ4-based immunocytokine may activate a different set of effector cells through binding to FcγRII, an activity that is not measured in standard ADCC assays. Most of the *in vitro* activity depends on NK cells expressing FcγRIII, which like FcγRI, has reduced binding for IgG4.

In immune competent mouse models the results show clear differences between the activity of Cγ1 and Cγ4 IL-2 immunocytokines [46]. Two different models were used, including the treatment of established s.c. CT26 colon carcinoma, as well as an established disseminated RENCA cell (renal carcinoma) lung metastasis model. Since the major cell type responsible for the anti-tumor effect in these syngeneic models is the CD8$^+$ T-cell (see above), it makes sense that the increased targeting of IL-2 to the tumor microenvironment (through the longer half-life) would improve the anti-tumor activity and that the effector functions such as ADCC would be unnecessary for this process. Anti-tumor efficacy was found to be significantly improved in both models through the use of the Cγ4-IL2, thus supporting the importance of improved IL-2 targeting, rather than effector function, in these tumor models.

Clinical perspectives

The immunocytokine field is rather small and encouraging pre-clinical data have emerged only in the last few years. Nonetheless, the proof of concepts established in mouse models are quite encouraging for the treatment of cancer patients with metastases in the setting of minimal residual disease. Although I have focused the majority of this review on IL-2 immunocytokines, it is also tempting to speculate that other cytokines, especially IL-12, could benefit from the approach of specific disease targeting approaches as a means of increasing the therapeutic index, alone or in combination with other immunocytokines. Immunocytokines could also be useful for non-cancer applications where it is desirable to localize cytokine bioactivity and increase the circulating half-life. Viral diseases are the most obvious application including, for example, the targeting of HIV viral reservoirs in patients undergoing triple drug therapy. Other clinical uses are likely to include the combination of therapeutic approaches. For example, vaccines are highly effective at initiating immune responses and often serve to prevent disease. In therapeutic vaccine settings, the use of an IL-2 based immunocytokine to further boost the response and expand reactive immune cells at the disease site could be a means of improving their efficacy. Such approaches could be used in conjunction with gene therapy, or antigen-pulsed dendritic cell vaccines. The two IL-2 immunocytokines discussed in this review have recently entered the clinic. It will now be possible to evaluate the potential role for these molecules in cancer immunotherapy.

References

1 Silverstein AM (1988) *In*: HB Jovanovich (ed.): *A History of Immunology*. Academic Press, San Diego, California
2 Gillies SD, Young D, Lo K-M, Foley SF, Reisfeld RA (1991) Expression of genetically engineered immunoconjugates of lymphotoxin and a chimeric anti-ganglioside GD2 antibody. *Hybridoma* 10: 347–356
3 Hoogenboom HR, Raus JC, Volckaert G (1991) Targeting of tumor necrosis factor to tumor cells: secretion by myeloma cells of a genetically engineered antibody-tumor necrosis factor hybrid molecule. *Biochim Biophys Acta* 1096: 345–354
4 Fell HP, Gayle MA, Grossmaire L, Ledbetter JA (1991) Genetic construction and characterization of a fusion protein consisting of a chimeric F (ab') with specificity for carcinomas and human IL-2. *J Immunol* 146: 2446–2452
5 Smith RA, Baglioni C (1987) The active form of tumor necrosis factor is a trimer. *J Biol Chem* 262: 6951–6954

6 Reisfeld RA, Gillies SD (1996) Recombinant antibody fusion proteins for cancer immunotherapy. *In*: U Guenthert, P Schlag, W. Birchmeier (eds): *Current topics in microbiology and immunology: attempts to understand metastasis formation III.* Springer-Verlag, Berlin, 27–53
7 Savage P, So A, Spooner RA, Epenetos AA (1993) A recombinant single chain antibody interleukin-2 fusion protein. *Brit J Cancer* 67: 304–310
8 Gillies SD, Reilly EB, Lo K-M, Reisfeld RA (1992) Antibody-targeted IL-2 stimulates the killing of autologous tumor cells. *Proc Natl Acad Sci USA* 89: 1428–1432
9 Gillies SD, Young D, Lo K-M, Roberts S (1993) Biological activity and *in vivo* clearance of antitumor antibody/cytokine fusion proteins. *Bioconjugate Chem* 4: 230–235
10 Tao M-H, Levy R (1993) Idiotype/granulocyte-macrophage colony-stimulating factor fusion protein as a vaccine for B-cell lymphoma. *Nature* 362: 755–758
11 Hornick JL, Kwali LA, Hu P, Lynch M, Anderson PM, Epstien AL (1997) Chimeric CLL-1 antibody fusion proteins containing granulocyte-macrophage colony-stimulating factor or interleukin 2 with specificity for B-cell malignancies exhibit enhanced effector functions while retaining tumor targeting properties. *Blood* 89: 4437–4447
12 Xiang J, Qi Y, Liu E (1993) Recombinant bifunctional molecule Fv/IFN-gamma possesses the anti-tumor Fv as well as the gamma interferon activities. *Cancer Biother* 8: 327–337
13 Xiang J, Qi Y, Cook D, Moyana T (1996) Targeting gamma interferon to tumor cells by a genetically engineered fusion protein secreted from myeloma cells. *Hum Antibod Hybridom* 7: 1–10
14 Gillies SD, Lan Y, Wesolowski JS, Qian X, Reisfeld RA, Holden S, Super M, Lo K-M (1998) Antibody-IL12 fusion proteins are effective in SCID mouse models of prostate and colon carcinoma metastases. *J Immunol* 160: 6195–6203
15 Gubler U, Chua AO, Schoenhaut DS, Dwyer CM, McComas W, Motyka R, Nabavi N, Wolitzky AG, Quinn PM, Familletti PC et al (1991) Coexpression of two distinct genes is required to generate secreted bioactive cytotoxic lymphocyte maturation factor. *Proc Natl Acad Sci USA* 88: 4143–4147
16 Pepe VH, Sonenshein GE, Yoshimura MI, Shulman MJ (1986) Gene transfer of immunoglobulin light chain restores heavy chain secretion. *J Immunol* 137: 2367–2372
17 Proost P, De Meester I, Schols D, Struyf S, Lambeir A-M, Wuyts A, Opdenakker G, De Clercq E, Scharpe S, Van Damme J (1998) Amino-terminal truncation of chemokines by CD26/dipeptidyl-peptidase. IV. Conversion of RANTES into a potent inhibitor of monocyte chemotaxis and HIV infection. *J Biol Chem* 273: 7222–7227
18 Challita-Eid PM, Abboud CN, Morrison SL, Penichet ML, Rosell KE, Poles T, Hilchey SP, Planelles V, Rosenblatt JD (1998) A RANTES-antibody fusion protein retains antigen specificity and chemokine function. *J Immunol* 161: 3729–3736
19 Melani C, Figini M, Nicosia D, Luison E, Ramakrishna V, Casorati G, Parmiani G, Eshhar Z, Canevari S, Colombo MP (1998) Targeting of interleukin 2 to ovarian carcinoma by fusion with a single-chain Fv of antifolate receptor antibody. *Cancer Res* 58: 4146–4154
20 Hank JA, Surfus JE, Gan J, Jaeger P, Gillies SD, Reisfeld RA, Sondel PM (1996) Activation of human effector cells by a tumor reactive recombinant anti-ganglioside GD2 interleukin-2 fusion protein (ch14.18-IL2). *Clin Cancer Res* 2: 1951–1959
21 Chua AO, Chizzonite R, Desai BB, Truitt TP, Nunes P, Minetti LJ, Warrier RR, Presky DH, Levine JF, Gately MK et al (1994) Expression cloning of a human IL-12 receptor component. A new member of the cytokine receptor superfamily with strong homology to gp130. *J Immunol* 153: 128–136
22 Harvill ET, Fleming JM, Morrison SL (1996) *In vivo* properties of an IgG3-IL-2 fusion prote*In*: a general strategy for immune potentiation. *J Immunol* 157: 3165–3170
23 Wysocka M, Kubin M, Vieira LQ, Ozmen L, Garotta G, Scott P, Trinchieri G (1995) Interleukin-12 is required for interferon-gamma production and lethality in lipopolysaccharide-induced shock in mice. *Eur J Immunol* 25: 672–676
24 Kendra K, Gan J, Ricci M, Surfus J, Shaker A, Super M, Frost JD, Rakmilevich A, Hank JA, Gillies SD, Sondel PM (1999) Pharmacokinetics and stability of the 14.18-IL2 fusion protein in mice. *Cancer Immunol Immunother* 48(5): 219–229
25 Hu P, Hornick JL, Glasky MS, Yun A, Milkie MN, Khawli LA, Anderson PM, Epstein AL (1996) A chimeric Lym-1/interleukin 2 fusion protein for increasing tumor vasculature permeability and enhancing antibody uptake. *Cancer Res* 56: 4998–5004
26 Gillies SD, Wesolowski JS (1990) Antigen binding and biological activities of engineered mutant chimeric antibodies with human tumor specificities. *Hum Antibod Hybridom* 1: 47–54

27 Sabzevari H, Gillies SD, Muelle BM, Pancook JD, Reisfeld RA (1994) A recombinant antibody interleukin 2 fusion protein suppresses growth of hepatic human neuroblastoma metastases in severe combined immunodeficient mice. *Proc Natl Acad Sci USA* 91 (20): 9626–9630
28 Pancook JD, Becker JC, Gillies SD, Reisfeld RA (1996) Eradication of established hepatic human neuroblastoma metastases in mice with severe combined immunodeficiency by antibody-targeted interleukin-2. *Cancer Immunol Immunother* 42: 88–92
29 Becker JC, Pancook JD, Gillies SD, Mendelsohn J, Reisfeld RA (1996) Eradication of human hepatic and pulmonary melanoma metastases in SCID mice by antibody-interleukin 2 fusion proteins. *Proc Natl Acad Sci USA* 93: 2702–2707
30 Haraguchi M, Yamashiro S, Yamamoto A, Furukawa K, Takamiya K, Lloyd KO, Shiku H, Furukawa K (1994) Isolation of GD3 synthase gene by expression cloning of GM3 α-2,8-sialtransferase cDNA using anti-GD2 monoclonal antibody. *Proc Natl Acad Sci USA* 91: 10 455–10 459
31 Becker JC, Pancook JD, Gillies SD, Furukawa K, Reisfeld RA (1996) T cell-mediated eradication of murine metastatic melanoma induced by targeted interleukin 2 therapy. *J Exp Med* 183: 2361–2366
32 Becker JC, Varki N, Gillies SD, Furukawa K, Reisfeld RA (1996) An antibody-interleukin 2 fusion protein overcomes tumor heterogeneity by induction of a cellular immune response. *Proc Natl Acad Sci USA* 93: 7826–7831
33 Becker JC, Varki NM, Gillies SD, Furukawa K, Reisfeld RA (1997) Long-lived and transferable tumor immuniy in mice after targeted interleukin-2 therapy. *J Clin Invest* 98: 2801–2804
34 Xiang R, Lode HN, Dolman CS, Dreier T, Varki NM, Qian X, Lo K, Lan Y, Super M, Gillies SD et al (1997) Elimination of established murine colon carcinoma metastases by antibody-interleukin-2 fusion protein therapy. *Cancer Res* 57: 4948–4955
35 Xiang R, Lode HN, Drieir T, Gillies SD, Reisfeld RA (1998) Induction of persistent tumor-protective immunity in mice cured of established colon carcinoma metastases. *Cancer Res* 58: 3918–3925
36 Lode HN, Dreier T, Xiang R, Varki NM, Kang AS, Reisfeld RA (1997) Gene therapy with a single chain interleukin 12 fusion protein induces T cell-dependent protective immunity in a syngeneic model of murine neuroblastoma. *Proc Natl Acad Sci USA* 95: 2475–2480
37 Lode HN, Xiang R, Dreier T, Varki NM, Gillies SD, Reisfeld RA (1998) Natural killer cell-mediated eradication of neuroblastoma metastases to bone marrow by targeted interleukin-2 therapy. *Blood* 91: 1706–1715. 1998
38 Dolman CS, Mueller BM, Lode HN, Xiang R, Gillies SD, Reisfeld RA (1998) Suppression of human prostate carcinoma metastases in severe combined immunodeficient mice by interleukin 2 immunocytokine therapy. *Clin Cancer Res* 4 (10): 2551–2557
39 Penichet ML, Harvill ET, Morrison SL (1998) An IgG3-IL-2 fusion protein recognizing a murine B cell lymphoma exhibits effective tumor imaging and antitumor activity. *J Interferon Cytokine Res* 18: 597–607
40 Liu S-J, Sher Y-P, Ting C-C, Liao K-W, Yu C-P, Tao M-H (1998) Treatment of B-cell lymphoma with chimeric IgG and single-chain Fv antibody-interleukin-2 fusion proteins. *Blood* 92: 2103–2112
41 Reisfeld RA, Gillies SD, Mendelsohn J, Varki NM, Becker JC (1995) Involvement of B lymphocytes in the growth inhibition of human pulmonary melanoma metastases in athymic nu/nu mice by an antibody-lymphotoxin fusion protein. *Cancer Res* 56: 1707–1712
42 Angiolillo AL, Sgadari C, Tosato G (1996) A role for the interferon-inducible protein 10 in inhibition of angiogenesis by interleukin-12. *Ann N Y Acad Sci* 795: 158–167
43 Scherf U, Benhar I, Webber KO, Pastan I, Brinkmann U (1996) Cytotoxic antitumor activity of a recombinant tumor necrosis factor-B1 (Fv) fusion protein on LeY antigen-expressing human cancer cells. *Clin Cancer Res* 2: 1523–1531
44 Trinchieri G (1995) Interleukin-12: A cytokine produced by antigen-presenting cells with immunoregulatory functions in the generation of T-helper cells type 1 and cytotoxic lymphocytes. *Blood* 84: 4008–4027
45 Voest EE, Kenyon BM, O'Reilly MS, Truitt G, D'Amato RJ, Folkman J (1995) Inhibition of angiogenesis *in vivo* by interleukin 12. *J Natl Cancer Inst* 87: 581–586
46 Gillies SD, Lan Y, Lo K-M, Super M, Wesolowski J (1999) Improving the Efficacy of Antibody-IL2 Fusion Proteins by Reducing their Interaction with Fc Receptors. *Cancer Res* 59 (9) 2159–2166

Further improvement of protein drugs

Recombinant Protein Drugs
ed. by P. Buckel

Improving protein therapeutics: the evolution of the modern pharmacopoeia

Paul A. Burke[1] and Scott D. Putney[2]

[1] *Department of Pharmaceutics and Drug Delivery, Amgen, MS 8-1-C, One Amgen Ctr. Dr., Thousand Oaks, CA 91320, USA*
[2] *Eli Lilly and Co., Lilly Corporate Center, Indianapolis, IN 46285, USA*

Introduction

Development of protein therapeutics is a long-standing focus of the biotechnology industry. Proteins currently marketed or undergoing clinical testing number in the hundreds [1, 2] and include monoclonal antibodies, growth factors, cytokines, soluble receptors, hormones and proteins to block the function of a variety of infectious agents. Proteins are specific, exert their effects at low concentrations, and their virtually limitless number enables their use to influence a large variety of biological processes. It is possible that this class of drugs will eventually constitute a significant part of the pharmacopoeia. Whereas proteins have many attractive properties, they also have disadvantages that may limit their widespread acceptance by patients and physicians. These include low oral and transdermal bioavailabilities, which have necessitated their delivery by injections or infusions [3]. Moreover, injections must be given frequently because the half-lives of proteins are short (Tab. 1).

One approach to reducing the requirement for frequent injections has been to alter the pharmacokinetic properties of the molecule. Serum half-lives can be extended through covalent attachment of biocompatible polymers such as poly(ethylene glycol) [10–12], or through genetic engineering approaches

Table 1. Half-lives in humans and approved dosing frequencies of several recombinant proteins

Protein	Serum half-life (hours)	Weekly dosing frequency [4]
α-interferon [5]	5.6	3
γ-interferon [6]	0.6	3
hGH [7]	0.3	7
Epo [8]	6	3
G-CSF [8]	5	7
GM-CSF [9]	2	7

such as increasing the levels of glycosylation or creating fusion constructs [13, 14]. Proteins thus modified may have other altered properties (such as toxicity [15], immunogenicity, or lower bioactivity) as well, however, and must be developed as completely new drugs. An alternative way to reduce the need for frequent injections is to create a dosage form that delivers the native protein continuously, thus maintaining the concentration within the therapeutic window for an extended period. Sustained-release formulations offer numerous advantages including: (i) protecting the protein over an extended period from degradation or elimination; (ii) increased patient comfort, convenience and compliance and (iii) the ability to deliver the protein locally to a particular site or body compartment, thereby lowering overall systemic exposure. In some cases, sustained administration results in a decrease in the required cumulative dose. More importantly, it can justify commercial development of proteins that, for a variety of reasons (e.g., very short half-lives or excessive systemic toxicity), could not be marketed in a solution form.

Sustained-release systems are a relatively commonplace method to deliver low molecular weight drugs. There are several well-established methods to accomplish continuous administration, including transdermal patches, injectable depots such as those in which the drug is embedded in a polymeric matrix or vesicles (e.g., liposomes) and various types of externally worn, implantable, or orally administered pressure-driven pumps [16]. Several of the many currently marketed examples include the orally administered pump which releases the anti-hypertensive nifedipine, the transdermal delivery of nitroglycerine to treat heart disease, or of scopolamine for motion sickness, subdermal silicon capsules to treat nicotine addiction and the ethylene vinyl acetate or polyanhydride polymeric systems for the intrauterine release of levonorgestrel or for the delivery of carmustine to treat brain tumors [4].

Efforts to develop sustained-release formulations of proteins have focused on incorporating the protein into microspheres made of biodegradable polymers such as poly(lactide-co-glycolide) (PLG) [17–19]. PLG is non-immunogenic and has a long safety record. In addition to its use for drug delivery, it is used to make biodegradable sutures, bandages and bone plates [20, 21]. After subcutaneous or intramuscular injection, the protein is released by a combination of diffusion and polymer erosion (Fig. 1). By varying the polymer composition and molecular weight, and by adding excipients that stabilize the protein and slow its release, the release rate can be adjusted to maintain the serum concentration within the therapeutic window.

Although the first report of sustained-release of a microencapsulated protein was published over 20 years ago [16], the first sustained-release formulation of a protein entered clinical testing in 1996 [22]. The difficulty in developing sustained-release protein systems has been due principally to their instability; processes that produce sustained-release forms of smaller, more stable compounds are too harsh for proteins. Unlike smaller compounds, proteins are large structures with complex architecture possessing secondary, tertiary and, in some cases, quaternary structure. They often have labile bonds and numer-

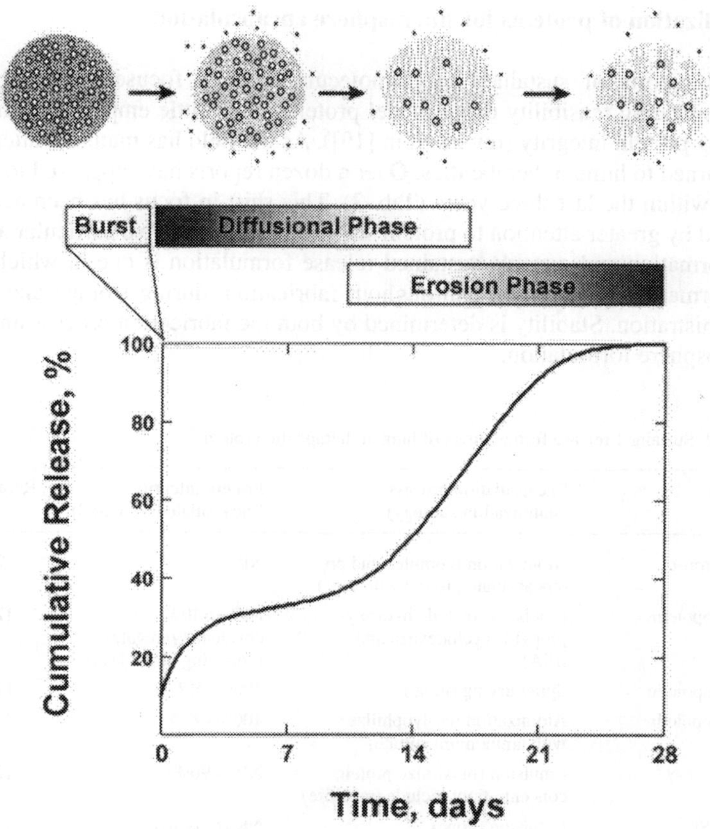

Figure 1. PLG microspheres, approximately 50 microns in diameter, contain solid protein particles (denoted as large circles). After injection, initial drug release (the "burst") results from dissolution of protein particles at the microsphere surface (to give soluble protein denoted as small circles). Sustained-release occurs as the protein diffuses from the interior of the microsphere through pores created by polymer degradation or by dissolution of encapsulated solids. Drug release can range from days to months. Degradation rates are determined by polymer molecular weight, lactide:glycolide ratio and the presence of hydrophobic end groups.

ous chemically reactive groups on their side chains. Disruption of these structures (e.g., denaturation or aggregation) or the modification of side chains can occur readily with many proteins and lead to loss of activity or immunogenicity. This can limit the efficacy of therapy or, worse, create safety concerns.

Development of depot formulations of proteins not only requires methods to maintain stability during manufacture and storage of the finished product (a requirement for any protein therapeutic), but the protein also must remain stable during encapsulation and for weeks or months after administration. These challenges have necessitated new methods of protein stabilization and encapsulation.

Stabilization of proteins for microsphere encapsulation

Initial reports of sustained macromolecule delivery focused primarily on demonstrating feasibility using model proteins, with little emphasis on maintaining protein integrity (reviewed in [19]). As the field has matured, attention has turned to human therapeutics. Over a dozen reports have appeared to date, most within the last three years (Tab. 2). This shift in focus has been accompanied by greater attention to protein stability. Proteins have a particular active conformation and a stable sustained-release formulation is one in which this conformation is maintained throughout fabrication, during storage and after administration. Stability is determined by both the fabrication process and the microsphere formulation.

Table 2. Sustained-release formulations of human therapeutic proteins*

Protein	Encapsulation process (stabilization strategy)	Protein integrity Encapsulated (released)	Reference
Interferon-α	Atomization (complex and co -encapsulate protein with zinc)	NR	[23]
Erythropoietin	Emulsion (include hydroxy-propyl-β-cyclodextrin and BSA)	84% (>40% covalent aggregates remaining at 32 days)	[24]
Erythropoietin	Spray drying (none)	100% (NR)	[25]
Erythropoietin	Atomization (co-lyophilize with ammonium sulfate)	100% (99%)	[26]
Interferon-γ	Emulsion (maximize protein concentration; include trehalose)	NR (>90%)	[27]
GM-CSF	Emulsion (none)	NR (bioactive protein released)	[28]
Growth hormone	Emulsion (co-lyophilize with trehalose and mannitol)	NR (100%)	[27]
Growth hormone	Emulsion (maximize protein concentration; include trehalose)	~95% (<75% at 30 days)	[29]
Growth hormone	Atomization (complex and co-encapsulate protein with zinc)	97% (98% at 28 days)	[30]
Interleukin-1α	Emulsion (include BSA)	NR (<50% bioactivity released over 20 days)	[31]
Nerve growth factor	Emulsion (include carboxy-methyl-dextran and BSA)	NR (<60%)	[32]
Nerve growth factor	Atomization (none)	NR (94%)	[33]
Vascular endothelial growth factor	Atomization (none)	100% (93% at day 21)	[34]

*All proteins were encapsulated with poly(lactide-co-glycolide). Percent integrity listed is % monomer (or native dimer if applicable) determined by size-exclusion chromatography, except in [24] and [32] where gel electrophoresis and ELISA, respectively, were used. Integrity of encapsulated protein was determined by extracting the protein from the microspheres and assaying under non-denaturing conditions. Integrity of released protein is that obtained after hydration of the microspheres. NR, not reported. BSA, bovine serum albumin.

Protein degradation or inactivation occurs in one or more of three ways: physical (conformational) inactivation, aggregation and chemical inactivation. The physical stability of a protein is maintained using two strategies [18]. The first is to prevent unfolding of the polypeptide chain which can lead to chemical inactivation (by exposing buried reactive groups) or to aggregation (which is generally caused by exposure and interaction of hydrophobic groups). The second is to prevent irreversible aggregation or inactivation if partial unfolding does occur, thus allowing the protein to refold to its native conformation. These strategies are pursued both by informed process design and by formulation development approaches.

Preserving integrity through the microsphere fabrication process

In essentially all processes microsphere fabrication requires exposure of the protein to organic polymer solutions. Some processes additionally require exposure to an organic extraction solvent. The extent to which a given process affects protein structure or activity is assessed by extracting the drug from the final product prior to storage or use. Aqueous protein solutions may be encapsulated directly by emulsifying the drug solution in an immiscible solution of polymer. PLG microspheres of small molecular weight drugs and peptides, such as the ten amino acid LHRH agonist [35, 36], have been made by an emulsion process, depicted in Figure 2. This process has been applied to both model and therapeutic proteins by several groups (Tab. 2). Protein solutions also have been encapsulated by single emulsion [37] and phase separation [38] processes. These methods share two important features: the presence of a water/oil interface, and the need to remove both the organic polymer solvent and the water of the protein solution [39].

Several approaches have been taken to stabilize proteins for emulsion methods (Tab. 2). The fraction of the drug in the surface-denatured layer is minimized by inclusion of exogenous surfactants in the protein phase [24, 32, 40], by coencapsulating surface-active albumin or gelatin along with the drug of choice [24, 31, 32, 41], or by maximizing the protein concentration in the encapsulated solution (>100 mg/mL) [27]. Some of these results suggest that the protein in the interfacial layer represents a fixed loss, with exchange between surface-denatured and native populations being reversible or nonexistent. Cleland and Jones [27] stabilized hGH and γ-interferon toward emulsification by incorporating trehalose and mannitol in the protein phase. These small molecule osmolytes are known stabilizers of proteins in bulk solution (via preferential hydration of the native form [42]). In addition, these compounds stabilize [43] proteins against the final stress encountered in emulsion processes, i.e., the removal of water (by evaporation or lyophilization) from the encapsulated protein solution.

Lyophilized or precipitated proteins may be encapsulated as dehydrated solids wherein the protein particles are exposed directly to the polymer sol-

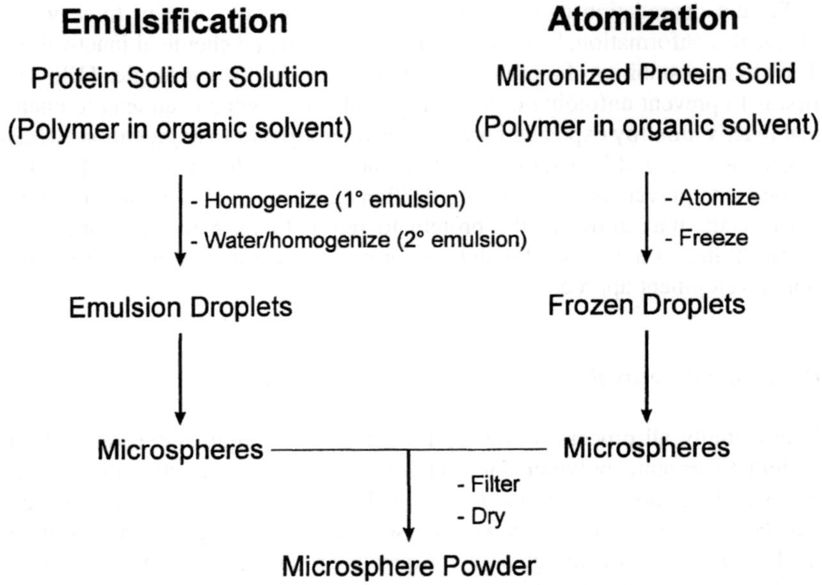

Figure 2. Two different processes to produce PLG microspheres. The emulsion process (left) is commonly used to encapsulate low molecular weight drugs and peptides, and the atomization process (right) is more suitable for proteins. Both begin with the polymer dissolved in an organic solvent (e.g., methylene chloride) in which the drug is insoluble. In the emulsion process the drug, in an aqueous solution or as a solid, is emulsified with the polymer solution. This gives small droplets or particles of drug contained in a larger droplet of polymer solution. Addition of water extracts the organic solvent and causes the PLG to precipitate around the drug particles, resulting in hardened microspheres, which are filtered and dried. In the atomization process, solid protein is suspended in the PLG solution and atomized using sonication or air atomization. The resultant droplets are frozen in liquid nitrogen. Addition of ethanol (at -80 °C), in which both the protein and the PLG are insoluble, extracts the organic solvent from the microspheres. Microspheres are injected after suspension in a slightly viscous aqueous vehicle.

vent. These conditions mimic the use of enzymes in organic solvents for synthetic applications [44]. The effect of organic solvents on protein powders has been probed spectroscopically; little additional denaturation results beyond that caused by lyophilization prior to organic solvent exposure [45, 46]. Moreover, enzymes exhibit remarkable thermostability in anhydrous solvents [47], an appealing feature for a commercial-scale process. The native protein structure is not favored thermodynamically in organic solvents. Nevertheless, conditions of limited molecular mobility – secured by a suitable solvent, a low-water environment, or low temperatures – provide a kinetic trap ensuring physical stability. Lyoprotectants also stabilize protein powders against organic solvent exposure [45]. Since no phase transitions are imposed on the protein particles during or after encapsulation, the incorporated drug particles will match the structure – and in theory the storage stability profile – of the starting material, as long as the kinetic trap is maintained.

While protein solids have been encapsulated by a variety of techniques, the most common is the spray-freeze atomization process depicted in Figure 2 [30, 48]. The process is essentially anhydrous, thereby minimizing water-induced conformational flexibility in the protein, which can result in unfolding [45, 49]. The polymer solvent is extracted with ethanol under conditions of low temperature (<–40 °C) and hence restricted motion.

Besides preserving protein integrity, the atomization process has several additional advantages. Because there are no immiscible phases, the process is free of surfactants, which are used in emulsion processes to reduce microsphere agglomeration and are difficult to remove. High (essentially quantitative) encapsulation efficiencies are obtained since the protein is insoluble throughout the process; up to 60% of the protein is lost to the external aqueous phase in emulsion techniques [29]. Also, the protein load in the microspheres is independent of the protein's solubility in water, in contrast to solution encapsulation methods.

Stability during storage and after administration

Stability within microspheres depends primarily on the formulation. Proteins differ significantly in their susceptibility to inactivation and in their inactivation pathways. Determining the optimal formulation is therefore a process of educated trial and error. Typically something is learned about the source of instability during development of a purification scheme or, if available, during development of a lyophilized formulation. Once the degradation pathways have been elucidated, various methods to prevent or inhibit these are investigated. This often requires the use of specific, pharmaceutically acceptable excipients (Tab. 2), which are added prior to lyophilization or as solids during microsphere formation. This keeps them in close proximity to the protein after microsphere administration.

An attractive way to maximize the physical stability of proteins in microspheres is to form a reversible, insoluble complex of the protein. Maintaining the protein in an undissolved, complexed form while in the microsphere both prevents or inhibits denaturation and protects the protein from enzymatic degradation or local pH changes. Many proteins form complexes with metal cations such as zinc [50], and zinc is present in pharmaceutical formulations of insulin [51]. Zinc has also been used to stabilize hGH in microspheres [30, 48] which mimics the natural means of storage of hGH in the pituitary [52]. Human growth hormone recovered from microspheres made with the atomization process was identical to the protein before encapsulation, as shown by reversed-phase, ion-exchange and size-exclusion chromatography, electrophoresis, bioactivity analysis and tryptic mapping [48]. Analysis in rhesus monkeys and transgenic mice expressing hGH showed that the hGH microspheres were no more immunogenic than hGH solution given as frequent injections [53].

In addition to being used to stabilize proteins toward organic solvents during microsphere fabrication, as discussed above, excipients can also stabilize the protein during storage by acting as glass formers or, in the case of some sugars, by forming hydrogen bonds with the protein after the removal of water [43]. Excipients such as buffers or ion-exchangers can be added to maintain the pH within the microspheres during degradation of the PLG polymer, although recent work has shown that the pH within the microsphere varies little during polymer degradation [54].

Uses of microspheres to deliver proteins

Just as improved delivery systems have enhanced the usefulness of low molecular weight drugs, sustained-release delivery of proteins has the potential to improve and expand the use of protein therapeutics. The most readily apparent use of sustained protein delivery is for proteins that are currently administered systemically. Examples of these (Tab. 2) range from proteins for replacement therapy to those given for autoimmune disorders, cancer and antiviral therapy. For proteins that are administered systemically, the goal is to maintain the serum concentration above the minimum therapeutic concentration. A Phase I clinical study of hGH in growth-hormone-deficient adults [22] showed that an elevated level of hGH is maintained for about three weeks by a single injection of microencapsulated protein (Fig. 3). Moreover, elevated levels of insulin-like growth factor (IGF-I) and IGF-binding protein 3 (IGFBP-3), both of which are induced by hGH, are maintained for a similar period of time. The biological effect of the sustained-release form (as measured by the increase in IGF-I and IGFBP-3) is notably greater than when the same dose is given as daily injections of the protein solution [30, 53].

Other applications of sustained-release include local delivery (such as delivery to sites that cannot be accessed by the blood stream) and vaccines. Such applications may eventually represent a large use of sustained-release protein formulations. Microsphere properties and performance, such as the duration of release, the protein load and microsphere size, can be adjusted to suit a particular application. The duration of release is determined principally by the polymer molecular weight and hydrophobicity. Microspheres as small as a few microns can be produced for certain applications, such as uptake by antigen-presenting cells, or for injection through very thin needles.

Local delivery

In many cases, proteins are administered systemically even though the desired site of action is a particular organ or tissue. It is generally not possible or practical to administer protein solutions directly to these sites because this would require invasive procedures and because the effective concentration would

A

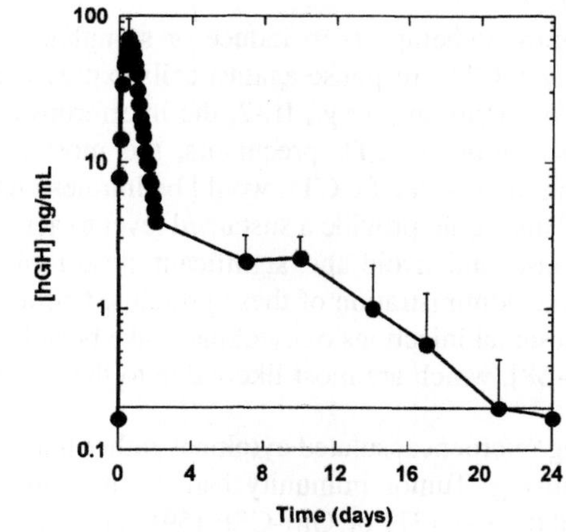

B

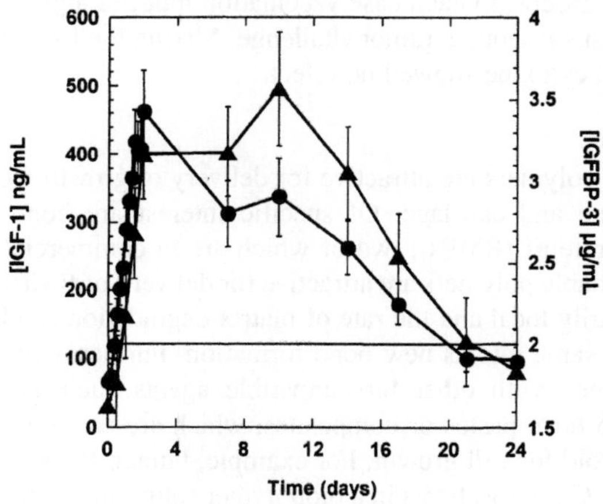

Figure 3. Serum protein concentrations induced by subcutaneous administration in human adults of a sustained-release formulation of hGH. A. Serum hGH levels following a single injection of hGH microspheres. B. Serum levels of IGF-I (triangles) and IGFBP-3 (circles) induced by the levels of hGH in (A). The horizontal line in (B) indicates the lower limit of normal for these proteins, and the line in (A) indicates the level of hGH (~0.2 ng/mL) that induces elevated levels of IGF-I and IGFBP-3. The hGH dose was 0.06 mg/kg. Data adapted from [22]. Values are means ± standard error.

quickly dissipate. Microsphere formulations would allow the effective concentration to be maintained locally for days to months, require significantly less protein and greatly reduce systemic exposure.

Immunotherapy of cancer

The goal of tumor immunotherapy is to induce or stimulate a CD8+ T-cell (cytotoxic T lymphocyte, CTL) response against cells expressing tumor-associated antigens. Because cytokines (e.g., IL-2, the interferons and GM-CSF) play a role in the activation of CTL precursors, the most straightforward approach to generating tumor-specific CTL would be intralesional administration of the cytokine. This would provide a sustained level to activate the developing immune response and avoid the significant dose-limiting toxicities resulting from systemic administration of these proteins. Unfortunately, clinical results with intralesional injections of cytokines have been limited to occasional responses [55–58], which are most likely due to the rapid clearance of the protein.

Initial studies using microencapsulated cytokines rather than gene transfection have been promising. Tumor immunity can be induced using microspheres containing either IL-1 [31] or GM-CSF [59]. The IL-1 microspheres were made using an emulsion method and the GM-CSF microspheres were formed by crosslinking chondroitin sulfate with glutaraldehyde. Although these methods of microsphere formation caused loss of activity of the IL-1 and are likely to have modified the GM-CSF by the reaction of glutaraldehyde with the free amino groups, in each case vaccination induced a protective immune response against subsequent tumor challenge. Mixing the irradiated cells with unencapsulated cytokine showed no effect.

Bones and joints

Biodegradable polymers are attractive for delivery of growth factors for engineering of bone and cartilage. Of specific interest are bone morphogenic (osteogenic) proteins (BMPs), two of which are in commercial development [60]. Biodegradable polymers are attractive for delivery of BMPs because their action is primarily local and the rate of matrix degradation can be adjusted to proceed at the same rate as new bone formation. Furthermore, microspheres can be combined with other biocompatible agents such as gels or other biopolymers to form pastes or composites, which are easily molded and can provide a scaffold for cell growth. For example, human BMP-2, administered as a paste of PLG microspheres in a biopolymer solution, is effective in repairing osseous defects in rats [61, 62]. BMPs have also shown promise for periodontal regeneration [63].

A related application is the treatment of joint disorders. In rheumatoid arthritis, the joints are sites of chronic inflammation, mediated by a variety of proinflammatory cytokines. Several cytokine antagonists (e.g., a soluble p55 TNF receptor [64], an anti-tumor necrosis factor (TNF) monoclonal, an IL-1 receptor antagonist and a soluble IL-1 receptor [65]) are being pursued in clinical trials as potential therapies, and a TNF receptor-Fc fusion protein (Enbrel, Immunex) has recently been approved [13]. All of these proteins share the dual need for chronic delivery (to neutralize perpetual proinflammatory signals arising from the synovium) and for levels sufficient to inhibit the target cytokine (which can require a large molar excess). Rheumatoid arthritis may prove susceptible to anti-angiogenic therapy as well. New vasculature is required to support the pathological growth of synovial cells in rheumatoid arthritis; levels of the angiogenic factor, vascular endothelial growth factor (VEGF), are elevated in rheumatoid synovial tissue [66].

Vasculature

In addition to being the most common avenue of drug delivery, the vasculature itself is a potential target of treatment. In an extrapolation of conventional intra-arterial drug administration, polymeric microspheres have been tested as chemoembolization anti-cancer agents. Targeted endovascular delivery results in occlusion, followed by release of the chemotherapeutic agent from the emboli. First demonstrated in humans over fifteen years ago, when mitomycin was delivered from ethylcellulose microcapsules [67], this approach to cancer treatment is still an active area of research.

Small microspheres (nanospheres) are also being explored for the prevention of post-angioplasty restenosis. PLG nanoparticles containing the anti-inflammatory dexamethasone were administered intraluminally by a brief infusion in a rat carotid model of balloon injury. The nanospheres effectively penetrated the arterial wall, persisting for up to two weeks [68]. Several additional agents have subsequently been tested [69]; a slow-release pluronic gel formulation of an antisense c-*myb* oligonucleotide inhibited smooth muscle cell accumulation in the carotid artery [70].

Microspheres containing angiogenic factors are also being considered for the treatment of coronary ischemia. Basic fibroblast growth factor (bFGF) was delivered from alginate microspheres when stabilized by the ligand heparin [71]. Heparin-alginate beads containing bFGF were administered extraluminally in a porcine model of chronic ischemia, resulting in improved coronary flow and reduction in infarct size [72]. A related approach to revascularization of the heart is currently being tested in humans.

Cancer therapy using angiogenesis inhibitors

From the earliest days of sustained-release of proteins from polymeric matrices, this technology has been pursued for delivery of anti-cancer proteins. An angiogenesis inhibitor, which deprives the tumor of growth-supporting vasculature, was found to inhibit tumor growth when delivered in a sustained, localized fashion [73]. To date many such factors have been identified [74] and several have been tested (with frequent administration of a protein solution) in clinical trials.

Antibodies to angiogenic factors have also been used [75]. With the concept that angiogenic factors, such as VEGF, are not simply growth enhancers but are required for maintenance of existing vasculature, such antibodies may hold additional promise for cancer therapy. This is shown by the regression of preformed blood vessels following administration of an antibody to VEGF [76]. This indicates a potential threat to normal vasculature by systemic delivery of these proteins and suggests that local delivery may not only be desirable but also necessary.

Protein delivery to the brain

Proteins are unable to access some tissues from the blood stream. An example is the brain which is protected from the vasculature by the blood-brain barrier. In this case the protein (or its gene) must be delivered using invasive techniques, and significant research has been done with gene delivery using recombinant viruses [77, 78] or transfected cells [79, 80]. An alternative would be to deliver a sustained-release microsphere formulation, and encapsulation and brain delivery of nerve growth factor (NGF) has been demonstrated [32, 81]. One report showed prevention of cholinergic degeneration in the nucleus basalis after cortical devascularization [82]. Recent studies of brain implants of PLG have verified the biocompatibility of these polymers [83].

Intraocular delivery

Another protected site is the retina, which is protected by the blood-retinal barrier. Consequently, numerous eye disorders (e.g., proliferative vitreoretinopathy, cytomegalovirus (CMV) retinitis, and endophthalmitis) must be treated by direct injection of the drug into the posterior (vitreal) chamber [84]. Due to risks of infection and retinal detachment and the invasive nature of intravitreal injections, a strong incentive exists for sustained-release dosage forms. In 1996 the first such product, Vitrasert, a non-erodible implant releasing ganciclovir over six months, was approved for the treatment of CMV retinitis [85]. This device is placed out of the line of vision and requires eventual retrieval. Initial reports of intravitreal injection of PLG microspheres have been made [86, 87] and, although they would presumably be free-floating within the vitreous, preliminary testing in rabbits suggests that microspheres are unlikely to interfere with vision [87].

Whereas the majority of research into sustained intraocular drug delivery involves small drugs, numerous opportunities exist for proteins. Inhibitors of neovascularization have long been considered as potential therapies of diabetic and proliferative retinopathy [88]. Cytokines are potential therapeutic agents for herpes simplex virus infection [89] and for choroidal neovascularization associated with age-related macular degeneration [90]. A wide variety of ophthalmological pathologies result from uncontrolled vascularization, and retinal neovascularization has been inhibited *in vivo* with intravitreal injection of a chimeric receptor of VEGF [91]. A human anti-CMV antibody is being developed for CMV retinitis and, although effective vitreal levels have been achieved in rabbits with systemic administration [92], direct administration to the posterior vitreal chamber would both greatly reduce systemic exposure and reduce the risk of antibody formation.

Vaccines

Vaccination to develop long-lasting immunity depends on continuous exposure to the protein antigen [93], and immune responses to numerous PLG-encapsulated viral and bacterial antigens have been demonstrated. Humoral (IgG and IgM) responses have been elicited by parenteral administration of PLG-encapsulated diphtheria toxoid tetanus toxoid and HIV gp120; mucusol immunity (IgA) was induced with *B. pertussis* after intranasal dosing and with SIV and Staphylococcal enterotoxin after oral administration [94]. These microsphere formulations were made using emulsion processes and, because antibody formation is the goal, the necessity to maintain protein integrity is less stringent than with therapeutic proteins. Unless the principal antigenic determinants are discontinuous and hence depend on a particular tertiary structure, a considerable degree of denaturation can be tolerated.

The most vigorous and long-lasting immunity is believed to be induced if antigen exposure is not only continuous but also if it occurs in two or more pulses (boosters) separated by several weeks or months [93]. Achieving such pulsatile delivery is considerably more challenging because this requires release at a predetermined time as well as maintaining the unreleased protein in an antigenic form for weeks or months. This has recently been achieved with tetanus toxoid in which pulses of release at 3 and 7 weeks were achieved by using different microsphere formulations consisting of PLG that degrade at different rates [95].

Summary

On the time-scale of the evolution of the modern pharmacopoeia, protein therapeutics are relatively new. However, because cellular functions are in large part carried out by proteins and because the knowledge of protein function is expanding due to genomic information, it is likely that therapeutic proteins will continue to be developed at an increasing rate. The ability to clone and express genes and cDNAs and produce virtually any protein in large quantities has allowed numerous proteins to be tested as drugs and many have reached the marketplace. The next step, development of more advanced protein delivery systems, such as injectable sustained-release systems, will improve the use and expand the application of protein therapeutics. Such advances are necessary to enable proteins to become as widespread and commonplace as other classes of drugs.

References

1 Struck MM (1994) Biopharmaceutical R and D success rates and development times: A new analysis provides benchmarks for the future. *Bio/Technology* 12: 674–677
2 Talmadge JE (1998) Pharmacodynamic aspects of peptide administration biological response modifiers. *Adv Drug Deliv Rev* 33: 241–252
3 Lee HJ (1995) Biopharmaceutical properties and pharmacokinetics of peptide and protein drugs. In: M Taylor, G Amidon (eds): *Peptide-based drug design.* American Chemical Society, Washington, D.C., 69–97
4 Arky R (1997) *Physician's desk reference.* Medical Economics Company, Montvale, NJ
5 Zhi J, Teller SB, Satoh H, Koss-Twardy SG, Luke DR (1995) Influence of human serum albumin content in formulations on the bioequivalency of interferon alfa-2a given by subcutaneous injection in healthy male volunteers. *J Clin Pharmacol* 35: 281–284
6 Mordenti J, Chen SA, Ferraiolo BL (1993) Pharmacokinetics of interferon-gamma. *In*: AHC Kung, RA Baughman, JW Larrick (eds): *Therapeutic proteins. Pharmacokinetics and pharmacodynamics.* W.H. Freeman, New York, 187–199
7 Harvey S (1995) Growth hormone metabolism. *In*: S Harvey, CG Scanes, WH Daughaday (eds): *Growth Hormone.* CRC Press, Boca Raton, FL, 285–301
8 Cohen AM (1993) Erythropoietin and G-CSF. *In*: AHC Kung, RA Baughman, JW Larrick (eds): *Therapeutic proteins. Pharmacokinetics and pharmacodynamics.* W.H. Freeman, New York, 165–186
9 Stute N, Furman WL, Schell M, Evans WE (1995) Pharmacokinetics of recombinant human granulocyte-macrophage colony-stimulating factor in children after intravenous and subcutaneous administration. *J Pharm Sci* 84: 824–828
10 Knauf MJ, Bell DP, Hirtzer P, Luo Z-P, Young JD, Katre NV (1988) Relationship of effective molecular size to systemic clearance in rats of recombinant interleukin-2 chemically modified with water-soluble polymers. *J Biol Chem* 263: 15 064–15 070
11 Clark R, Olson K, Fuh G, Marian M, Mortensen D, Teshima G, Chang S, Chu H (1996) Long-acting growth hormones produced by conjugation with polyethylene glycol. *J Biol Chem* 271: 21 969–21 977
12 Tsutsumi Y, Kihira T, Tsunoda S, Kamda H, Nakagawa S, Kaneda Y, Kanamori T, Mayumi T (1996) Molecular design of hybrid tumor necrosis factor-alpha III: Polyethylene glycol-modified tumor necrosis factor-alpha has markedly enhanced antitumor potency due to longer plasma half-life and higher tumor accumulation. *J Pharmacol Exp Ther* 278: 1006–1011
13 Moreland LW, Baumgartner SW, Schiff MH, Tindall EA, Fleischmann RM, Weaver AL, Ettlinger RE, Cohen S, Koopman WJ, Mohler K et al (1997) Treatment of rheumatoid arthritis with a recombinant human tumor necrosis factor receptor (p75)-Fc fusion protein. *N Engl J Med* 337: 141–147
14 Macdougall IC, Gray SJ, McEvoy O, Breen C, Jenkins B, Browne J, Egrie J (1999) Pharmacokinetics of novel erythropoiesis stimulating protein (NESP) compared with epoetin alfa in dialysis patients. *J Amer Soc Nephrol* 10: 2392–2397
15 Bendele A, Seely J, Richey C, Sennello G, Shopp G (1998) Short communication: Renal tubular vacuolation in animals treated with polyethylene-glycol-conjugated proteins. *Toxicol Sci.* 42: 152–157
16 Langer R (1990) New methods of drug delivery. *Science* 249: 1527–1533
17 Cleland JL (1996) Protein delivery from biodegradable microspheres. *In*: L Sanders, W Hendren (eds): *Protein delivery – physical systems.* Plenum Publishing, New York, 1–43
18 Schwendeman SP, Cardomone M, Brandon MR, Klibanov A, Langer R (1996) Stability of proteins and their delivery from biodegradable polymer microspheres. *In*: S Cohen, H Bernstein (eds): *Microspheres/microparticles: characterization and pharmaceutical application.* Marcel Dekker, New York, 1–49
19 Pitt CG (1990) The controlled parenteral delivery of polypeptides and proteins. *Int J Pharm* 59: 173–196
20 Austin PE, Dunn KA, Elly-Cofield K, Brown CK, Wooden WA, Bradfield JF (1995) Subcuticular sutures and the rate of inflammation in noncontaminated wounds. *Ann Emerg Med* 25: 328–330
21 Pihlajamaki H, Bostman O, Hirvensalo E, Tormala P, Rokkanen P (1992) Absorbable pins of self-reinforced poly-L-lactic acid for fixation of fractures and osteotomies. *J Bone Joint Surg* 74: 853–857

22 Vance ML, Woodburn CJ, Putney S, Grouse J, Lee HJ, Johnson OL (1997) Effects of sustained release growth hormone on serum GH, IGF-I and IGFBP-3 concentration in GH deficient adults. *Endocrinol Metab* 4 (suppl A): 75
23 Tracy MA, Bernstein H, Khan M (1998) *US Patent 5,711,978*
24 Morlock M, Koll H, Winter G, Kissel T (1997) Microencapsulation of rh-erythropoietin, using biodegradable poly(d,l-lactide-co-glycolide): protein stability and the effects of stabilizing excipients. *Eur J Pharm Biopharm* 43: 29–36
25 Bittner B, Morlock M, Koll H, Winter G, Kissel T (1998) Recombinant human erythropoietin (rhEPO) loaded poly(lactide-co-glycolide) microspheres: Influence of the encapsulation technique and polymer purity on microsphere characteristics. *Eur J Pharm Biopharm* 45: 295–305
26 Zale SE, Burke PA, Bernstein H, Brickner A (1996) Composition for sustained release of non-aggregated erythropoietin. *US Patent 5,674,534*
27 Cleland JL, Jones AJS (1996) Stable formulations of recombinant human growth hormone and interferon-gamma for microencapsulation in biodegradable microspheres. *Pharmacol Res* 13: 1464–1475
28 Pettit D, Pankey S, Nightlinger N, Disis M, Gombotz W (1996) GM-CSF encapsulated in PLGA microspheres for vaccine adjuvancy. *Proc Int Symp Control Rel Bioact Mat* 23: 857–858
29 Cleland JL, Mac A, Boyd B, Yang J, Duenas ET, Yeung D, Brooks D, Hsu C, Chu H, Mukku V et al (1997) The stability of recombinant human growth-hormone in poly(lactic-co-glycolic acid) (PLGA) Microspheres. *Pharmacol Res* 14: 420–425
30 Johnson OL, Cleland JL, Lee HJ, Charnis M, Duenas E, Jaworowicz W, Shepard D, Shahzamani A, Jones AJS, Putney SD (1996) A month-long effect from a single injection of microencapsulated human growth hormone. *Nat Med* 2: 795–799
31 Chen L, Apte RN, Cohen S (1997) Characterization of PLGA microspheres for the controlled delivery of IL-1 alpha for tumor immunotherapy. *J Control Release* 43: 261–272
32 Krewson CE, Dause R, Mak M, Saltzman WM (1996) Stabilization of nerve growth factor in controlled release polymers and in tissue. *J Biomater Sci-Polym Ed* 8: 103–117
33 Cleland JL, Duenas ET (1997) Controlled delivery of nerve growth factor for local treatment of neuronal diseases. *Proc Int Symp Control Rel Bioact Mat* 24: 823–824
34 Cleland JL, Duenas ET, Kahn J, Park A, Daugherty A, Cuthbertson A (1997) Local controlled delivery of vascular endothelial growth factor provides neovascularization. *Proc Int Symp Control Rel Bioact Mat* 24: 85–86
35 Sanders LM, Kell BA, McRae GI, Whitehead GW (1986) Prolonged controlled release of nafarelin, a luteinizing hormone-releasing hormone analogue from biodegradable polymeric implants: influence of composition and molecular weight of polymer. *J Pharm Sci* 75: 356–360
36 Ogawa Y, Yamamoto M, Okada H, Yashiki Y, Shimamoto T (1988) A new technique to efficiently entrap leuprolide acetate into microcapsules of polylactic acid or copoly(lactic/glycolic) acid. *Chem Pharm Bull* 36: 1095–1103
37 Tabata Y, Takebayashi Y, Ueda T, Ikada Y (1993) A formulation method using D,L-lactic acid oligomer for protein release with reduced initial burst. *J. Cont. Rel.* 23: 55–64
38 Lewis DH (1990) Controlled release of bioactive agents from lactide/glycolide polymers. *In*: M Chasin, R Langer (eds): *Biodegradable Polymers as Drug Delivery Systems.* Marcel Dekker, New York, 1–41
39 Putney SD, Burke PA (1998) Improving protein therapeutics with sustained-release formulations. *Nat Biotechnol* 16: 153–157
40 Mittal S, Cohen A, Maysinger D (1994) *In vitro* effects of brain derived neurotrophic factor released from microspheres. *NeuroReport* 5: 2577–2582
41 Mendez A, Camarata PJ, Suryanarayanan R, Ebner TJ (1997) Sustained intracerebral delivery of nerve growth factor with biodegradable polymer microspheres. *Meth Neurosci* 21: 150–167
42 Arakawa T, Timasheff S (1985) The stabilization of proteins by osmolytes. *Biophys J* 47: 411–414
43 Pikal MJ (1996) Freeze drying of proteins: process, formulation and stability. *In*: JL Cleland, R Langer (eds): *Formulation and Delivery of Proteins and Peptides*. American Chemical Society, Washington, 120–133
44 Klibanov AM (1989) Enzymatic catalysis in anhydrous organic solvents. *Trends Biochem Sci* 14: 141–144
45 Burke PA, Griffin RG, Klibanov AM (1992) Solid-state NMR assessment of enzyme active center structure under nonaqueous conditions. *J Biol Chem* 267: 20 057–20 064
46 Griebenow K, Klibanov AM (1996) On protein denaturation in aqueous-organic mixtures but not

in pure organic solvents. *J Amer Chem Soc* 118: 11 695–11 700

47 Volkin DB, Staubli A, Langer R, Klibanov AM (1991) Enzyme thermoinactivation in anhydrous organic solvents. *Biotechnol Bioeng* 37: 843–853

48 Johnson OL, Jaworowicz W, Cleland JL, Bailey L, Charnis M, Duenas E, Wu CC, Shepard D, Magil S, Last T et al (1997) The stabilization and encapsulation of human growth-hormone into biodegradable microspheres. *Pharmacol Res* 14: 730–735

49 Hageman M (1992) Water sorption and solid-state stability of proteins. *In*: TJ Ahern, MC Manning (eds): *Stability of protein pharmaceuticals, part A; chemical and physical pathways of protein degradation*. Plenum Press, New York, 273–309

50 Coleman JE (1992) Zinc Proteins: Enzymes, storage proteins, transcription factors, and replication proteins. *Annu Rev Biochem* 61: 897–946

51 Steiner DF, Bell GI, Tager HS, Rubenstein AH (1995) Chemistry and biosynthesis of the islet hormones: insulin, islet amyloid polypeptide (amylin), glucagon, somatostatin, and pancreatic polypeptide. *In*: LJ Degroot (ed.): *Endocrinology*. W.B. Saunders, Philadelphia, 1296–1328

52 Cunningham BC, Mulkerrin MG, Wells JA (1991) Dimerization of human growth hormone by zinc. *Science* 253: 545–548

53 Lee HJ, Riley G, Johnson O, Cleland JL, Kim N, Charnis M, Bailey L, Duenas E, Shahzamani A, Marian M et al (1997) *In vivo* characterization of sustained-release formulations of human growth-hormone. *J Pharmacol Exp Ther.* 281: 1431–1439

54 Burke PA (1996) Determination of internal pH in PLGA microspheres using 31p NMR spectroscopy. *Proc Int Symp Control Rel Bioact Mat* 23: 133–134

55 Cortesina G, Destefani A, Galeazzi E, Cavallo G, Jemma C, Giovarelli M, vVai S, Forni G (1991) Interleukin 2 injected around tumour draining lymph nodes in head and neck cancer. *Head Neck* 13: 125–131

56 Ozzello L, Habif D, DeRosa C, Cantell K (1992) Cellular events accompanying regression of skin recurrences of breast carcinomas treated with intralesional injections of natural interferons alpha and gamma. *Cancer Res* 52: 4571–4581

57 Vlock D, Snyderman C, Johnson J, Myers E, Eibling RJ, Kirkwood J, Dutcher J, Adams G (1995) Phase 1b trial of the effect of peritumoural and intranodal injections of IL-2 in pateints with advanced squamous cell carcinoma of the head and neck; An Eastern Co-operative Oncology Group Trial. *J Immunol* 115: 134–139

58 Wussow P, Block B, Hartmann F, Deicher J (1988) Intralesional interferon alpha in advanced malignant melanoma. *Cancer* 61: 1071–1074

59 Golumbek PT, Azhari R, Jaffee EM, Levitsky HI, Lazenby A, Leong K, Pardoll DM (1993) Controlled release, biodegradable cytokine depots: a new approach in cancer vaccine design. *Cancer Res* 53: 5841–5844

60 Reddi AH (1994) Symbiosis of biotechnology and biomaterials: Applications in tissue engineering of bone and cartilage. *J Cell Biochem* 56: 192–195

61 Kenley R, Marden LJ, Turek T, Jin L, Ron E, Hollinger JO (1994) Osseous regeneration in the rat calvarium using novel delivery systems for recombinant human bone morphogenetic protein-2 (rhBMP-2). *J Biomed Mater Res* 28: 1139–1147

62 Lee SC, Shea M, Battle MA, Kozitza K, Ron E, Turek T, Schaub RG, Hayes WC (1994) Healing of large segmental defects in rat femurs is aided by rhBMP-2 in PLGA matrix. *J Biomed Mater Res* 28: 1149–1156

63 Ripamonti U, Reddi AH (1994) Periodontal regeneration: potential role of bone morphogenetic proteins. *J Periodont Res* 29: 225–235

64 Eliaz R, Wallach D, Kost J (1996) Long-term protection against the effects of tumor necrosis factor by controlled delivery of the soluble p55 TNF receptor. *Cytokine* 8: 482–487

65 Feldmann M, Brennan FM, Maini RN (1996) Role of cytokines in rheumatoid-arthritis. *Annu Rev Immunol* 14: 397–440

66 Fava RA, Olsen HM, Spencer-Green G, Yeo K-T, Yeo T-K, Berse B, Jackman RW, Senger DR, Dvorak HF, Brown LF (1994) Vascular permeability factor/endothelial growth factor (VPF/VEGF): accumulation and expression in human synovial fluids and rheumatoid synovial tissue. *J Exp Med* 180: 341–346

67 Kato T, Nemoto R, Mori H, Takahashi M, Tanakawa Y, Horada M (1981) Arterial chemoembolization with microencapsulated anticancer drug. *J Amer Med Assoc* 245: 1123

68 Guzman LA, Labhasetwar V, Song CX, Jang YS, Lincoff AM, Levy R, Topol EJ (1996) Local intraluminal infusion of biodegradable polymeric nanoparticles – A novel approach for prolonged

drug delivery after balloon angioplasty. *Circulation* 94: 1441–1448
69 Song CX, Labhasetwar V, Murphy H, Qu X, Humphrey WR, Shebuski RJ, Levy RJ (1997) Formulation and characterization of biodegradable nanoparticles for intravascular local drug delivery. *J Control Release* 43: 197–212
70 Simons M, Edelman ER, DeKeyser JL, Langer R, Rosenberg RD (1992) Antisense *c-myb* oligonucleotides inhibit intimal arterial smooth muscle cell accumulation *in vivo*. *Nature* 359: 67–70
71 Edelman ER, Mathiowitz E, Langer R, Klagsbrun M (1991) Controlled and modulated release of basic fibroblast growth factor. *Biomaterials* 12: 619–626
72 Harada K, Grossman W, Friedman M, Edelman ER, Prasad PV, Keighley CS, Manning WJ, Sellke FW, Simons M (1994) Basic fibroblast growth factor improves myocardial function in chronically ischemic porcine hearts. *J Clin Invest* 94: 623–630
73 Langer R, Conn H, Vacanti J, Haudenschild C, Folkman J (1980) Control of tumor-growth in animals by infusion of an angiogenesis inhibitor. *Proc Natl Acad Sci USA* 77: 4331–4335
74 Folkman J (1995) Angiogenesis in cancer, vascular, rheumatoid and other disease. *Nat Med* 1: 27–31
75 Kim KM, Li B, Winer J, Armanini M, Gillett N, Phillips GS, Ferrara N (1993) Inhibition of vascular endothelial growth factor-induced angiogenesis suppresses tumour growth *in vivo*. *Nature* 362: 841–844
76 Yuan F, Chen Y, Dellian M, Safabakhsh N, Ferrara N, Jain RK (1996) Time-dependent vascular regression and permeability changes in established human tumor xenografts induced by an anti-vascular endothelial growth factor vascular permeability factor antibody. *Proc Natl Acad Sci USA* 93: 14 765–14 770
77 Ridet JL, Privat A (1995) Gene therapy in the central nervous system: direct *versus* indirect gene delivery. *J Neurosci Res* 42: 287–293
78 Blomer U, Naldini L, Verma IM, Trono D, Gage F (1996) Applications of gene therapy to the CNS. *Hum Mol Genet* 5: 1397–1404
79 Lindner MD, Kearns CE, Win SR, Frydel B, Emerich DF (1996) Effects of intraventricular encapsulated hNGF-secreting fibroblasts in aged rats. *Cell Transplant* 5: 205–223
80 Kordower JH, Win SR, Li Y, Mufson EF, Sladek JR, Hammang JP, Baetge EE, Emerich DF (1994) The aged monkey basal forebra*ln*: rescue and sprouting of axotomized basal forebrain neurons after grafts of encapsulated cells secreting human nerve growth factor. *Proc Natl Acad Sci USA* 91: 10 898–10 902
81 Camarata PJ, Suryanarayanan R, Turner DA, Parker RG, Ebner TJ (1992) Sustained release of nerve growth factor from biodegradable polymer microspheres. *Neurosurgery* 30: 313–319
82 Maysinger D, Jalsenjak I, Cuello AC (1992) Microencapsulated nerve growth factor: Effects on the forebrain neurons following devascularizing cortical lesions. *Neurosci Lett* 140: 71–74
83 Kou JH, Emmett C, Shen P, Aswani S, Iwamoto T, Vaghefi F, Cain G, Sanders L (1997) Bioerosion and biocompatibility of poly(d,l-lactic-co-glycolic acid) implants in brain. *J Control Release* 43: 123–130
84 Peyman HA, Ganiban GJ (1995) Delivery systems for intraocular routes. *Adv Drug Deliv Rev* 16: 107–123
85 Smith TJ, Pearson PA, Blandford DL, Brown JD, Goins KA, Hollins JL, Schmeisser ET, Glavinos P, Baldwin LB, Ashton P (1992) Intravitreal sustained-release ganciclovir. *Arch Ophthalmol* 110: 255–258
86 Moritera T, Ogura Y, Honda Y, Wada R, Hyon S-H, Ikada Y (1991) Microspheres of biodegradable polymers as drug delivery system in the vitreous. *Invest Ophthalmol Visual Sci* 32: 1785–1790
87 Giordano GG, Chevez-Barrios P, Refojo MF, Garcia CA (1995) Biodegradation and tissue reaction to intravitreous biodegradable poly(D,L-lactic-co-glycolic)acid microspheres. *Curr Eye Res* 14: 761–768
88 Patz A, Brem S, Finkelstein D, Chen CH, Lutty G, Bennett A, Coughlin WR, Gardner J (1978) A new approach to the problem of retinal neovascularization. *Ophthalmology* 85: 626–637
89 Geiger K, Howes EL, Sarvetnick N (1994) Ectopic expression of gamma interferon in the eye protects transgenic mice from intraocular herpes simplex virus type 1 infections. *J Virol* 68: 5556–5567
90 Chan CK, Kempin SJ, Noble SK, Palmer GA (1994) The treatment of choroidal neovascular membranes by alpha interferon: an efficacy and toxicity study. *Ophthalmology* 101: 289–300
91 Aiello LP, Pierce EA, Foley ED, Takagi H, Chen H, Riddle L, Ferrara N, King GL, Smith LEH

(1995) Suppression of retinal neovascularization *in vivo* by inhibition of vascular endothelial growth factor (VEGF) using soluble VEGF-receptor chimeric proteins. *Proc Natl Acad Sci USA* 92: 10 457–10 461
92 Ostberg L, Queen C (1995) Human and humanized monoclonal antibodies: preclinical studies and clinical experience. *Biochem Soc Trans* 23: 1038–1043
93 Janeway CA, Travers P (1994) *Immunobiology: The immune system in health and disease.* Current Biology, Ltd., London
94 Cleland JL (1995) Design and production of single-immunization vaccines using polylactide-polyglycolide microsphere systems. *In*: MF Powell, MJ Newman (eds): *Vaccine Design: The Subunit and Adjuvant Approach.* Plenum Press, New York, 439–462
95 Sanchez A, Gupta RK, Alonso MJ, Siber GR, Langer R (1996) Pulsed controlled-release system for potential use in vaccine delivery. *J Pharm Sci* 85: 547–552

Recombinant Protein Drugs
ed. by P. Buckel

Principles of gene transfer and foreign protein expression for human gene therapy

Theodore Friedmann

Center for Molecular Genetics, UCSD School of Medicine and Program in Human Gene Therapy, La Jolla, CA 92093, USA

Introduction

The conceptual and technical bases for human gene therapy are maturing rapidly. At its inception in the early 1970s, gene therapy presumed the eventual development of efficient and targeted vectors to deliver therapeutic foreign genetic elements into defective cells for the purpose of complementing underlying genetic defects responsible for human genetic disease. The initial models for this approach were the single-gene Mendelian defects associated with classical "inborn errors of metabolism". It was a relatively simple task to demonstrate early that normal alleles could be introduced into defective cells, that newly expressed gene products could complement genetic defects and that aspects of complex disease phenotypes could be reversed in *in vitro* and animal model systems.

For some time, the technological march to human clinical application seemed relatively straightforward, although technically challenging. The great clinical need for improved treatment for many dire human diseases, together with the optimism and zeal of many investigators, led to a series of early clinical studies in human patients during the late 1980s and early 1990s that proved, unfortunately, that therapeutically useful levels of gene transfer and foreign gene expression in human tissues would be more difficult and more elusive than many had expected. These early studies were useful in their demonstration that foreign genes could be introduced into intact humans and other mammals by a variety of *ex vivo* and *in vivo* methods and that such foreign transgenes could indeed, under some conditions, be expressed for prolonged periods of time *in vivo*. Unfortunately, and to many people's surprise, the studies also demonstrated that the efficiency and stability of gene expression from initial classes of gene transfer vectors, both viral and non-viral, were too low and the methods for gene introduction too promiscuous and too nonspecific to produce a clinically useful effect in real patients with real disease.

During the past several years, the concepts and tools required for clinically applicable gene therapy have advanced very quickly. Improved vector systems have been and continue to be developed and new techniques for gene transfer and for transplantation of genetically modified cells and tissues are appearing with blinding speed. With this maturation and evolution of the field over the past several decades, the genetic approach to therapy has come to be applied to diseases characterized by Mendelian genetic defects, by acquired genetic defects such as those represented by most human cancers, multigenic and multifactorial disorders such as many kinds of cardiovascular and degenerative disease and, finally, even to largely non-genetic disorders such as AIDS and other infectious diseases. A large number of clinical trials are underway worldwide for most of these classes of disease and it seems very likely that clinical efficacy will be demonstrated in a number of these systems in the very near future.

Interestingly, as the road to somatic cell gene modification is becoming smoother, the road to other applications of gene transfer technology is becoming less well delineated. Looming ahead are still largely imponderable problems associated with germ-line genetic modification, enhancement of non-disease traits and the vague but inevitable confluence of gene transfer technology with advances in reproductive technology, exemplified by cloning and other oocyte nuclear transplantation applications. The near future will thrill us through the development of truly effective gene therapy for many terrible diseases while it challenges us in ways previously reserved for science fiction.

The concept of human gene therapy dates back to the early 1970s and was initially based on the notion that the introduction of a wild-type allele of a disease-related gene into the appropriate target cell could complement a defective gene product and correct a disease phenotype [1]. The earliest target diseases were the single-gene defects represented by the "inborn errors of metabolism", as defined by Archibald Garrod [2]. From the very outset, implementation of the concept of gene therapy rested on the need for a number of technical advances, including the development of efficient and safe vectors for transferring therapeutic genes, the design of methods for specific and efficient vector delivery to the diseased tissue, and the assurance of stable, prolonged and/or appropriately regulated gene expression at physiologically appropriate levels in the diseased tissue *in vivo*. During the ensuing several decades, great advances have been made toward all these goals.

Gene transfer vectors

Virus vectors

It was realized early in the development of gene therapy that engineered and disabled viruses would constitute one class of effective gene transfer vectors, since many kinds of mammalian viruses have evolved to carry out precisely the task required in gene therapy – the efficient and stable insertion of foreign genes into cells in a way that does not damage the host cells but that permits stable, long-term expression of the newly introduced gene. The prototype vectors, and the first efficient gene transfer agents, were the retrovirus vectors, developed in the early 1980s [3, 4]. While these agents have significant advantages, including their genetic simplicity and their ability to integrate into the host cell genome to provide stable, long-term expression, they suffer from a number of deficiencies, including their relatively low titers, their instability *in vivo* and their inability to infect non-replicating cells. Several of these difficulties have been eased to some extent by the discovery that the murine retroviruses can be engineered to contain foreign envelope proteins such as the G protein of vesicular stomatitis virus (VSV-G) on their surfaces to allow purification to higher titers, increased stability *in vivo* and expanded and potentially targeted cell tropism [5–8]. The difficulties with retrovirus vectors have recently been solved still further by the development of vectors derived from the lentivirus class of retroviruses [9–12], as represented by HIV that causes AIDS and related viruses such as feline lentivirus [12, 13]. The general strategy for the design and use of these vectors is similar to the other retrovirus vectors, but their use is facilitated by their ability to infect non-replicating cells such as neurons and fully differentiated hepatocytes *in vivo* [12].

Other classes of virus vectors have become available that obviate some of the deficiencies of retrovirus- and lentivirus vectors and that make gene transfer into virtually all mammalian cell types quite efficient. Vectors derived from adenoviruses can be made to titers of 10^{12} or more, at least two to three orders of magnitude higher than the retrovirus vectors [14–16]. They infect non-replicating cells with great efficiency but do not integrate into the host cell genome, thereby making prolonged transgene expression unlikely in many replicating target cells. Early generations of adenovirus vectors have been hampered by their potent immunogenicity and their powerful adjuvant effect that also can produce a host immune response to the transgene product [16]. Newer generations of further engineered adenovirus vectors and, in particular, the recent development of replication-dependent "gutless" adenovirus vectors promise to reduce markedly, but possibly not completely eliminate, the host immune response to these vectors [17]. Nevertheless, in fact, prolonged and potentially therapeutic levels of transgenes in several disease models have been achieved with various classes of adenovirus vectors [16].

Vectors derived from the human adeno-associated parvovirus (AAV) have also become a very important gene vector system [18]. The AAV vectors combine some of the attractive features of retroviruses and adenoviruses since they are generally non-pathogenic and apparently non-immunogenic. They are able to infect non-replicating cells, can also integrate into the host genome to permit prolonged and stable expression and can be made to high titers [18]. The use of AAV vectors is currently providing very high, stable and potentially therapeutic levels of gene products in animal model systems of several metabolic diseases, including hemophilia B [19, 20]. A number of additional important virus vector systems are being examined, including vectors derived from herpes viruses, alpha viruses, papovaviruses, baculoviruses, vaccinia, influenza virus, poliovirus, Epstein-Barr virus and even bacteriophage [21]. Finally, while most viral transduction systems have taken advantage of replication-defective variants of the vectors, a replication-competent vector system has recently been applied to the specific destruction of tumor cells *in vivo*, based on designs of adenovirus variants that produce cell lysis preferentially in cells deficient in the tumor suppressor gene p53 [22]. Direct injection of one such virus mutant into the tumor mass in patients with some kinds of cancer, particularly head and neck cancers, has been reported to produce a clinically beneficial result.

Naked DNA, non-viral vectors and receptor-mediated gene delivery

In addition to virus vectors, a number of non-viral gene transfer systems for therapeutic gene delivery have recently undergone an impressive evolution and improvement, both *in vitro* and *in vivo*. These systems include the development of liposomes, cationic lipids, polylysine conjugates and even naked plasmid transfection methods [23–25]. The potential use of naked plasmid DNA for therapeutic gene transfer is made possible by the surprising fact that plasmid DNA is unexpectedly stable in some tissues *in vivo*, for instance in skeletal muscle. Furthermore, the efficiency of *in vivo* gene expression after plasmid delivery by a variety of routes, including intramuscular, intradermal, intravenous and intrasplenic injection, is sufficiently high to permit effective use of DNA to express new proteins *in vivo*, as demonstrated by their effectiveness as vaccines for immunization against a variety of infectious diseases such as influenza and others [26].

In applications other than as DNA vaccines, the *in vivo* delivery of plasmid DNA has been reported to produce direct effects in a number of other pathological settings, as for instance in the apparent therapeutic effect in patients with severe peripheral vascular occlusive disease. In those studies, the intramuscular injection of a plasmid vector encoding vascular endothelial growth factor (VEGF) has been reported to induce neovascularization and salvage of limbs destined for amputation [27, 28].

The addition of compacting agents and of an endosmolytic agent such as adenovirus markedly improves gene transfer by naked DNA [24]. In addition, the development of methods to link compacted DNA with the endosomolytic adenovirus has increased the efficiency of naked gene transfer still further [24]. Finally, the inclusion of targeting ligands to foreign DNA complexes seems to provide promise for eventual tissue specificity, increased *in vivo* stability and improved gene transfer by naked DNA [24].

Liposomes and cationic lipids represent the next step up from naked DNA in the complexity of gene transfer vectors. Liposomes might even be thought of as a first step in the design of a virus vector. These particles consist of a structurally constrained or compacted segment of DNA associated with a protective layer of lipid to mediate cell entry. Liposomes and cationic lipid-DNA complexes deliver their genetic information into mammalian cells by fusion with the lipid bilayer of a target cell. However, the instability of such structures *in vivo* and the absence of ligands for interaction with tissue-specific receptors make the uptake into cells and the delivery of a therapeutic agent inefficient and promiscuous. Nevertheless, despite this overall inefficiency of liposome-mediated gene transfer and their notorious instability *in vivo*, liposomes were among the first vector systems to be used in a clinical setting *in vivo* for gene transfer in a cancer gene therapy study. Additional applications for cancer, cardiovascular disease and metabolic diseases such as cystic fibrosis have demonstrated levels of gene transfer sufficient to complement the CFTR defect of cystic fibrosis [29], to induce a host immune response in patients with malignant melanoma and other forms of cancer against their own tumor cells [30, 31] and to transfer potentially therapeutic genes into the cardiovascular system [32–34].

The further design of these lipid-DNA conjugates to allow them to function with the higher efficiency typical of virus vectors has been suggested by the recent demonstration that at least one viral envelope protein, the G protein of VSV, can be introduced into the liposome lipid envelope [35]. Such VSV-G-liposome particles demonstrate an insensitivity to inactivation by serum and an increased ability to transfer foreign genes into recipient cells, making them virus vector-like in their ability to enter cells by interacting with a specific cellular receptor rather than non-specifically entering cells through membrane fusion. The further modification of this system to include cell-specific ligands (see below) in VSV-G or in other viral envelope proteins would be expected to produce a particle able to deliver a therapeutic gene directly into a target tissue *in vivo*. This development would therefore represent the successful construction of a virus vector from first principles.

Vector targeting

One of the major goals for all vector-mediated gene transfer and especially for *in vivo* gene delivery is the modification of the vectors to define their entry to a specific cell type. The general strategy for accomplishing this vector targeting is to incorporate ligands into the virus particle that recognize tissue-specific receptors or other target cell membrane molecules and thereby restrict infection only to those cells expressing the receptor. If appropriate ligands, such as single-chain antibodies or small peptides, are incorporated into suitable sites in the receptor-binding domain of the appropriate viral protein, the ability of the virus to interact with its normal receptor might be abrogated or reduced and replaced with a new interaction to define a totally new vector tropism.

Such re-targeted vectors have been reported with retroviruses and adenovirus vectors [36–41]. In a number of studies, investigators have created chimeric viral envelope proteins by introducing proteins, single-chain antibodies or tissue-specific homing peptides into the envelope of the ecotropic

Moloney murine leukemia virus (MLV) envelope protein or into the fiber protein of adenovirus vectors. With various degrees of success, the vectors have demonstrated an altered tropism that reflects the new ligand-receptor interactions. In the case of the targeted MLV vectors, however, there has so far been little success in full replacement of the native envelope protein with the chimeric envelope, with the result that the vector demonstrated either poor infectivity or retained the tropism determined by the native envelope protein. This difficulty suggests that many of the chimeric envelope proteins are poorly expressed, poorly transported to the cell surface for virus assembly, cannot trimerize adequately in assembled virus particles, display the new ligand inefficiently in the context of the chimeric protein or have not adequately retained the fusiogenic functions required for virus infection. All these issues represent potentially soluble technical problems, and the general approach toward vector targeting seems feasible.

Routes of gene delivery

There are two major routes for therapeutic gene transfer – the *ex vivo* and the *in vivo* routes. In the *ex vivo* method, cells derived from the patient are exposed *in vitro* to the gene transfer vector. After the therapeutic gene is introduced *in vitro* into cells, the genetically modified cells are then returned to the patient to provide the new function *in vivo*. In the *in vivo* route, the gene transfer vector is introduced directly into the patient *in vivo*, either into the diseased organ, in the form of a targeted vector that can be directed specifically to the defective cells, or as a more or less promiscuous vector that can provide a therapeutic function from a variety of cells. Both of these schemes are being used in a large number of human clinical studies.

Ex vivo

This approach has been used in a number of studies intended to restore or correct expression of disease-related genes or to introduce new genes that might modify a disease phenotype. This is the approach that has been imagined to be ideal for readily accessible tissues such as the bone marrow. Unfortunately, the obviously great potential for gene therapy of many genetic and hematological diseases through modification of bone marrow stem cells has proven to be elusive because of difficulties in identifying and purifying the stem cells and the inefficiency of virtually all gene transfer methods to introduce genes into such cells without inducing the cells into differentiation pathways. Nevertheless, other tissues have proven to be more accessible for the *ex vivo* approach to gene therapy. Theoretically, the simplest strategy is the one involved in the studies aimed at correction of the genetic defects in inborn errors such as adenosine deaminase (ADA) deficiency [42, 43] and low-density lipoprotein receptor (LDLR) deficiency [44]. In those studies, the appropriate cells (peripheral blood T-cells for ADA deficiency, hepatocytes for LDLR deficiency) have been obtained from patients, genetically modified in culture *in vitro*, expanded as appropriate and returned to the patients. A large number of studies are currently underway that use the *ex vivo* approach for immunotherapy of cancer. The rationale for this approach is the knowledge that the development of cancer in a patient may be at least partly the result of a failure of one of the arms of the host immune response to destroy newly arisen cancer cells. In those therapeutic approaches, immune stimulatory functions, such as cytokines or co-stimulatory molecules, are introduced *in vitro* into cancer cells derived from patients. The genetically modified cells are then irradiated or otherwise rendered incapable of replication and then returned to the patient as a vaccine to induce a new host immune response against the tumor or to strengthen an inadequate immune response. Encouraging results are beginning to be reported in several of these systems, including the immunotherapy of solid tumors such as malignant melanoma [30, 45] and neuroblastoma [46, 47], as well as some leukemias [48–50] and other hematological malignancies.

In vivo

With improvements in vector titers, purity, targeting and *in vivo* stability has come an increased interest in the feasibility of *in vivo* gene delivery for gene therapy. Important technical advances toward this goal have included the improvement of retrovirus titers and stability [5–8, 51], the development of the lentivirus and adeno-associated vectors [12, 18], major improvements in the design of adenovirus vectors [16] and the now rapidly developing technology of vector targeting (see above). Some of the most promising current results are being obtained with the adeno-associated vectors in the treatment of the factor IX deficiency of hemophilia B. With this system, it has recently been possible to demonstrate in animal models potentially therapeutic levels of a foreign factor IX gene for very prolonged periods of time after *in vivo* delivery of the vector to the liver or skeletal muscle of factor IX-deficient animals [19, 20]. High levels of the factor VIII gene have also been demonstrated at high and persistent levels in animal models of hemophilia A. Furthermore, the newer generations of adenoviruses have shown effectiveness in expressing therapeutic levels of normal genes in animal models for alpha 1 antitrypsin deficiency, factor VIII deficiency and in the hypercholesterolemia resulting from defects in LDLR and in apoE [52–56]. Many other additional *in vivo* studies are underway for a variety of disease models.

A variant of the direct *in vivo* vector delivery approach is represented by studies aimed at more efficient transfer of potentially therapeutic genes to solid tumors, such as glioblastomas of the brain. In this case, the tumor is injected not with a vector but rather with cells that produce retrovirus vectors expressing "suicide" genes such as the thymidine kinase gene of the herpes virus simplex type 1. In principle, the replicating cells in the tumor will be exposed constantly to a locally high concentration of vectors and will be transduced efficiently. Other cells in the vicinity, such as normal neurons and other resident cells of the central nervous system (CNS), will be transduced much less efficiently because most are replicating slowly, if at all, and therefore not susceptible to retrovirus infection. Subsequent treatment of the patient with the prodrug ganciclovir will result in the production of the toxic phosphorylated metabolite only in the transduced tumor cells, thereby killing them while sparing non-tumor cells in surrounding normal brain tissue. While elegant in principle, this method has proven to be inefficient and largely ineffective to date and is increasingly receiving less attention than the other approaches involving direct vector delivery.

Gene correction

All the methods described above are based on the concept that genetic correction requires the addition of therapeutic genetic information to augment a genome containing disease-causing alleles. In the very long term, of course, methods will become available to make specific and targeted changes in the sequence of the target disease-related genes themselves. The earliest groping attempts toward this goal are now being made [57]. While these early studies are unlikely to represent definitive or clinically applicable sequence-correction techniques, it would be reasonable to predict that such methods based on targeted homologous recombination will be developed. When that occurs, definitive therapy of disease will occur through correction of underlying mutations rather than by addition of additional genetic information.

Human applications for therapy and enhancement

There are currently several hundred clinical gene therapy studies underway in the US, Europe, Japan and elsewhere. They are all based on the new expression of a gene product *in vivo* to complement a defect in a resident gene product or to add a new function that can modify an existing disease phenotype. While there are few, if any, convincing examples of true therapeutic benefit to patients by these genetic manipulations, there are many indications that initial demonstrations of true benefit to patients are imminent. It will come first in small-scale studies through applications that may not lend themselves readily to large-scale use. The pace of application will then obviously accelerate and will be further catalyzed by the powerful role that the biotechnology and pharmaceutical sectors are already playing in the research and implementation of the tools of gene therapy, including their production, distribution and marketing. These are the areas in which academic institutions do not play their principal roles.

In addition, pressures and opportunities for genetic approaches to many disorders will grow rapidly because of information and materials that will fall out of the cornucopia of the human genome project. Many new disease-related genes will quickly become available in many new kinds of disease, and the impetus for delivery of gene transfer technologies to the bedside will be more and more irresistible. Without a doubt, however, there will also be an increasing potential for genetic modification of a variety of human traits that may not represent true "disease" phenotypes but that do present opportunities for "enhancement" genetic modification for quasi-medical, cosmetic or social purposes. The genetic components for many human emotional, cognitive and personality traits are beginning to be recognized and characterized, and opportunities will therefore arise for altering them at a genetic level. For instance, the memory defects of Alzheimer's disease will increasingly be understood and treated pharmacologically, as they should be. Of course, new knowledge of the genetic basis for memory acquisition and retention will also present an irresistible target for correction, leading inevitably to pharmacological and genetic modification of memory even in normals. Similarly, gene transfer-based enhanced hair growth will be applied in a justifiably therapeutic sense, for instance, to patients undergoing cancer chemotherapy, but eventually also in"normals" for cosmetic purposes. Other physical and mental human traits including physical stature, skin color, aggressiveness, etc., will all, in the long term, become targets for genetic modification. Equally imponderable is the role that germ-line genetic modification will eventually play in therapeutic or enhancement gene modification [58]. However, the recent unconfirmed reports of the isolation of human embryonic stem cells bring the possibilities for germ-line modification closer to reality.

Addendum

Since the preparation of the original manuscript, there have been several pivotal events in the field of gene therapy that are having a great impact on the directions of the technology, on public perceptions and on the procedures used for review and regulation of human clinical studies.

Ironically, two sets of events have served to demonstrate how far we still are from truly efficient gene transfer technology and wide clinical application while, at the same time, providing the first convincing evidence for real therapeutic benefit of gene transfer technology in real patients with real human disease. The death of Mr. Jesse Gelsinger in the autumn of 1999 in a clinical study of ornithine transcarbamylase deficiency at the University of Pennsylvania served to highlight the great unknowns that still plague human clinical research in general and gene therapy in particular. Our inadequate knowledge of the pharmacodynamic and pharmacokinetic properties of vectors, their in vivo fate, the nature and mechanisms of host response to vectors and transgene products and the mechanisms for review and regulation of human experiments in this new field of medicine have been made painfully evident. These problems have resulted in loss of public confidence in this field and in the human genetics community, in the shutdown of some gene therapy programs, harsh sanctions against investigators and major changes in the roles of the federal regulatory agencies overseeing gene transfer studies in humans in the United States. The new review and regulatory procedures are aimed at greater emphasis on clinical training of investigators performing gene transfer studies in humans, on more effective reporting of adverse clinical events, on reducing the potential conflicts of interests in investigators that may interfere with clinical judgement and on improved methods of open and public review of proposed studies.

At the same time, recent results from two research groups have shown that patients with an immunological disorder (X-linked severe combined immunodeficiency disease) and a form of hemophilia (factor IX deficiency) are apparently benefitting in clinically significant ways from the restored expression of virus-delivered genes. These results represent the first, rigorous and convincing evidence for therapeutic benefit to patients in gene transfer studies. It seems very likely that these highly encouraging results, together with the renewed emphasis in the field on rigorous pre-clinical studies, on more attention to the design and performance of human clinical studies as well as to the qualifications of investigators, will allow more and more clinical studies to move to the stage of demonstrating some clinical benefit to experimental subjects and patients.

It is a very encouraging time in human gene therapy research and clinical application. It is a time not to step back from human clinical applications in this difficult area of medicine, but rather to develop broader and more comprehensive programs built on rigor in pre-clinical studies, better design and performance of clinical studies and improved governmental and institutional procedures for review and regulation. It must be only the most pessimistic viewers who can look at this landscape and not see enormous cause for optimism. The goal that we have all sought for so long, i.e., definitive control of human disease at the most basic level of the underlying genetic defect, is now in our grasp – loosely but without too much doubt.

References

1 Friedmann T, Roblin R (1972) Gene therapy for human genetic disease? *Science* 175: 949–955
2 Garrod AE (1923) *Inborn errors of metabolism*, Oxford: Oxford University Press,
3 Wei C, Gibson M, Spear PG, Scolnick EM (1981) Construction and isolation of a transmissible retrovirus containing the src gene from Harvey murine sarcoma virus and the thymidine kinase gene from herpes simplex virus type 1. *J Virol* 39: 935–944
4 Shimotohno K, Temin HM (1981) Formation of infectious progeny virus after insertion of herpes simplex thymidine kinase gene into DNA of an avian retrovirus. *Cell* 26: 67–77
5 Emi N, Friedmann T, Yee J-K (1991) Pseudotype formation of murine leukemia virus with the G protein of vesicular stomatitis virus. *J Virol* 65: 1202–1207
6 Burns JC, Matsubara T, Lozinski G et al (1994) Pantropic retroviral vector-mediated gene transfer, integration, and expression in cultured newt limb cells. *Develop Biol* 165: 285–289
7 Chen ST, Iida A, Guo L, Friedmann T, Yee JK (1996) Generation of packaging cell lines for pseudotyped retroviral vectors of the G protein of vesicular stomatitis virus by using a modified tetracycline inducible system. *Proc Natl Acad Sci USA* 93: 10 057–10 062
8 Friedmann T (1995) Pseudotyped retroviral vectors for studies of human gene therapy. *Nat Med* 1: 275–277
9 Naldini L, Blömer U, Gallay P et al (1996) *In vivo* gene delivery and stable transduction of non-dividing cells by a lentiviral vector. *Science* 272: 263–267
10 Poeschla E, Corbeau P, Wong-Staal F (1996) Development of HIV vectors for anti-HIV gene therapy. *Proc Natl Acad Sci USA* 93: 11 395–11 399
11 Naldini L, Blömer U, Gage FH, Trono D, Verma IM (1996) Efficient transfer, integration, and sustained long-term expression of the transgene in adult rat brains injected with a lentiviral vector. *Proc Natl Acad Sci USA* 93: 11 382–11 388
12 Naldini L, Verma IM (1999) Lentiviral vectors. *In*: T Friedmann (ed.): *The development of human gene therapy.* Cold Spring Harbor Laboratory Press, Cold Spring Harbor, 47–60
13 Poeschla EM, Wong-Staal F, Looney DJ (1998) Efficient transduction of nondividing human cells by feline immunodeficiency virus lentivirus vectors. *Nat Med* 4: 354–357
14 Smith AE (1995) Viral vectors in gene therapy. *Annu Rev Microbiol* 49: 807–838
15 Kovesdi I, Brough DE, Bruder JT, Wickham TJ (1997) Adenoviral vectors for gene transfer. *Curr Opin Biotechnol* 8: 583–589
16 Wivel NA, Gao G-P, Wilson JM (1999) Adenovirus vectors. *In*: T Friedmann (ed.): *The development of human gene therapy.* Cold Spring Harbor Laboratory Press, Cold Spring Harbor, 87–110
17 Kafri T, Morgan D, Krahl T, Sarvetnick N, Sherman L, Verma I (1998) Cellular immune response to adenoviral vector infected cells does not require *de novo* gene expression: implications for gene therapy. *Proc Natl Acad Sci USA* 95: 11 377–11 382
18 Samulski RJ, Sally M, Muzyczka N (1999) Adeno-associated viral vectors. *In*: T Friedmann (ed.): *The development of human gene therapy.* Cold Spring Harbor Laboratory Press, Cold Spring Harbor, 131–172

19 Herzog RW, Hagstrom JN, Kung SH et al (1997) Stable gene transfer and expression of human blood coagulation factor IX after intramuscular injection of recombinant adeno-associated virus. *Proc Natl Acad Sci USA* 94: 5804–5809
20 Snyder RO, Miao CH, Patijn GA et al (1997) Persistent and therapeutic concentrations of human factor IX in mice after hepatic gene transfer of recombinant AAV vectors. *Nat Genet* 16: 270–276
21 Jolly DJ (1999) Emerging viral vectors. *In*: T Friedmann (ed.): *The development of human gene therapy.* Cold Spring Harbor Laboratory Press, Cold Spring Harbor, 209–240
22 Heise C, Sampson-Johannes A, Williams A, McCormick F, Von Hoff DD, Kirn DH (1997) ONYX-015, an E1B-attenuated adenovirus, causes tumor-specific cytolysis and anti-tumoral efficacy that can be augmented by standard chemotherapeutic agents. *Nat Med* 3: 639–645
23 Felgner PL, Zelphati O, Liang X (1999) Advances in synthetic gene-delivery system technology *In*: T Friedmann (ed.): *The development of human gene therapy.* Cold Spring Harbor Laboratory Press, Cold Spring Harbor, 241–260
24 Cotten M, Wagner E (1999) Receptor-mediated gene delivery strategies. *In*: T Friedmann (ed.): *The development of human gene therapy.* Cold Spring Harbor Laboratory Press, Cold Spring Harbor, 261–277
25 Wolff JA (1999) Naked DNA gene transfer in mammalian cells. *In*: T Friedmann (ed.): *The development of human gene therapy.* Cold Spring Harbor Laboratory Press, Cold Spring Harbor, 279–307
26 Ulmer JB, Liu MA (1999) Delivery systems and adjuvants for DNA vaccines. *In*: T Friedmann (ed.): *The development of human gene therapy.* Cold Spring Harbor Laboratory Press, Cold Spring Harbor, 309–330
27 Baumgartner I, Pieczek A, Manor O et al (1998) Constitutive expression of phVEGF165 after intramuscular gene transfer promotes collateral vessel development in patients with critical limb ischemia. *Circulation* 97: 1114–1123
28 Isner JM (1998) Therapeutic angiogenesis: a new frontier for vascular therapy. *Vasc Med* 1: 79–87
29 Zabner J, Cheng SH, Meeker D et al (1997) Comparison of DNA-lipid complexes and DNA alone for gene transfer to cystic fibrosis airway epithelia *in vivo. J Clin Invest* 100: 1529–1537
30 DeBruyne LA, Chang AE, Cameron MJ et al (1996) Direct transfer of a foreign MHC gene into human melanoma alters T cell receptor usage by tumor-infiltrating lymphocytes. *Cancer Immunol Immunother* 43: 49–58
31 Nabel GJ, Gordon D, Bishop DK et al (1996) Immune response in human melanoma after transfer of an allogeneic class I major histocompatibility complex gene with DNA-liposome complexes. *Proc Natl Acad Sci USA* 93: 15 388–15 393
32 Dzau VJ, Mann MJ, Morishita R, Kaneda Y (1996) Fusigenic viral liposome for gene therapy in cardiovascular diseases. *Proc Natl Acad Sci USA* 93: 11 421–11 425
33 Laitinen M, Pakkanen T, Donetti E et al (1997) Gene transfer into the carotid artery using an adventitial collar: Comparison of the effectiveness of the plasmid-liposome complexes, retroviruses, pseudotyped retroviruses and adenoviruses. *Hum Gene Ther* 8: 1645–1650
34 Stephan DJ, Yang ZY, San H et al (1996) A new cationic liposome DNA complex enhances the efficiency of arterial gene transfer *in vivo. Hum Gene Ther* 7: 1803–1812
35 Abe A, Miyanohara A, Friedmann T (1998) Enhanced gene expression with fusogenic liposomes containing vesicular stomatitis virus G glycoprotein. *J Virol* 72: 6159–6163
36 Reynolds PN, Curiel DT (1999) Strategies to adapt adenoviral vectors for gene therapy applications: targeting and integration. *In*: T Friedmann (ed.): *The development of human gene therapy.* Cold Spring Harbor Laboratory Press, Cold Spring Harbor, 111–130
37 Russell SJ, Hawkins RE, Winter G (1993) Retroviral vectors displaying functional antibody fragments. *Nucl Acid Res* 21: 1081–1085
38 Kasahara N, Dozy AM, Kan YW (1995) Tissue-specific targeting of retroviral vectors via ligand-receptor interactions. *Adv Drug Deliv Rev* 17: 227–234
39 Somia NV, Zoppé M, Verma IM (1995) Generation of targeted retroviral vectors by using single-chain variable fragment: An approach to *in vivo* gene delivery. *Proc Natl Acad Sci USA* 92: 7570–7574
40 Schnierle BS, Moritz D, Jeschke M, Groner B (1996) Expression of chimeric envelope proteins in helper cell lines and integration into Moloney murine leukemia virus particles. *Gene Ther* 3: 334–342
41 Chu T-HT, Dornburg R (1997) Toward highly efficient cell-type specific gene transfer with retroviral vectors displaying single-chain antibodies. *J Virol* 71: 720–725

42 Blaese RM, Culver KW, Miller AD et al (1995) T lymphopcyte-directed gene therapy for ADA-SCID: Initial trial results after 4 years. *Science* 270: 475–480
43 Bordignon C, Notarangelo LD, Nobili N et al (1995) Gene therapy in peripheral blood lymphocytes and bone marrow for ADA-immunodeficient patients. *Science* 270: 470–475
44 Grossman M, Rader DJ, Muller DWM et al (1995) A pilot study of *ex vivo* gene therapy for homozygous familial hypercholesterolemia. *Nat Med* 1: 1148–1154
45 Stopeck AT, Hersh EM, Akporiaye ET et al (1997) Phase I study of direct gene transfer of an allogeneic histocompatibility antigen, HLA-B7, in patients with metastatic melanoma. *J Clin Oncol* 15: 341–349
46 Bowman L, Grossman M, Rill D et al (1998) Il-2 adenovector-transduced autologous tumor cells induce an anti-tumor immune response in patients with neuroblastoma. *Blood* 92: 1941–1949
47 Bowman LC, Grossman M, Rill D et al (1998) Interleukin 2-gene modified allogenic tumor cells for treatment of relapsed neuroblastoma. *Hum Gene Ther* 9: 1303–1311
48 Brenner MK (1997) Hematological malignancies. *FASEB J* 11: 640–648
49 Zhao RCH, McIvor RS, Griffin JD, Verfaillie CM (1997) Gene therapy for chronic myelogenous leukemia (CML): A retroviral vector that renders hematopoietic progenitors methotrexate-resistant and CML progenitors functionally normal and nontumorigenic *in vivo*. *Blood* 90: 4687–4698
50 Dilloo D, Brown M, Roskrow M et al (1997) CD40 ligand induces an anti-leukemia immune response *in vivo*. *Blood* 90: 1927–1933
51 Yee J-K (1999) Retroviral vectors. *In*: T Friedmann (ed.): *The development of human gene therapy*. Cold Spring Harbor Laboratory Press, Cold Spring Harbor, 21–45
52 Teng BB, Ishida B, Forte TM et al (1997) Effective lowering of plasma, LDL, and esterified cholesterol in LDL receptor knockout mice by adenovirus-mediated gene delivery of ApoB mRNA editing enzyme (Apobec1). *Arterioscler Thromb Vasc Biol* 17: 889–897
53 Van Dijk KW, van Vlijmen BJ, Van der Zee A et al (1998) Reversal opf hypercholesterolemia in apolipoprotein E2 and apolipoprotein E3-Leiden transgenic mice by adenovirus-mediated gene transfer of the VLDL receptor. *Arterioscler Thromb Vasc Biol*18: 7–12
54 Gerard RD, Chan L (1996) Adenovirus-mediated gene transfer: strategies and applications in lipoprotein research. *Curr Opin Lipidol* 7: 105–111
55 Kashyap VS, Santamarina-Fojo S, Brown DR et al (1995) Apolipoprotein E deficiency in mice: Gene replacement and prevention of atherosclerosis using adenovirus vectors. *J Clin Invest* 96: 1612–1620
56 Stevenson SC, Marshall-Neff J, Teng B, Lee CB, Roy S, McClelland A (1995) Phenotypic correction of hypercholesterolemia in ApoE-deficient mice by adenovirus-mediated *in vivo* gene transfer. *Arterioscler Thromb Vasc Biol* 15: 479–484
57 Kren BT, Bandyopadhyay P, Steer CJ (1998) *In vivo* site-directed mutagenesis of the factor IX gene by chimeric RNA/DNA oligonucleotides. *Nat Med* 4: 285–290
58 Walters L, Palmer JG (1997) *The ethics of human gene therapy*. Oxford University Press, Oxford

Short biographies

George G. Brownlee is Professor of Chemical Pathology at the Sir William Dunn School of Pathology, University of Oxford, and Fellow of Lincoln College, Oxford (UK). His first degree, from the University of Cambridge (Natural Sciences), was followed by a Ph.D. under the direction of Fred Sanger at the MRC Laboratory of Molecular Biology, Cambridge (UK). In 1966 Brownlee became a MRC staff member and continued to work on fundamental problems of molecular biology in Cambridge until 1980. He then joined the University of Oxford where he became interested in the application of molecular methods to disease. After studying factor IX gene-defective in haemophilia B, he is now focussing on influenza virus research. Professor Brownlee has received various important prizes – particularly for his research on haemophilia. He is a Fellow of the Royal Society and the Academy of Medical Sciences.

Peter Buckel studied Biology at the Ludwig-Maximilians University in Munich (Germany). He received his Ph.D. in Microbiology at the University Regensburg. His postdoctoral studies in Regensburg and Munich focussed on the genetic isolation and expression of recombinant proteins. With this background, Peter Buckel joined Boehringer Mannheim in Tutzing (1977) and built up the Pharmaceutical Biotechnology department with a major focus on research, development and production of therapeutic recombinant proteins. He held Senior Vice President positioning as head of Biotechnology and global pharmaceutical R&D at Boehringer Mannheim and as head of Molecular Medicine at Roche Pharma. Peter Buckel is Professor at the University Munich and besides several scientific and industrial board positions he is Chairman of the Scientific Advisory Board in the Human Genome Project of the German Ministry of Education and Research. Currently, he is Chief Executive Officer (CEO) of Xantos Biomedicine GmbH, a young functional genomics drug discovery company.

Paul Burke is Associate Director of Pharmaceutics at Amgen (Thousand Oaks, California), where he leads a group responsible for the development of sustained release parenteral formulations of proteins and peptides, and other novel formulations. He is a member of the development team for Abarelix Depot, the first sustained release formulation of GnRH antagonist to complete commercial development. From 1993 to 1997 Dr. Burke was at Alkernes, where he contributed to the development of the ProLease® delivery technology, designing microsphere formulations of several protein therapeutics including a multiweek formulation of erythropoietin. Dr. Burke received his Ph.D. in chemistry from the Massachusetts Institute of Technology (MIT) in 1992.

Désiré Collen is Professor at the Faculty of Medicine, Katholieke Universiteit (KU) of Leuven and Director of the Center for Molecular and Vascular Biology and of the Center for Transgene Technology and Gene Therapy in Leuven (Belgium). Since he became M.D. (1968) as well as a Ph.D. in Chemistry (1974) at the KU Leuven, Collen has authored and co-authored over 530 research papers in peer-reviewed international journals and over 130 review articles. Due to his important findings and developments in the molecular biology and pathophysiology of homeostasis and thrombosis as well as in transgenesis, gene targeting and gene transfer of the cardiovascular system, Collen was made Member of the Royal Academy of Medicine of Belgium in 1985. He received renowned awards such as the Prix Louis Jeantet de Médecine, the Five-yearly Prize of Fundamental Medical Sciences of the Belgian Government and the Bristol-Myers-Squibb Award for Cardiovascular Research (together with M. Verstraete).

Theodore Friedmann is Professor of Pediatrics and Director of the Gene Therapy Program at the University of California, San Diego. After completion of his studies in Chemistry (A.B.) and medicine (M.D.) at the University of Pennsylvania, Friedmann gained extensive practical and research experience in the Children's Hospital Medical Center in Boston, Massachusetts (where he also worked as a Teaching and later Research Fellow at Harvard University), the National Institutes of Health (Bethesda, Maryland) and The Salk Institute for Biological Studies in La Jolla, California. In 1976 he joined Fred Sanger's team at the University of Cambridge (UK) and George Brownlee's pathology team at the University of Oxford (UK) in 1983. Theodore Friedmann has published innumerable articles in pediatrics and later in gene therapy and molecular genetics and is the author and editor of several books on this subject.

Paul L.F. Giangrande received his B.Sc. from the University in Manchester (UK) in Pharmacology and graduated with Honours in Medicine in 1979. His practical and scientific career led him to the Cantonal Hospital in Basel (Switzerland) and to the Westminster Hospital and Medical School, where he worked as a Lecturer in Haematology. After several years as a Research Fellow at the Royal Free Hospital in London and at the Haemophilia and Thrombosis Centre in Milan (Italy), Giangrande is now Director of the Oxford Haemophilia Centre in Oxford (UK), and Vice-President of the World Federation of Haemophilia in 2000.

Stephen D. Gillies graduated at Rutgers University/UMDNJ in Animal Virology. After receiving his Ph.D. in Microbiology in 1981, he became a Fellow of Damon Runyon in the laboratory of Susumu Tonegawa. In 1984, he took a position as Director of Molecular Biology at Damon Biotech. Eight years later, he joined Fuji ImmunoPharmaceuticals Corp. (now Lexigen) where he serves as President and Director of Research. Since Lexigen became part of EMD Pharmaceuticals in 1999, he also serves as Vice-President of Basic Research, North America for EMD Pharmaceuticals. During his career, he made important discoveries in the mechanisms of immunoglobulin gene regulation and the development of novel antibodies and antibody fusion proteins for cancer detection and therapy.

Peter Hans Hofschneider received his Ph.D. from the University in Heidelberg (Germany) and his M.D. from the University of Tübingen. Following a postdoctoral fellowship at the Max-Planck Institute for Biochemistry in Munich, his appointment to the Chair of the German Society of Genetics and the Max-Planck Institute for Biochemistry, his participation in the founding of Biogen as member of its Scientific Board, and his chairmanship of the Scientific Council of the Max Planck Society are only some of major milestones in his long career. Hofschneider has co-edited important publications on Microbiology and Immunology and Virology in particular. His important works earned him – among others – the membership of EMBO, the Medallion for Civic Initiative of the German Cancer Aid Society, the First Class Order of Merit of the Federal Republic of Germany, the Jacob Henle Medal and the Bavarian Order of Merit. Since 1966/67 Hofschneider is Professor of the Medical Faculty of the University of Munich and Director at the Max-Planck Institute for Biochemistry in Martinsried (Germany).

H. Roger Lijnen received his M.Sc. in Chemistry in 1974 and his Ph.D. in Biochemistry in 1978 at the University of Leuven (Belgium). He focussed on the research areas of molecular biology and pathophysiology of haemostasis and thrombosis. His important discoveries during his scientific career at the University of Leuven and over 200 research papers, books and survey articles in peer-reviewed international journals earned him international prizes as well as the Chair of the Scientific Program Committee of the XIIth International Congress of Fibrinolysis in 1994. Lijnen is now Professor at the Faculty of Medicine at the University of Leuven and Member of the Senior Advisory Council of the Scientific and Standardization Committee (SSC) of the International Society on Thrombosis and Haemostasis (ISTH).

Kenneth Murray began his scientific career at the University of Birmingham (UK), where he obtained a B.Sc. and Ph.D. degree in Chemistry in 1959. After postdoctoral work at Stanford University, he returned to England to a further postdoctoral position with Fred Sanger at the MRC Laboratory of Molecular Biology in Cambridge (UK). In 1967 he moved to the University of Edinburgh, where he was appointed to the Chair of Molecular Biology in 1976. From 1979 to 1982 he was a member of the scientific staff at the European Molecular Biology Laboratories in Heidelberg. On returning to Edinburgh, he resumed his position as Head of the Department of Molecular Biology until 1984, when he took over a Chair in Molecular Biology sponsored by Biogen which he had co-founded in 1978. In 1983 he founded the Darwin Trust of Edinburgh and continues as Chairman of the Trustees of the Darwin Trust. He was interim director of research at Biogen's Geneva laboratories from 1985 to 1987 and continues to be a member of Biogen's Board of Directors and Scientific Advisory Board. Murray looks back on an extensive list of honours and awards; he was knighted for his services to science in 1993 and awarded a Royal Medal of the Royal Society of Edinburgh in 2000.

Erich Platzer is a board certified hematologist and medical oncologist, graduated from the university of Erlangen, Germany, where he also was an attending physician and associate professor of medicine until 1991. In the 1980s, he had worked several years as an experimental scientist in academia, including at Memorial Sloan-Kettering Cancer Center, New York. During that time he had a prime role in the team succeeding in the first purification of natural human G-CSF, which lead up to the development of Neupogen® by Amgen. In 1991, Platzer joined F. Hoffmann LaRoche Ltd. Headquarters in Basel, as Medical Director in oncology. After various positions in Development and Marketing he became Therapeutic Area Head Oncology. Platzer left Roche in 1999 and now works on the boards of a number of biotech start up companies: Novuspharma SpA (Monza, I), Micromet GmbH (Martinsried, D), and Collabra Pharma (South San Francisco, USA)

Scott Putney is Group Leader in the Laboratory for Protein Engineering at Lilly Research Laboratories, Indianapolis, USA. From 1991–1998, he was Vice-President of the Protein and Molecular Biology branch at Alkermes, Inc., where he led the development of a sustained-release formulation of human growth hormone, the first such marketed delivery system of a protein drug. From 1983–1991 he was Vice-President of the Molecular Biology branch at RepliGen Corporation, where he led an effort to develop a vaccine for HIV-1. Putney received his Ph.D. and post-doctoral training from the Massachusetts Institute of Technology (MIT).

Charles Weissmann is Professor emeritus at the University of Zürich, Switzerland, and Senior Research Scientist of the MRC Prion Unit at St. Mary's Hospital in London, UK. He received his M.D. in Medicine and Ph.D. in Organic Chemistry from the University in Zürich before he began his scientific career as Postdoctoral Fellow at the New York University School of Medicine where – only four years later – he became Associate Professor at the Department of Molecular Biology. In 1967 Weissmann returned to the University of Zürich where he took a position as Professor, Department of Molecular Biology, and as Director of the Institute of Molecular Biology. Weissmann received countless awards and honours from reputed universities and institutions, including that of Foreign Member of the Royal Society and the Robert-Koch Medal.

Karl Welte is Head of the Department of Pediatric Hematology and Oncology at the Hannover Medical School (Germany) since 1996. He studied Medicine in Tübingen and Berlin and became a pediatrician in 1984. Between 1981 and 1987 Welte extensively researched the purification and characterization of cytokines at the Sloan-Kettering Memorial Cancer Center in New York (USA) where he became Assistant Professor and head of the Laboratory of Cytokine Biology in 1985. In 1987 Welte returned to Germany and became Professor of Pediatrics at the Medical School in Hannover. He performed the first European studies with GM-CSF and G-CSF in patients with chronic neutropenia and co-founded an international registry for chronic neutropenia. Welte has received many awards, including the Kind-Philipp-Prize for Leukemia Research (1986), the Johann-Georg-Zimmermann-Prize for Cancer Research in 1989, the Prix Galien de Recherche Pharmaceutique (1992), and the Award for Excellency at the International Symposium on Molecular Biology of Hematopoieses in 2000.

List of approved "recombinant protein drugs"

List of approved recombinant therapeutics. From Signals online magazine, June 2000, http://www.signalsmag.com

Product name	Company(s) [developer, marketer]	Product category	First indication approved by FDA	Date of first FDA approval	Additional FDA-approved indication(s)	Date(s) of additional FDA approval(s)
Actimmune	InterMune Pharmaceuticals (Connetics; licensed from Genentech)	Recombinant interferon gamma-1b	Management of chronic granulomatous disease	12/90	To delay the time to disease progression in severe malignant osteopetrosis	2/00
Activase	Genentech (Roche)	Recombinant tissue plasminogen activator	Acute myocardial infarction	11/87	1. acute massive pulmonary embolism	6/90
					2. acute myocardial infarction (accelerated infusion)	4/95
					3. ischemic stroke within 3 h of symptom onset	6/96
Avonex	Biogen	Recombinant interferon beta-1a	Relapsing multiple sclerosis	5/96	—	—
BeneFIX	Genetics Institute (American Home Products [AHP])	Recombinant human Factor IX	Treatment of hemophilia B	2/97	—	—
Betaseron	Chiron; Berlex Laboratories (Schering AG)	Recombinant interferon beta-1b	Relapsing, remitting multiple sclerosis	7/93	—	—
Cerezyme	Genzyme	Recombinant glucocerebrosidase	Gaucher's disease	5/94	—	—
Enbrel	Immunex; Wyeth-Ayerst (AHP)	Dimeric fusion protein; recombinant soluble p75 tumor necrosis factor receptor (TNFr) linked to Fc portion of human IgG1	Moderate-to-severe active rheumatoid arthritis (RA) (monotherapy in patients who have failed other therapies [DMARDS]); also for use in combination with methotrexate	11/98	1. Moderate-to-severe active juvenile RA	5/99
					2. Reducing signs & symptoms and delaying structural damage in moderately to severely active RA (adults); first-line treatment	6/00

continued on next page

List of approved recombinant therapeutics (continued)

Product name	Company(s) [developer, marketer]	Product category	First indication approved by FDA	Date of first FDA approval	Additional FDA-approved indication(s)	Date(s) of additional FDA approval(s)
Engerix-B	SmithKline Beecham; Merck (licensed from Biogen)	Recombinant hepatitis B virus (HBV) vaccine (contains HbSAg)	HBV infection	9/89	Adults with chronic hepatitis C virus (HCV) infection	8/98
Epogen	Amgen	Recombinant human erythropoietin	Anemia associated with chronic renal failure including dialysis & non-dialysis patients; also anemia in Retrovir-treated HIV patients	6/89	1. Anemia caused by chemotherapy in patients with non-myeloid malignancies	4/93
					2. Prevention of anemia associated with surgical blood loss	12/96
					3. Anemia in children with chronic renal failure undergoing dialysis	11/99
GlucaGen	Zymo-Genetics; Novo Nordisk	Glucagon; recombinant DNA	Treatment of hypoglycemia; also for use as diagnostic aid	6/98	—	—
Herceptin	Genentech (Roche)	Humanized monoclonal antibody to HER2 growth factor receptor	Treatment of HER-2 overexpressing metastatic breast cancer	9/98	—	—
Humulin	Eli Lilly (licensed from Genentech)	Recombinant human insulin	Diabetes	10/82	—	—
Infergen	Amgen; Yamanouchi Pharmaceutical Co.	Consensus interferon; non-natural recombinant type 1 alpha interferon	HCV infection (chronic)	10/97	—	—

continued on next page

List of approved recombinant therapeutics (continued)

Product name	Company(s) [developer, marketer]	Product category	First indication approved by FDA	Date of first FDA approval	Additional FDA-approved indication(s)	Date(s) of additional FDA approval(s)
Intron A	Schering-Plough (licensed from Biogen)	Recombinant human interferon alfa-2b	Hairy cell leukemia	6/86	1. Genital warts	6/88
					2. AIDS-related Kaposi's sarcoma	11/88
					3. HCV infection	2/91
					4. HBV infection	7/92
					5. Malignant melanoma	12/95
					6. Follicular lymphoma in conjunction with chemotherapy	11/97
					7. HBV infection in pediatric patients	8/98
Kogenate	Bayer (licensed from Genentech)	Recombinant antihemophilic factor (Factor VIII)	Hemophilia A	2/93	—	—
Leukine	Immunex	Recombinant granulocyte macrophage-colony stimulating factor (GM-CSF)	Autologous bone marrow transplant (BMT)	3/91	1. Neutropenia resulting from chemotherapy in acute myelogenous leukemia	9/95
					2. Allogeneic BMT	11/95
					3. Peripheral blood progenitor cell mobilization & transplantation	12/95
Mylotarg	Wyeth-Ayerst (AHP); Celltech Group	Humanized anti-CD33 monoclonal antibody, conjugated with calicheamicin (chemotherapy)	Relapsed acute myeloid leukemia in CD33+ patients who are 60+ years old and are not candidates for cytotoxic chemotherapy	5/00	—	—

continued on next page

List of approved recombinant therapeutics (continued)

Product name	Company(s) [developer, marketer]	Product category	First indication approved by FDA	Date of first FDA approval	Additional FDA-approved indication(s)	Date(s) of additional FDA approval(s)
Neumega	Genetics Institute; Wyeth-Ayerst (AHP)	Recombinant human interleukin-11 (platelet growth factor)	Chemotherapy-induced thrombocytopenia (platelet depletion)	11/97	—	—
Neupogen	Amgen; Kirin Brewery Co.	Recombinant granulocyte colony stimulating factor (G-CSF)	Chemotherapy-induced neutropenia	2/91	1. Autologous or allogeneic bone marrow transplantation (BMT)	6/94
					2. Chronic severe neutropenia	12/94
					3. To support peripheral blood progenitor cell transplantation	12/95
					4. Acute myelogenous leukemia	4/98
Novolin	Zymo-Genetics; Novo Nordisk	Recombinant human insulin	Insulin-dependent diabetes	7/91	—	—
NovoSeven	Zymo-Genetics; Novo Nordisk	Recombinant factor VIIa	Treatment of bleeding episodes in hemophilia A or B patients with inhibitors (antibodies) to factor VIII or factor IX	3/99	—	—
Nutropin	Genentech (Roche)	Recombinant human growth hormone (hGH)	Growth failure in children due to chronic renal insufficiency; growth hormone inadequacy in children	3/94	1. Turner's syndrome	12/96
					2. Growth hormone inadequacy in adults	12/97
Nutropin AQ	Genentech (Roche)	Recombinant hGH (liquid)	Growth failure in children due to chronic renal insufficiency; growth hormone inadequacy in children	12/95	1. Turner's syndrome	12/96
					2. Growth hormone inadequacy in adults	12/97

continued on next page

List of approved recombinant therapeutics (continued)

Product name	Company(s) [developer, marketer]	Product category	First indication approved by FDA	Date of first FDA approval	Additional FDA-approved indication(s)	Date(s) of additional FDA approval(s)
Nutropin Depot	Alkermes; Genentech (Roche)	Recombinant hGH (sustained-release)	Growth hormone deficiency in children	12/99	—	—
Orthoclone OKT3	Ortho Biotech (J&J)	Murine monoclonal antibody to CD3 receptor	Reversal of acute kidney transplant rejection	6/86	Reversal of heart and liver transplant rejection	6/93
Proleukin	Chiron; Ligand (Canada)	Recombinant human interleukin-2	Renal cell carcinoma	5/92	Metastatic melanoma	1/98
Protropin	Genentech (Roche)	Recombinant hGH	hGH deficiency in children	10/85	—	—
Pulmozyme	Genentech (Roche)	Recombinant human DNase	Reduction of incidence of respiratory tract infections in patients with cystic fibrosis (CF)	12/93	1. Treatment of CF in severely ill patients (less than 40% lung function) 2. Treatment of CF in infants and young children	12/96 3/98
Recombinate	Genetics Institute (AHP); Baxter Healthcare	Recombinant antihemophilic factor (rAHF); recombinant Factor VIII	Prevention & control of bleeding in Hemophilia A	12/92	—	—
Recombivax HB	Merck & Co. (licensed from Chiron)	Recombinant HBV vaccine	Prevention of HBV infection	7/86	—	—
Refacto	Genetics Institute; Wyeth-Ayerst (AHP) (purchased rights from Pharmacia & Upjohn in 8/97)	Recombinant factor VIII SQ; albumin-free	Hemophilia A; also, short-term prophylaxis to reduce frequency of spontaneous bleeding episodes	3/00	—	—

continued on next page

List of approved recombinant therapeutics (continued)

Product name	Company(s) [developer, marketer]	Product category	First indication approved by FDA	Date of first FDA approval	Additional FDA-approved indication(s)	Date(s) of additional FDA approval(s)
Regranex Gel	Chiron; Ortho-McNeil Pharmaceuticals (J&J) (licensed from ZymoGenetics)	Recombinant human platelet-derived growth factor-beta	Lower extremity diabetic neuropathic ulcers	12/97	—	—
Remicade	Centocor (J&J); Schering-Plough	Chimeric monoclonal antibody to tumor necrosis factor-alpha	Moderate-to-severe Crohn's disease (including fistulizing Crohn's disease)	8/98	Rheumatoid arthritis in patients who have had inadequate response to methotrexate	11/99
ReoPro	Centocor (J&J); Lilly	Chimeric monoclonal antibody fragment to GPIIb/IIIa platelet receptor	Anti-platelet; prevention of blood clots in the setting of high-risk percutaneous transluminal coronary angioplasty (PCTA)	12/94	Refractory unstable angina when PCTA intervention is planned	11/97
Retavase	Centocor (J&J) (acquired rights from Boehringer Mannheim & DuPont Merck Pharmaceuticals)	Recombinant tissue plasminogen activator	Treatment of acute myocardial infarction	10/96	—	—
Rituxan	Idec Pharmaceuticals; Genentech; Hoffmann-La Roche	Chimeric pan-B monoclonal antibody that targets CD20 antigen on B cell surface	Treatment of relapsed or refractory low-grade or follicular CD20-positive B-cell non-Hodgkin's lymphoma	11/97	—	—
Roferon-A	Hoffmann-La Roche (licensed from Genentech); Gilead Sciences (for HCV)	Recombinant interferon alfa-2a	Hairy cell leukemia	6/86	1. AIDS-related Kaposi's sarcoma 2. Chronic myelogenous leukemia 3. HCV infection	11/88 11/95 11/96

continued on next page

List of approved recombinant therapeutics (continued)

Product name	Company(s) [developer, marketer]	Product category	First indication approved by FDA	Date of first FDA approval	Additional FDA-approved indication(s)	Date(s) of additional FDA approval(s)
Synagis	MedImmune; Abbott Laboratories	Humanized monoclonal antibody that binds to the F (fusion) protein on surface of respiratory syncytial virus (RSV)	Prevention of serious lower respiratory tract disease caused by RSV in high-risk pediatric patients	6/98	—	—
TNKase	Genentech (Roche); Boehringer Ingelheim Pharma KG	Tenecteplase; Recombinant tissue plasminogen activator (2nd-generation); single-bolus; can be admin over 5 seconds in 1 dose	Acute myocardial infarction in adults	6/00	—	—
Zenapax	Protein Design Labs; Hoffmann-La Roche	Humanized monoclonal antibody (SMART Anti-TAC) that binds to the interleukin-2 receptor on activated T-cells	Prevention of acute kidney transplant rejection	12/97	—	—

Subject index

Actimmune 191
Activase 191
Adams, Dan 6, 13
adeno-associated parvovirus (AAV), human 171
adeno-associated vector 175
adenosine deaminase (ADA) 81
adenosine deaminase gene 80
adenovirus 171–174
adenovirus vector 171, 173, 174
AIDS/HIV 73, 79, 98, 171
Alafi, Moshe 13, 16, 18
albumin, human 82, 84
allelic variant 27
allergic reaction 72
American Cancer Society 10, 15, 19, 34
anaphylactic reaction 31, 83
Andreopoulos, Spyros 21
androgen response element (ARE) 72
angiogenesis inhibitor 161
angiogenesis inhibitor, in cancer therapy 161
angiogenic factor 161
antibody, fibroblast interferon 17
antibody, inhibitory 72, 83, 84
antibody engineering 129
antibody fragment (Fab) 132
antibody-cytokine fusion protein 130
antibody-dependent cellular cytotoxity (ADCC) 136
anti-cancer agent 19
anti-tumour activity 19
antiviral activity 16, 27
arterial occlusion, peripheral 119
arthritis 73
Asilomar Conference 6
Avonex 191

B16 melanoma 139
B19 parvovirus 82
baby hamster kidney (BHK) 77, 80
B-domainless factor VIII 82
BeneFIX 79, 84, 191
Betaseron 191
Biogen 7–10, 13, 16, 18–20, 33, 35–38, 45, 60
Biogen, Scientific Board 7–9, 13, 16, 18, 19, 36, 37
Biogent 38
„bloody nose" 35
Boll, Werner 12
bone marrow transplantation (BMT) 95
bone morphogenic protein (BMP) 160
bovine cell 32
bovine factor IX, mRNA 76
bovine spongiform encephalitis (BSE) 79
Boyer, Herb 6
British Genetic Manipulation Advisory Group 9
Burke, Derek 13

C1q 144
cancer, immunotherapy of 160
Cantell, Kari 9, 10, 12, 15, 17, 34
γ-carboxyglutamic acid (Gla) 78
γ-carboxyglutamic acid (Gla), domain 71
γ-carboxyglutamic acid (Gla), residues 78
γ-carboxylase 78

carboxylase, vitamin K-dependent 77
γ-carboxylation 77
carcinoma, renal cell 35
Cawthorne, Rob 20, 35
cDNA 16, 73, 80
cDNA clone 23
cDNA library 76
cDNA, β-globin 11
cDNA, interferon 9, 11–13, 15–17, 19, 21, 22, 24, 28
cDNA, interferon α2 28
Cerezyme 191
Cetus 20
CG doublet 71, 72
CH2 domain of the H chain 130
CH3 domain of the H chain 130
chaperone 80
chimeric viral envelope protein 173
chinese hamster ovary (CHO) cell 76, 78, 80, 81
Christmas disease 67, 72
chromatography, immuno-affinity 77, 81
chromatography, ion-exchange 81
chronic neutropenia, severe 97
clinical trial 20, 30, 34
clotting cascade 68, 69
clotting cascade, initiating pathway 68
clotting cascade, sustaining pathway 68
clotting factor, half-life 83, 85
co-expression, factor VIII and vWF 80
cold 34, 35
colony hybridisation assay 17
complement-dependent cytotoxity (CDC) 136
congenital androgen insensitivity 69
containment laboratory, P4 46
COS-1, monkey kidney 80
Creutzfeldt-Jakob disease (CJD) 79
Curtis, Peter 6, 10, 11
cytopathic effect 16
cytopathic effect assay 15
cytopathic effect reduction assay 17
cytotoxic lymphocyte (CTL) 140
cytotoxicity, antibody-dependent cell-mediated 23

Daudi cell 23
Davies, Julian 35–37
2'-deoxycoformycin 81
depot formulation 153
Desmodus salivary plasminogen activator (DSPA) 117
dihydrofolate reductase (DHFR) 80
DNA complex, cationic lipid 172
DNA polymerase I, *E. coli* 75
DNA, chromosomal 26
DNA, cloned 24, 26
DNA, naked 172
DNA, plasmid 11
Dupont 13

Ecsödi, Josef 11, 28, 33
electron cryomicroscopy 58, 59
Enbrel 191
encapsulation 152
endoplasmatic reticulum (ER) 71
Engerix-B 192
envelope proteins, chimeric viral 173
epidermal growth factor (EGF), domain 71
epithelial antigen, EpCAM 140
Epogen 192
Escherichia coli 15–18, 20, 21–23, 27–31, 36, 73
Escherichia coli, DNA polymerase I 75

factor V 80
factor VIIa 83
factor VIII, assay 85
factor VIII, B-domainless 82
factor VIII, domain 70
factor VIII, gene 69
factor VIII, human 79

factor VIII, plasma-derived 82
factor VIII, porcine 79
factor VIII, SQ 82
factor IX, biologically active 77
factor IX, domain 70
factor IX, inhibitor 84
factor IX, mRNA 74
factor IX, plasma-derived 82, 83
factor IX, polymorphism 76
factor IX, post-translational modification 77
factor IX, promoter 72
factor IX, recovery 85
factor X 68, 71
factor XI 68
Fc receptor (FcR) 136
febrile neutropenia 93
Federal Institute of Technology (FIT) 36
Fernandez, Lou 37
fibrinogen 68
fibrin-specificity 117, 118
fibroblast 23, 27
fibroblast, interferon 11, 13, 14, 23, 27
fibroblast interferon antibody 17
Fiers, Walter 7, 27, 36, 38
fifth disease 82
Fildes, Bob 20
filgrastim 89
"first-generation" recombinant product 82
Flavell, Dick 32, 36–37
formulation development 155
founder effect 72
Fountoulakis, M. 30
furin 78, 82
fused protein 9, 11, 20, 129

β-galactosidase 28
β-galactosidase gene 28
ganglioside GD2 137
Garrod, Archibald 170
gel electrophoresis, conformation sensitive 70
gel electrophoresis, denaturing-gradient 70
Gelsinger, Jesse 177
gene, inversion 70, 71
gene conversion 27
gene correction 176
gene delivery, *ex vivo* 174
gene delivery, *in vivo* 174
gene delivery, receptor-mediated 172
gene delivery, route 174
gene duplication 71
gene therapy 85, 169–177
gene therapy, history 169–170
gene therapy, vector 171, 172
gene transfer 169
Genentech 6, 7, 13, 18, 22, 28
genetic defect, acquired 170
genetic defect, Mendelian 170
germ-line genetic modification 177
Gilbert, Walter 6, 7, 9, 11, 13, 19, 20, 35–37
Glaxo 37
β-globin, cDNA 11
globin, gene 19
globin, mRNA 11, 73
GlucaGen 192
glycan, *N*-linked 78
glycan, *O*-linked 78
glycosylation 16, 23
GM-CSF 133
Goeddel, David 28, 36
G-protein, vesicular stomatitis virus (VSV-G) 171, 173
growth hormone 9

H chain isotype 144
haemangioma 35
haemarthrosis 67
haemophilia 67
haemophilia, acquired 83, 84
haemophilia, prophylactic therapy 73
haemophilia A 67, 74, 83
haemophilia B 67, 74, 83
haemophilia B Leiden 72

hairy cell leukaemia 34, 35
Haley, Jim 16–18
half-life, circulating fusion protein 130
Hall, Alan 16
Hartley, Brian 7, 9, 28
Helixate 84
Helsinki 12
hepatic nuclear factor 4 72
hepatitis, serum 45, 50
hepatitis, virus 19
hepatitis A 79
hepatitis B 34–36, 79
hepatitis B, chronic 35
hepatitis B, vaccines 36
hepatitis B virus (HBV) 43
hepatitis B virus, cell-mediated immune response to 57
hepatitis B virus, escape mutant 56
hepatitis B virus, geographical distribution 44
hepatitis B virus, T-cell epitopes 57, 59
hepatitis B virus, vaccination against 54, 56
hepatitis B virus core antigen (HBcAg) 43, 49, 52, 53, 56–58
hepatitis B virus core antigen, vaccination with 53, 56
hepatitis B virus core antigen activity 49
hepatitis B virus core antigen epitope 57
hepatitis B virus core antigen fusion protein 57, 58
hepatitis B virus core antigen particle 52, 58
hepatitis B virus *e* antigen (HBeAg) 43
hepatitis B virus genome 49
hepatitis B virus pathology 51, 53
hepatitis B virus polymerase 45
hepatitis B virus serotype *adyw* 46
hepatitis B virus surface antigen (HBsAg) 43, 49, 51
hepatitis B virus surface antigen, expression in yeast 51
hepatitis B virus surface antigen PreS sequence 49
hepatitis B virus x antigen (HBxAg) 50
hepatitis C 35, 73, 79
hepatitis C, chronic 35
hepatocellular carcinoma (HCC) 43, 56
hepatocellular carcinoma, vaccination against 56
hepatoma, human 77
hepatoma, rat 77
Herceptin 192
heteroduplex analysis 70
heteroduplex mapping 25
Hiscott 28
HIV/AIDS 73, 79, 98, 171
Hoffmann La Roche 38
Hofschneider, Peter Hans 7
Hood, Lee 13, 15, 22
human albumin 82, 84
human factor VIII 79
human growth hormone (hGH) 157
human growth hormone, mRNA 73
human hepatoma (HepG2) 77
human insulin, mRNA 73
human interferon activity 20
human interferon α 9, 30
human interferon α1 gene 27
human interferon γ, glycosylated 36
human leukocyte interferon 28
human lymphokine-activated killer (LAK) 139
Humulin 192
Hunkapiller, Michael 15, 22
hybridisation assay 11, 12
hybridization translation 6
hybridisation-translation analysis 14, 16
hybridization-translation assay 12, 15
β-hydroxyaspartate 78, 79

immune response, cell-mediated 57
immunocytokine 130
immunodiffusion analysis 48
immunoglobulin, mRNA 73, 74
immunoglubulin-binding protein (BiP) 80
immunological defence 31
immunological screening 46
immunotherapy of cancer 160
inactivation, viral 73
Inco 6, 13, 19
Infergen 192
influenza 74
inhibitory antibody 72, 83, 84
insulin 7, 9
insulin, human, mRNA 73
interferon 3, 9–17, 19–23, 27–35
interferon, biologically active 27
interferon, cloning 21, 22
interferon, fermentation 22, 28
interferon, fibroblast 11, 13, 14, 23
interferon, human leukocyte 28, 31
interferon, human 20
interferon, hybrid 31, 32
interferon, leukocyte 15, 17, 19, 22, 23, 27, 30, 31, 34
interferon, leukocyte, Cantell's 34
interferon, leukocyte, natural 34
interferon, lymphoblastoid 15, 31, 34
interferon, mature 22, 29
interferon, mRNA 3, 9–11, 13, 15
interferon, natural 20, 22, 34
interferon, purification 22, 30
interferon, recombinant 30, 34
interferon activity 17, 18, 23
interferon α 16, 23, 30, 33, 35
interferon α, duplication 27
interferon α, human 9, 30
interferon α, mouse 9
interferon α, pegylated 35
interferon α gene 25, 26
interferon α gene, mouse 32
interferon α gene family 27
interferon α1 23, 24, 27, 34
interferon α1, human, gene 27
interferon α2 23, 27, 34
interferon α2, crystallisation 31
interferon α2, methionyl- 29
interferon α2, recombinant 34, 35
interferon α2 cDNA 28
interferon β 23, 36
interferon β, human recombinant 38
interferon β1, fibroblast 27
interferon β2 27
interferon γ 36, 133
interferon γ, glycosylated human 36
interferon cDNA 9, 11–13, 15–17, 19, 21, 22, 24, 28
interferon cDNA plasmid 17
interferon determination 15
interferon expression 28
interferon gene 18, 22, 24, 27, 32
interferon gene family 32
interferon pseudogene 24, 25
interferon treatment 31
interferon-like protein 22, 27
interferon-producing cell 27
interferon-related gene 24
interleukin-2 130
interleukin-6 27
interleukin-12 133, 134
interleukin-12 p35 subunit 134
interleukin-12 p40 subunit 134
intervening sequence 27
intraocular delivery 162
Intron A 34, 35, 193
isotype, H chain 144

Johnsrud, Lorraine 11–13, 15

Kaposi sarcoma 35
knockout mouse, PrP 16
Kogenate 82, 84, 193
Kourilsky, Philippe 7
Krim, Mathilde 34

lac promoter 28
β-lactamase 28
β-lactamase gene 11, 48
lanoteplase 117

Lengyel, Peter 9, 16, 32
lenograstim 89
leukaemia, chronic myeloid 35
leukaemia, hair cell 34
leukaemia, murine 34
Leukine 193
leukocyte 10, 11, 13
leukocyte, mRNA 34
leukocyte, RNA 11
leukocyte, poly(A)$^+$ RNA 13
leukocyte, virus-induced 9
leukocyte culture 20
leukocyte interferon 15, 17, 19, 22, 23, 27, 30, 31, 34
leukocyte interferon, Cantell's 34
leukocyte interferon, human 31
leukocyte interferon, natural 34
leukocyte interferon gene 27
leukocyte migration inhibition, mitogen-induced 23
licensing 83
life expectancy 72
lipid, cationic 172
lipid-DNA conjugate 173
liposome 172
local delivery 158
lymphoblastoid cell 10, 22, 27, 34
lymphoblastoid, interferon 15, 31, 34
lymphoma, non-Hodgkin's 35
lymphotoxin 130

Mach, Bernard 13
Maddox, John 22
Maniatis, Tom 9, 23, 28
Massachusetts Institute of Technology (MIT) 18, 19
melanoma 35
melanoma, B16 139
metastase, neuroblastoma 139
methotrexate 81
5'-methylcytosine 71
microencapsulated protein 152
Miller, Jeffrey 22
missense defect 72
modification, post-translational 71
Mogenson 17
molgramostim 90
Moloney murine leukemia virus (MLV) 174
monkey kidney, COS-1 80
mouse cell 27, 28, 32
mouse interferon α 9
mRNA, bovine factor IX 76
mRNA, factor IX 74
mRNA, globin 11, 73
mRNA, human growth hormone 73
mRNA, human insulin 73
mRNA, immunoglobulin 73, 74
mRNA, interferon 3, 9–11, 13, 15
mRNA, leukocyte 34
mRNA, ovalbumin 73, 74
multiple sclerosis 38
murine leukaemia 34
Murray, Ken 7, 19, 36
mutation, frameshift 71
mutation, missense 71
mutation, nonsense 71
mutation, point 72
mutation, regulatory 72
mutation, splice 71
mutation hotspots 72
myeloid cell 34
myeloid leukaemia, chronic 35
myeloma, multiple 34
myelosuppression 91
Mylotarg 193
myocardial infarction, acute 107–119

Nagabushan, T.L. 31
Nagata, Shigekazu 11, 13, 15, 16, 24, 30, 33, 36
National Cancer Institute 10
natural killer cell 23
Nature 22
Neumega 194
Neupogen 194
neuroblastoma metastase 139
neutropenia, febrile 93

neutropenia, severe chronic 97
nonsense defect 72
Novolin 194
NovoSeven 83, 84, 194
nucleocapsid 59
Nutropin 194
Nutropin AQ 194
Nutropin Depot 195

occlusion, peripheral arterial 119
OKT3 195
oligonucleotide 73–75, 79
oocyte 10–12
oocyte supernatant 15
Orthoclone 195
osteosarcoma 10, 34
ovalbumin, mRNA 73, 74

paired basic amino acid cleaving enzyme (PACE) 78
partial linkage map 25
parvovirus 79
parvovirus, adeno-associated (AAV) 171
parvovirus, B19 82
penicillin 31
peripheral blood progenitor cells (PBPC) 96
peripheral blood progenitor cells, transplantation of 96
Pestka, Sydney 13
phage λ vector 24
phosphorylation 78, 79
pig growth hormone 36
plaque reduction assay 15
plasma-derived factor VIII 82
plasma-derived factor IX 82, 83
plasmid, hybrid 15, 16, 29
plasmid, interferon cDNA 17
plasmid pBR322 11, 28
plasminogen activation 111, 112
plasminogen activator, tissue-type (t-PA) 107–119
plasminogen activator inhibitor (PAI) 107
plasminogen activator inhibitor-1 (PAI-1) 113, 115, 116
poly(A)$^{+}$ RNA 10–13, 15
poly(A) signal 76
poly(lactide-co-glycolide)(PLG) 152
polymerase chain reaction (PCR) technique 29, 73
porcine factor VIII 79
post-translational modification 71, 79
post-translational modification, carbohydrate 78
post-translational modification, factor IX 77
prion 73, 79, 82
proinsulin 11
Proleukin 195
protein C 71
protein expression, foreign 169
protein stabilization 153, 154
prothrombin 68
Protropin 195
pseudogene 27
Ptashne, Mark 23
puberty 72
Pulmozyme 195

QβRNA 11, 16
quasi-species, viral 16
Quesada, Jorge 34

RANTES 135
rat hepatoma 77
Recombinant DNA Guidelines 11, 28
recombinant product, "first generation" 82
recombinant product, "second generation" 79
recombinant tissue-type plasminogen activator (rt-PA) 119
Recombinate 82, 84, 195
recombination 70, 71

Recombivax HB 195
Refacto 82, 84, 85, 195
Regranex Gel 196
Remicade 196
reocclusion 115
ReoPro 196
Retavase 196
reteplase 115, 116
retrovirus 171, 173
retrovirus, murine 171
retrovirus vector 171, 173
Revel, Michel 13, 27
reverse genetics 32
reverse transcriptase 74, 75
rhesus monkey 30
ribavirin 35
Rituxan 196
RNA, double-stranded 5
RNA, leukocyte 11
RNA, poly(A)$^+$ 10–13, 15
RNA-DNA hybrid 3
Roche 34
Roferon 34
Roferon-A 196
Rudnick, Seth 37

Sanger, Fred 7
sarcoma, Kaposi 35
sargramostim 90
Schäfer, Ray 6, 7
Schaller, Heinz 7
Schein, Cathy 28
Schellekens, Huub 30
Schering-Plough 13, 19, 28, 30, 31, 34, 36, 37
SCID mouse, immunodeficient 139
"second generation" recombinant product 79
sequencing, Maxam & Gilbert method 73, 76
sequencing, Sanger method 73
serine protease 70
serum hepatitis 45, 50
Sharp, Phil 6, 7, 9, 19, 36
signal sequence 15, 20, 28
single-chain FV molecule (scFV) 129
single-chain urokinase-type PA (scu-PA) 117
Southern blotting 69, 72, 73
splicing defect 72
SQ, factor VIII 82
squirrel monkey 28
Stanford University 21
staphylokinase 118
Strander, Hans 10, 34
Streuli, Michel 11, 15, 16, 23, 33
sulphation 78, 79
sustained-release formulation 152
Synagis 197

Taira, Hideharu 16, 17
Taniguchi, Tada 6, 11, 14, 20, 23, 27, 28, 36
T-cell epitope 57, 59
testosterone 72
thrombin 68
thrombin activatable fibrinolysis inhibitor (TAFI) 112
thrombolysis 113, 117, 119
thrombolytic therapy 113, 115
tissue factor 68
TNKase 197
TNK-rt-PA 116
transplantation, bone marrow 95
transplantation, peripheral blood progenitor cells 96
tumor, solid 34
tumor load 31
tumor microenvironment 130
tumor necrosis factor α (TNF-α) 130
tumor necrosis factor β (TNF-β) 130
tumor-infiltrating lymphocyte (TIL) 132
Turner's syndrome 69

vaccination, against cancer (HCC) 56

vaccination, against HBV 54, 56
vaccine, subunit 43
variant Creutzfeldt-Jakob disease (vCJD) 79
vascular endothelial growth factor (VEGF) 172
vector, adeno-associated 175
vector, adenovirus 171, 173, 174
vector, non-viral 172
vector, re-targeted 173
vector, retrovirus 171, 173
vector targeting 173
vesicular stomatitis virus, G-protein (VSV-G) 171, 173
Vincent, Jim 37, 38
viral inactivation 73
vitamin K 78
vitamin K, carboxylase activity 77
von Rotz, Rose-Marie 33
von Willebrand factor (vWF) 69, 80

Wade, Nicholas 21
Wellcome 34
West Coast entrepreneurs 20

X chromosome 69
xenograft 139
X-inactivation 69

Zenapax 197
Zoon, Cathy 15, 22, 23

MIX
Papier aus verantwortungsvollen Quellen
Paper from responsible sources
FSC® C105338

If you have any concerns about our products,
you can contact us on
ProductSafety@springernature.com

In case Publisher is established outside the EU,
the EU authorized representative is:
Springer Nature Customer Service Center GmbH
Europaplatz 3, 69115 Heidelberg, Germany

Printed by Libri Plureos GmbH
in Hamburg, Germany